SOCIAL AND EMOTIONAL SKILLS TRAINING FOR CHILDREN

Selected Works from the Authors

Social and Emotional Skills Training for Children

The Fast Track Friendship Group Manual

Karen L. Bierman, Mark T. Greenberg,
John D. Coie, Kenneth A. Dodge,
John E. Lochman, and Robert J. McMahon

THE GUILFORD PRESS
New York   London

The authors have checked with sources believed to be reliable in their efforts to provide information that is complete and generally in accord with the standards of practice that are accepted at the time of publication. However, in view of the possibility of human error or changes in behavioral, mental health, or medical sciences, neither the authors, nor the editor and publisher, nor any other party who has been involved in the preparation or publication of this work warrants that the information contained herein is in every respect accurate or complete, and they are not responsible for any errors or omissions or the results obtained from the use of such information. Readers are encouraged to confirm the information contained in this book with other sources.

Library of Congress Cataloging-in-Publication Data is available from the publisher.

ISBN 978-1-4625-3172-1 (paperback)

Poster illustrations and agenda pictures by Michael Brahosky.
Baxter story illustrations by Andrew Heckathorne.
All other illustrations by Nate Kling.

About the Authors

Karen L. Bierman, PhD, is Evan Pugh University Professor, Professor of Psychology and Human Development and Family Studies, and Director of the Child Study Center at The Pennsylvania State University. Since the 1980s, her research has focused on social-emotional development and children at risk, with an emphasis on the design and evaluation of school-based programs that promote social competence, school readiness, and positive peer relations, and that reduce aggression and related behavior problems. She also directs a predoctoral training program in the interdisciplinary educational sciences. Dr. Bierman has served as an educational advisor to a number of organizations devoted to improving early education for disadvantaged children, including Head Start and Sesame Workshop.

Mark T. Greenberg, PhD, holds the Bennett Endowed Chair in Prevention Research in the College of Health and Human Development at The Pennsylvania State University, where he is Founding Director of the Edna Bennett Pierce Prevention Research Center. He is the author of more than 300 journal articles and book chapters on developmental psychopathology, well-being, and the effects of prevention efforts on children and families. Dr. Greenberg is a recipient of numerous awards, including the Urie Bronfenbrenner Award for Lifetime Contribution to Developmental Psychology in the Service of Science and Society from the American Psychological Association. One of his current interests is how to help nurture awareness and compassion in our society.

John D. Coie, PhD, is Professor Emeritus of Psychology: Social and Health Sciences at Duke University. He is a past chair of the National Institute of Mental Health grant review panel on prevention research. Dr. Coie's research has primarily focused on the development and prevention of serious antisocial behavior. He retired from Duke in 2000, but continues to be involved with the Fast Track program and has developed and co-managed a program in Santa Barbara, California, for providing non-English-speaking Hispanic children with computer-based English language and reading training. He continues to be active in programs designed to reduce violence and recidivism in the community.

Kenneth A. Dodge, PhD, is the William McDougall Professor of Public Policy and Professor of Psychology and Neuroscience at Duke University, and Director of the Duke Center for Child and Family Policy. His research focuses on how problem behaviors such as chronic violence, school failure, drug use, and child abuse develop across the lifespan; how these problems can be prevented; and how communities can implement policies to prevent these outcomes and instead promote children's healthy development. He has developed, implemented, and evaluated several intervention programs that are based on this research. Dr. Dodge currently leads the Durham Family Initiative to prevent child abuse in Durham, North Carolina.

John E. Lochman, PhD, APBB, is Professor and Doddridge Saxon Chairholder in Clinical Psychology at the University of Alabama, where he is Director of the Center for Prevention of Youth Behavior Problems, and Adjunct Professor of Psychiatry and Behavioral Sciences at the Duke University Medical Center. He has authored more than 400 scientific articles, chapters, and books on the causes and consequences of highly aggressive behavior in childhood, and on the effects of intervention with this behavior. His current focus is dissemination research. Dr. Lochman has served as editor-in-chief of the *Journal of Abnormal Child Psychology* and is a former president of the Society for Child and Family Policy and Practice (Division 37 of the American Psychological Association) and of the American Board of Clinical Child and Adolescent Psychology. He is a recipient of the Distinguished Career Award from the Society of Clinical Child and Adolescent Psychology (Division 53 of the American Psychological Association).

Robert J. McMahon, PhD, is Professor of Psychology at Simon Fraser University in Burnaby, British Columbia, Canada, where he is also BC Leading Edge Endowment Fund Leadership Chair in Proactive Approaches to Reducing Risk for Violence among Children and Youth. To carry out the work of the Chair, he directs the Institute for the Reduction of Youth Violence. He is also a senior scientist at the BC Children's Hospital Research Institute in Vancouver. Dr. McMahon's primary research and clinical interests concern the assessment, treatment, and prevention of conduct problems and other problem behavior in children and youth, especially in the context of the family. He is author or editor of numerous books, scientific articles, chapters, and reviews. He is a past editor-in-chief of *Prevention Science* and serves on the editorial boards of four other journals.

Acknowledgments

The development of the original Fast Track Friendship Group program was supported by National Institute of Mental Health (NIMH) Grant Nos. R18MH48043, R18MH50951, R18MH50952, and R18MH50953. The Center for Substance Abuse Prevention and the National Institute on Drug Abuse also provided support for Fast Track through memoranda of agreement with NIMH. This work was also supported in part by Department of Education Grant No. S184U30002 and by NIMH Grant Nos. K05MH00797 and K05MH01027. In addition, the Friendship Group program was further developed and refined in the context of projects funded by NIMH Grant No. R34MH085889, the Pennsylvania Department of Health, and Institute of Education Sciences Grant No. R305A150488.

For their close collaboration in developing this program, we are grateful to the Altoona Area School District, Bellefonte Area School District, Durham Public Schools, Harrisburg School District, Highline Public Schools, Juniata County School District, Middletown Area School District, Mifflin County School District, Metropolitan Nashville Public Schools, State College Area School District, Seattle Public Schools, Steelton–Highspire School District, Tyrone Area School District, York City School District, Hull Services of Canada, Barnardos Children's Charity of Ireland, and Barnardos Children's Charity of the United Kingdom. We greatly appreciate the hard work and dedication of the many staff members who implemented the project, provided feedback and suggestions, collected the evaluation data, and assisted with data management and analyses. We are especially thankful for the contributions made by Sandra Stewart and Janet Welsh, who each provided extensive feedback and suggestions.

Contents

COMMONLY USED MATERIALS IN FRIENDSHIP GROUP

FRIENDSHIP GROUP MANUAL: EARLY ELEMENTARY SESSIONS

Introduction to the Friendship Group Manual

CHAPTER 1

Overview

This chapter provides an overview of the conceptual foundations and research base that inform the design of the Friendship Group program. It reviews the importance of positive peer relations for social-emotional development, and the negative impact of chronic peer rejection on behavior and mental health. It describes the developmental progression of skills that support social competence in early and middle childhood, and the corresponding developmental framework that underlies the organization of Friendship Group program sessions.

THE IMPORTANCE OF POSITIVE PEER RELATIONS

Friendships play an important role in social and emotional development, beginning in preschool and extending through life. Positive peer interactions provide companionship, support the development of social skills, and foster feelings of competence and self-esteem. With peers, children are able to practice and refine their communication, negotiation, and problem-solving skills. In the context of their friendships, children learn to understand and respect others' feelings, developing empathy and a commitment to fairness. These lessons have lifelong value. Children who develop competence and confidence in social interactions are advantaged in later years in areas of school, work, adult relationships, and mental health.

Conversely, children who are rejected by peers and excluded from play in childhood are at heightened risk for future problems, ranging from severe emotional distress to antisocial behaviors in adolescence and adulthood. Peer-rejected children are often lonely, anxious, angry, and sad, and they are more likely than others to be bullied or victimized by peers. In addition, children who are excluded or disliked by peers miss out on the positive social experiences they need to develop the more complex social skills that support social integration later in life.

The Friendship Group Program

Friendship Group, a unique, evidence-based program for peer-rejected children, is based on over 20 years of research. It incorporates proven strategies that build children's prosocial and play skills and strengthen their self-control, anger coping, and interpersonal problem-solving skills. Unlike other programs that focus primarily on shaping and managing behaviors, Friendship Group promotes the social and emotional skills that motivate and support friendships, such as empathy and caring. As detailed in Chapter 5, Friendship Group has been tested in rigorous studies. The program promotes friendships, decreases peer rejection, improves peer communication skills and cooperative behavior, and decreases impulsive and aggressive behaviors.

Friendship Group can be delivered during school (as a "pullout" program) or after school, as a school-based intervention or mental health service. The sessions are organized developmentally, with a program for early elementary students (26 lessons, ages 5–8, grades K–2) and a program for advanced elementary students (14 lessons, ages 8–11, grades 3–5). Following a standard format for coaching programs, each session focuses on a set of target skills. Discussions, modeling stories, and coach role plays are used to teach social skill concepts. Social skills are then practiced in the context of student role plays, structured activities, and collaborative group activities.

In the next sections of this chapter, we describe the developmental foundations of the Friendship Group program, and the principles of the "coaching model" of social skill training used in the program. Additional chapters focus on the administration of the Friendship Group program (Chapter 2), therapeutic processes (Chapter 3), behavior management (Chapter 4), and the Fast Track model of synchronized home–school intervention (Chapter 5). The case examples provided to illustrate common child characteristics and responses are based on composites; all identifying information about individual children has been removed or disguised.

Who Needs Friendship Group?

All children experience "ups" and "downs" in their peer relations as they encounter occasional conflicts or exclusion. However, when children have ongoing difficulties gaining acceptance by classroom peers or if they experience chronic social exclusion or victimization, it is important for teachers and parents to take action, because chronic peer rejection is harmful.

Children can have trouble getting along with peers for a number of reasons. Many rejected children are aggressive and impulsive, disruptive in the classroom and the peer group. Some are bullies who use aggression to coerce other children, and many are victims as well.

Socially anxious children may also experience chronic peer problems, although not all do so. Many shy children develop a small group of friends and feel comfortable interacting with peers at school and in the community. In such cases, shyness is not a social problem of concern. However, when shy children feel anxious and uncomfortable at school, and when they have difficulty making friends and gaining acceptance by peers, they are at heightened risk for chronic exclusion and victimization by peers.

Students with learning disabilities, attention deficits, autism spectrum characteristics, or related developmental challenges are also at risk for social isolation and peer rejection. These children are often awkward and insensitive in social settings, because they are slow to pick up on subtle social cues, read body language, and understand "implicit" social routines or expectations. Peers often find them to be "odd" or even "rude" and treat them accordingly, excluding them from play or, worse, teasing them.

Regardless of the nature of the behavioral, developmental, or emotional roots of the peer problems, children are likely to benefit from Friendship Group if they lack the social skills that would allow them to improve their peer relations and achieve high-quality friendships. Social skills include specific behaviors and culturally validated routines, such as polite manners (e.g., chew with your mouth closed, and introduce yourself to someone new). Social skills also include more intangible social finesse—the ability to behave in ways that are socially sensitive and culturally appropriate.

To apply positive social skills, children need to recognize socially appropriate and inappropriate behaviors, but knowing what to do is not enough. Often, children know what to do and can explain what should be done in a given situation—yet, they behave differently. For example, a child may know that cheating at a game is wrong, yet still cheat. Such failures in self-regulation (e.g., being overwhelmed by feelings or impulses in social situations) can undermine social success as much as a lack of skill knowledge.

Social skills include both proactive behaviors (e.g., friendly initiations, cooperative behaviors, communication skills) and self-regulation skills (e.g., emotion regulation, impulse control, anger management). Socially skillful interaction requires behavioral skills (e.g., being able to enact socially skillful behavior), thinking skills (e.g., being able to think flexibly about how to respond when faced with various social challenges or conflicts), and emotion skills (e.g., being sensitive to one's own and others' emotions, being able to regulate one's emotion and respond to another's).

It is often assumed that children "pick up" social skills naturally and automatically by observation and occasional adult direction. Children without social skills sometimes suffer harsh judgment, as children and other adults find them to be ill-mannered or discourteous. In reality, not all children absorb social skills by observation and osmosis; some children need explicit instruction and support. The good news is that children *can* be taught social skills. Social skill training promotes the development of social sensitivity and social competence, in order to help children gain peer acceptance, make and sustain close friendships, and avoid isolation or victimization by peers.

Individual versus Group Intervention Models

Although one-on-one sessions can be used to teach children social skills, group sessions offer more opportunities for practicing and consolidating social-emotional skills. Peer pairs or small peer groups provide children with opportunities to practice skills in the context of collaborative social activities that mirror naturalistic social challenges—but at lower levels of intensity than the larger peer group. In a small-group context, adults can create a safe and supportive peer context. They can slow down the pace of the social interaction and provide feedback to help children attend and respond to social cues, thus supporting their ability to engage in increasingly complex social interactions. In addition, collaborative interactions with peers offer practice in negotiation and social problem-solving skills, and stimulate the development of the cognitive skills that underlie effective social exchange, including self-control and perspective taking. For these reasons, Friendship Group advocates the inclusion of peer partners in group sessions.

DEVELOPMENTAL FOUNDATIONS OF FRIENDSHIP GROUP

As early as the toddler years, most children show a marked interest in other children and make efforts to initiate contact. However, it is not until the preschool years that most children begin to engage in sustained and ordered play with other children, and begin to use the word *friend* in a meaningful way. Social skills then develop very rapidly during the preschool years (ages 3–5) and prepare children for the social demands of formal school entry, such as getting along in a group, forming friendships, following rules and routines, and controlling impulses. The early elementary sessions of the Friendship Group program are designed to help children who enter early elementary school (grades K–2) without these foundational social skills in place. The Advanced Elementary Sessions (grades 3–5) address the more complex aspects of peer relations that emerge in the later elementary school years. The developmental progression of social skills that guides the organization of the program is reviewed briefly in the following sections.

Social Skill Development in Early Childhood

The foundations of effective social interaction develop in two intertwined domains: (1) positive play skills that emerge and mature to support effective social engagement, and (2) self-control skills that develop to support emotion regulation and the control of aggressive impulses. Play skills develop sequentially, beginning first with *parallel play*, when children play side by side, watching and imitating each other. *Cooperative play* emerges next, when children share materials, take turns, and help each other. Next, *coordinated play* emerges, when children make a plan and organize their play together, engaging in reciprocal role taking (playing mother and baby, or teacher and student) and dividing resources (toys, art materials) into equivalent shares for each play partner. Sustained, coordinated play is supported by the child's developing language skills, perspective-taking abilities, and attention and memory skills.

To support this increasingly complex play, children must learn to manage their feelings and control their impulses. To do so, children must develop the verbal, emotional, and social skills that allow them to inhibit their first impulses, comply with social protocol, and "use their words" to voice dissatisfaction and resolve disagreements.

Social Skill Development in Middle Childhood

In early elementary school, play interactions become more organized, elaborate, and rule-governed. Children more often play in larger peer groups, and competitive games increase in frequency and complexity. Understanding fair play and handling the pressures of competitive play are key to successful participation in grade school games. In general, children are moving from preschool to elementary play structures between the ages of 5 and 7, with more structured play characterizing the majority of large-group peer interactions by the ages of 7–8.

Correspondingly, self-control skills become more valued, including the capacity to regulate emotion and control impulses. Peers increasingly censure children who show dysregulated behavior, particularly children who exhibit reactive/outburst anger and/or norm-breaking behaviors such as rule violations, cheating, and poor sportsmanship. By second grade, aggressive-disruptive and hyperactive/inattentive behaviors become the primary predictors of peer rejection.

Around age 8 (third grade, on average), children's social cognitions mature, and they begin to understand the social world with greater sophistication. In particular, they begin to make social comparisons and to compare themselves with their peers. These new thinking skills have both positive and negative consequences for peer relations. On the one hand, children become increasingly capable of accurately reporting their social behavior and its effects on others, and of taking the perspective of others. They also become more competent at planning and social problem solving, generating multiple solutions to social problems and evaluating the appropriateness of each prior to acting. They are more able to understand and respect diverse points of view, and can work together more collaboratively to accomplish group decision making and conflict resolution. Children begin to differentiate *best friends* from *good friends* and *acquaintances*—recognizing that each type of relationship conveys a different degree of affection for and commitment toward each other. Their advanced social reasoning skills allow children to withstand disagreements and sustain friendships over time, as they continue to develop a sense of loyalty and commitment to their friends. In addition, *conversation* becomes a more central focus of peer interactions, and play becomes increasingly goal-oriented, as children strive to improve their skills in team sports or games.

The negative side of this growing social sophistication is that, by third grade, children are aware of the general group status of their classmates and can identify those who are liked or disliked by peers. Correspondingly, social status becomes more crystallized, and peer acceptance and peer rejection become quite stable from year to year. The intentional victimization or social exclusion of targeted peers emerges as a distinct feature of peer relations during the later school years. With advanced social reasoning, children are able to sustain negative reputational biases, harbor grudges against disliked peers, and organize campaigns of peer exclusion. Children who are emotionally volatile, isolated, and submissive are at increased risk for peer victimization. Table 1.1 summarizes this overview of developmental characteristics.

A Developmentally Informed Intervention Design

Friendship Group is organized in alignment with these naturally occurring progressions in children's social and emotional skills. The manual is divided into two broad developmental levels. The early elementary sessions are designed for children in the 5–8 age range (grades K–2). Advanced sessions target more complex peer problems and are designed for children in the 8–11 age range (grades 3–5). The social games and activities that comprise the sessions are organized developmentally, moving from easier play activities at the beginning of the program (e.g., parallel play) to increasingly complex social play later in the year (e.g., competitive games with rules), providing children with opportunities to consolidate simpler skills (reaching automaticity) before moving on to more advanced social challenges.

TABLE 1.1. Developmental Characteristics of Social Skill Development in Children Ages 3–11

Age (years)	Social skill development
Preschool (3–5)	• Children initiate interaction and engage comfortably in parallel play. • Cooperative play emerges and becomes more frequent. • Children can share materials and work together on a common activity. • Coordinated pretend play with complementary roles emerges. • Simple group games are enjoyed.
Early elementary school (5–8)	• Coordinated pretend play continues and grows in complexity. • Organized and competitive games with rules become more common. • Aggressive behavior decreases. • Fair play and good sportsmanship are valued. • Empathy and altruism increase. • Negotiation and conflict management skills emerge.
Later elementary school (8–11)	• Can make social comparisons and consider social values. • "Best friendships" often emerge. • Conversation increases as a form of interaction. • Social understanding and recognition of different perspectives increases. • Decision making is more collaborative. • Problem solving and conflict are often managed without adult support. • Social reputations crystallize, social mobility is more limited. • Intentional victimization and social exclusion emerge.

Friendship Group Early Elementary School Sessions

There are six units in the early elementary (K–2) Friendship Group program, ordered developmentally. See Table 1.2. The curriculum begins with strategies for initiating friendships and establishing common ground (Unit I), and moves on to promoting cooperation and self-control skills (Unit II). Initial practice activities and games involve parallel and cooperative play. Next, the program introduces negotiation skills, with activities that call for coordinated and complementary roles (Unit III), followed by a focus on competitive play (good sportsmanship), including social problem solving to resolve conflicts (Unit IV). In Unit V, effective communication and listening skills are reviewed, along with more complex play activities that require more advanced social coordination, negotiation, and teamwork. The final set of sessions emphasizes strategies for sustaining friendships, including managing disappointments and coping with provocation (Unit VI).

TABLE 1.2. Summary of Unit Contents for Early Elementary Sessions

Unit focus	Early elementary sessions (grades K–2; ages 5–8)
Unit I. Establishing Common Ground	• Social participation and joining in; initiating friendships • Sharing information (telling about you) • Asking questions and listening (listening to your friend) • Recognizing and expressing basic emotions; sharing feelings
Unit II. Caring and Controlled Behavior	• Caring and cooperation; helping and sharing • Impulse control; calming down and thinking before you act • Expressing concerns (saying the problem and how you feel) • Fair play; finding a fair solution
Unit III. Negotiating with Friends	• Planning together • Negotiation skills • Compromise (making a deal) • Fair strategies for decision making (voting, taking turns, flipping a coin)
Unit IV. Handling Competitive Play	• Taking turns and following rules • Good sportsmanship (good things to say when you win or lose) • Resisting the temptation to cheat • Treating your friends with respect
Unit V. Communicating Effectively	• Expressing your point of view • Listening to and respecting the other's perspective • Attending to body language; noticing others' feelings • Working together as a team
Unit VI. Coping with Tough Stuff	• Coping with provocation and bullying • Managing disappointments • Closing Friendship Group

Friendship Group Advanced Elementary School Sessions

The advanced sessions focus on social skills training during the later elementary years (grades 3–5). See Table 1.3. Many of the social and self-regulatory skills introduced during the early elementary years continue to be important in these later elementary years, and several of the advanced intervention group sessions are designed to review, reinforce, and support the maintenance and generalization of these skills. Specifically, there is a continuing emphasis on teamwork, cooperation and communication skills, fair play, and effective conflict management and social problem solving. In addition, some new issues and skills are introduced. These new skills build upon the increased cognitive abilities of older elementary students, including the capacity for greater self-reflection, social comparison, and social reasoning. They also tackle some of the more complex social dynamics that older elementary students face in the peer group, including navigating social networks, dealing with social aggression and other forms of social exclusion or bullying, and coping with feelings of social anxiety and insecurity. New skills also include setting personal goals, positive thinking, and making responsible decisions.

In general, the sessions at the advanced elementary level anticipate that children will have more well-developed attention, cognitive, and verbal skills than the sessions at the early elementary level. Whereas the early elementary sessions move at a faster pace, including more "hands-on" activities with brief discussions, the Advanced Elementary Sessions include longer and more in-depth discussions and role plays. In addition, the Advanced Elementary Sessions tackle more difficult self-regulatory and conflict management skills, focusing on managing stress and regulating social anxiety. Group activities challenge the older children in areas of team planning, group collaboration, verbal discussion, and social problem solving.

Note that the age guidelines that differentiate the early and Advanced Elementary Sessions are just general heuristics. In some cases, the demands of the Advanced Elementary Sessions may be too high for children (particularly some 8- to 9-year-olds). If this is the case for children in your group, consider using sessions from the early elementary program that are designed for children with less advanced verbal, attentional, and social skills.

TABLE 1.3. Summary of Unit Contents for Advanced Elementary Sessions

Unit focus	Advanced elementary sessions (grades 3–5; ages 8–11)
Unit I. Cooperation and Conversation Skills	• Making new friends; meeting and greeting • Having a conversation; asking questions and listening • Initiating interactions; inviting others to play, joining in • Sustaining conversations and interactions
Unit II. Understanding and Respecting Others	• The Golden Rule; good sportsmanship • Cooperation and negotiation (working it out, making a deal) • Managing conflict; perspective taking and compromise • Social problem-solving skills; overcoming conflicts
Unit III. Coping with Social Stress	• Managing stress (keeping your cool) • Appraising social situations; positive thinking • Coping with teasing and bullying
Unit IV. Responsible Decision Making	• Generating alternatives; advanced social problem solving • Setting personal goals • Committing to positive change

CHAPTER 2

Program Administration

In this chapter, we review the "coaching method" that informs the Friendship Group intervention design and describe how it promotes social skill development and improves children's social competence. We discuss the important decisions that must be made when planning a Friendship Group intervention, including (1) the location, number, and length of group sessions; (2) the selection of children for the group and the evaluation of their social skills and difficulties; (3) tailoring sessions to accommodate individual differences; (4) group size and composition, along with the staffing plan; and (5) the inclusion of peer partners. This chapter also reviews the "nuts and bolts" of session administration, including issues to consider when planning the space to be used for the group program, the management of the materials, use of the manual, and roles of the Friendship Group coaches (leader and co-leader).

THE FRIENDSHIP GROUP COACHING MODEL

Social skill training programs became popular as an intervention strategy to promote children's social competence and positive peer relations in the 1970s and 1980s. Many of the original social skill training programs were quite short in duration (10–12 sessions), and didactic in nature. Children were provided with instructions and models of positive social behaviors, and given the opportunity to practice those skills in brief role plays. These early programs had limited impact because they emphasized skill knowledge (learning what you are supposed to do), but spent insufficient time on skill practice (being able to perform the skills in social interactions). In addition, they often focused on discrete social behaviors (e.g., how to introduce yourself to someone new), rather than on the more complex interaction skills that characterize natural peer play and conversation. They did not provide the amount or kind of practice necessary to help children develop more substantial social competence.

We now understand that *social competence requires more than social knowledge and the ability to enact discrete behaviors.* Competent social interaction involves the rapid coordination of thought, emotion, and action, with much of the process guided by appraisal and decision responses that operate below conscious awareness. In other words, socially skillful children are able to operate on "automatic pilot" in many social situations, except when unexpected problems or novel challenges arise. They are able to do so because, through their extended experience with social interaction, skillful responses have become habitual and effortless. To reach this level of automaticity, extended skill practice is required. A good analogy is learning to play the piano. Knowing how a piece should be played is not the same as practicing sufficiently to play the piece well. Furthermore, extended practice of multiple pieces at one level of skill difficulty is often necessary to gain the general fluidity of competence to move forward and learn piano pieces at the next level of difficulty. Similarly, extended and supported practice opportunities are needed to remediate social skill deficits and promote fluid and skillful social interaction.

The coaching model that guides the Friendship Group program includes behavioral instructions and support. However, in addition, the program addresses emotional features of social behavior (emotion understanding and regulation) and the thinking skills that underlie effective interaction (play-planning skills, negotiation, conflict management, and related social problem-solving skills). In addition, the Friendship Group incorporates extended practice in multiple play and conversation contexts to strengthen children's social performance capabilities. The next section describes the coaching process in more detail and how the coaching model is utilized in the Friendship Group program.

KEY COMPONENTS OF EFFECTIVE COACHING

The coaching process provides (1) explicit instruction in social skills; (2) structured and supportive opportunities to practice those skills; (3) feedback that allows the child to adjust and improve skill performance; (4) opportunities for self-regulation that promote social awareness and sensitivity; and

---

Components of Effective Social Skill Training Sessions

1. **Skill presentations** use instruction, modeling, and discussions to clarify the social skill concepts and provide examples of positive and negative skill performance.

2. **Skill practice activities** offer opportunities to practice and refine skill performance in the context of strategic and structured games and activities.

3. **Performance feedback** provides specific praise to reinforce skill performance, with noncritical reactions from adults and peers to support social awareness and sensitivity.

4. **Self-regulation support** includes emotion coaching, induction strategies, and the use of problem-solving dialogue to empower children to solve their own social problems.

5. **Generalization programming** includes practice in multiple game and activity formats with peer partners, and efforts to coordinate support for peer interaction with teachers and parents.

(5) support to generalize social skills to "real-life" peer interactions. To accomplish these goals, each session is divided into core components (friendship circle, construction station, optional snack, collaborative challenges, closing circle).

Friendship Circle

Each session begins with a friendship circle, which includes explicit instruction in social skills. Children select a "feeling face" and share their feelings. The session plan is presented using a set of agenda pictures. The coach then introduces the skill for the day, using a story, role play, or other discussion starter. These brief, interactive lessons illustrate positive and negative examples of the skill (e.g., what to do and what not to do), and encourage active child engagement and discussion of the skills. Often, there is also a brief group activity or game following this discussion that exercises working memory and/or inhibitory control skills.

Construction Station

Next, each session includes tabletop activities or structured games that provide children with opportunities to practice the target skills. In the early elementary sessions, the construction station activities usually include manipulatives (e.g., arts and crafts, blocks). In the Advanced Elementary Sessions, the activities more often include role-play challenges, and also include three sessions in which "friendship movies" are taped and reviewed.

Optional Snack

In some situations (usually when groups are held after school or on weekends), Friendship Group also includes a snack period, which offers opportunities to practice conversation skills, as well as cooperative planning and teamwork. During initial sessions, basic cooperative planning is done at snack (e.g., determining who will do the various snack jobs, such as passing out cups and napkins, pouring juice). In later sessions, "sharing snacks" are introduced to foster practice in problem-solving and negotiation skills, as group members must decide how to divide snack materials fairly and work together to distribute them.

Collaborative Challenges

Each session also includes physically active games or team challenges that require the more general use of target skills. These challenges foster the practice of impulse control; motivate group engagement; and encourage practice in planning, communication skills, and group problem solving.

Closing Circle

Each session ends with a closing circle and performance feedback. Positive feedback reinforces skill performance and motivates future efforts. Throughout each session, coaches offer specific praise that identifies skillful behaviors and efforts. In addition, during the final session, group members share compliments, and coaches formally recognize skillful behaviors observed during the session.

Integrated Supports for Self-Regulation

Across the different components of each session, coaches use therapeutic strategies to support the development of child social-emotional skills. For example, coaches offer clarifying feedback, helping children to understand the social consequences of their behaviors. Young children often engage in impulsive behaviors (e.g., grabbing a toy, pushing ahead in line) to reach their goals, without taking note of the negative impact on peers. Clarifying feedback helps children understand how these behaviors make peers feel, so that they understand that peer complaints are not about *who they are*, but are the controllable consequences of *what they did*. Adult feedback plays a critical role in helping children recognize the way their behavior affects peers and the power they have to change that behavior. The manner in which this feedback is provided is important, as the goal is not to reprimand the child for misbehavior, but rather to help the child reflect on what happened in a way that promotes greater social awareness and more sensitive responding in the future (e.g., "When you grab the ball, it makes your friend sad, and he doesn't want to play with you. When you wait your turn, everyone has fun"). Friendship Group includes group planning and reflection discussions to help children consider the behaviors that helped them have fun together (and those that interfered with group success).

When children experience social problems in the group sessions, such as conflict with peers or exclusion, it is often tempting for coaches to jump in with directives or suggestions to solve the problem and set things right in the group. However, except in situations involving dangerous or otherwise unacceptable behavior, Friendship Group emphasizes the use of therapeutic strategies that empower children to correct their own behavior and solve their own social problems (emotion coaching, induction strategies, and social problem-solving dialogue, described in Chapter 3).

Generalization Programming

Naturalistic social interactions are complex and often require the child to respond flexibly to subtle social interaction cues in the context of high emotional arousal. Hence, to make sure that the skills trained in coaching sessions generalize to real-life settings, Friendship Group includes practice in increasingly complex social games and activities over time. The goal is to help children move from structured social opportunities that provide maximal support for skill acquisition to activities that gradually increase the level of difficulty and naturalistic challenge. In addition to coaching children in social skills, the inclusion of peer partners in the group sessions or the use of peer-pairing activities to strengthen peer interactions outside of group sessions is strongly encouraged (strategies for including peers are discussed in more detail later in this chapter).

PROGRAM FORMAT AND GROUP ORGANIZATION

Location, Number, and Length of Sessions

The Friendship Group program includes 26 sessions developed for the early elementary years (grades K–2) and 14 sessions for the advanced elementary years (grades 3–5). The sessions are written for a 60-minute period, with a time for snack and informal conversation built into each session. Sessions can be condensed into 45-minute sessions by dropping the snack period. The sessions are designed for weekly administration, but the early elementary program can also be run as twice-weekly sessions. When the time allotted for Friendship Group does not allow for administration of all the sessions, and group leaders must select a subset of sessions for administration, *it is important to preserve the developmental progression of skill presentation*. However, group leaders may choose to move more quickly through certain skill domains by condensing or skipping some sessions within units, in order to focus time on sessions that target the skills that are most salient for the children in a particular group. Decisions about program duration and the number and length of sessions will often be constrained by the intervention setting. The impact on the written program and any necessary adjustments should be considered in advance, in order to tailor the group content to most closely target the skill deficits of the participating children.

When constraints make it necessary to shorten Friendship Group and utilize only a subset of the sessions, it is important to be realistic about the amount of skill acquisition that can be accomplished in a shortened program. Research on social skill training suggests that short programs (e.g., 12–14 sessions) may be sufficient to promote positive behavior change and improve sociometric ratings when children primarily need to acquire new ways of interacting—for example, if the children in the group are primarily socially withdrawn. However, when children also have to "unlearn" problematic behaviors, such as aggression, or when developmental challenges reduce the speed with which new competencies are acquired, longer programs are needed to promote meaningful changes in social skills and peer acceptance. Effective coaching programs for children who are aggressive, learning disabled, or have attention-deficit/hyperactivity disorder (ADHD) are longer, in the range of 25–30 sessions. Longer programs give children the opportunity to practice and achieve mastery of each skill. Although there are only 14 sessions in the advanced elementary program, these can be extended for children with more substantial social skill delays in two ways: (1) by supplementing them with lessons on fair play, self-control, and negotiation skills from the early elementary sessions; and (2) by slowing the pace of delivery of the advanced elementary sessions, using optional activities and repeating activities in order to give children more time to practice and master target skills. To maximize children's gains from Friendship Group, it is important for children to work at skill level that is appropriate for them developmentally, so that they are actively engaged in sessions and demonstrating skill acquisition. It is also important for them to participate in a sufficient number of sessions to learn new skills and develop comfort and automaticity in skill performance.

In terms of the organization and location of group sessions, Friendship Group has been run effectively in a number of different ways: (1) as a "pullout" program during the school day, (2) as an extracurricular school-based program with sessions held after school or on the weekend, or (3) as a "freestanding" program offered by a community service agency or mental health provider. Each of these options is described briefly below.

Providing Friendship Group as a pullout program during the school day has a number of advantages. Children's peer difficulties are often most prominent in the school context, and promoting positive peer relations at school often has secondary benefits, including reduced behavior problems and enhanced learning engagement and achievement. In addition, a school-based program provides easy access to peer partners, which facilitates intervention effectiveness and generalization. The challenge of providing Friendship Group during the school day is that sessions must typically be shorter in length than in an extracurricular setting (usually no more than 45 minutes), and the space and schedule demands may be difficult to negotiate, depending on the school situation. Given the concurrent academic difficulties experienced by many rejected children, it is important to schedule school-based programs in ways that complement and do not conflict with academic programming.

Friendship Group can also be provided as a school-based extracurricular program, with sessions held at the school during an after-school or weekend period. This was the organization used in the original Fast Track project (see Chapter 5). The chief advantage of providing Friendship Group as an extracurricular program (rather than in-school program) is that sessions can last longer (60–90 minutes) and do not interfere with academic activities. When extracurricular groups are held at the school, particularly if they are held after school, it is often possible to include peer partners in sessions, fostering skill acquisition and generalization. Transportation difficulties sometimes arise and can create a challenge for some parents. Extracurricular sessions make it possible to run concurrent, collateral programs for parents.

Friendship Group can also be provided as a mental health service, with sessions held in an office location or community-based center. In such settings, the major challenge is (1) creating a positive group dynamic, given that normative peer partners are usually not included; and (2) fostering the generalization of developing social skills to the child's peer interactions at home and school.

Selecting Children for Friendship Group

Developmental research has made it clear that children can have difficulty gaining peer acceptance for different reasons. Coaching programs are most effective when they focus on unaccepted children who display deficits in the social skills that are targeted in the skill training program. The Friendship Group program focuses on promoting social competencies in areas of prosocial skills, play skills, communication skills, emotion regulation, impulse control, negotiation skills, and social problem-solving skills. Hence, children are most likely to benefit from this program when they are having difficulties with peers (e.g., low levels of acceptance by peers and elevated rejection), and when those difficulties are accompanied by deficits in one or more of the targeted skill areas. These children may (or may not) have additional behavioral, developmental, or emotional problems, such as aggressive or impulsive behaviors, social avoidance, or awkward or intrusive social behaviors. This program is helpful for children who share the "common ground" features of peer difficulties and social skill deficits, and who may demonstrate a range of different, concurrent adjustment difficulties.

Note that not all aggressive children have social skill deficits or peer problems. **Friendship Group is not a good intervention for children in the older elementary grades who have adequate social skills and established friendships, yet still show aggressive and antisocial behaviors.** These children will likely not benefit from Friendship Group (because they do not need the social skill remediation), and they may be a disruptive element in the group (because they are not motivated to forge new friendships). Conversely, aggressive children who are isolated, anxious, and who have social skill deficits are likely to benefit from Friendship Group because the social skill building and friendship formation focus fits their needs.

When selecting children for Friendship Group, we recommend that you get input from classroom teachers and parents to assess the quality of each child's peer relations, prosocial competencies, emotion regulation skills, attention skills, and behavior problems. These ratings will provide information that will guide you in identifying the needs of individual children, as well as informing decisions about group composition.

Tailoring Sessions to Accommodate Individual Differences

The original version of the Friendship Group program was developed for the Fast Track project (see Chapter 5), which served children who entered kindergarten showing high rates of aggressive-disruptive behavior. Since that original study, Friendship Group has also been used in prevention studies to help children entering kindergarten with high rates of impulsive and hyperactive behavior. The Friendship Group program has also been used by mental health service providers and in after-school therapeutic recreation programs. In those contexts, children are referred by parents, school personnel, or other service providers because they need help developing social skills and positive peer relations and hence represent a much wider range of child characteristics. For example, in addition to impulsive or aggressive children, other children who experience peer problems and social skill deficits include socially withdrawn and anxious children, children with significant attention deficits, and children with developmental challenges (including autism spectrum characteristics, pervasive developmental disorder).

Developmental Delays or Disabilities

Because the Friendship Group program was originally developed for and evaluated with children who had externalizing problems (e.g., aggressive-oppositional or hyperactive–impulsive behavior), the program includes an extended emphasis on self-control and negotiation skills, but assumes typical developmental levels of verbal skills. If you are using Friendship Group to address the social skill needs of children who are developmentally challenged, particularly children with delays in verbal skills, attention focus, or processing speed, you will need to tailor the program by adjusting the pace of activities and selectively using (or skipping) some of the activities, and/or providing individualized support for the children with those skill delays.

Low Verbal Skills or Attention Problems

In our experience, the program as written works well for many aggressive, impulsive, or socially withdrawn children. However, particularly at the younger ages, the pace of the program can overwhelm children with delayed verbal skills, slower processing speed, and/or reduced attention skills. Reducing the group size (e.g., to a peer pair or triad) is very helpful to these children, because it reduces the complexity and speed of social interaction. In addition, repeating skill sessions is often very helpful, because it gives them a chance to consolidate the information. Because children only benefit from sessions when they are actively engaged, it is better to progress more slowly in the program, repeating sessions or activities as needed, in order to maintain children's active engagement and skill mastery, rather than move forward more quickly with material that is too difficult. For the same reason, if you are working with older elementary children who have significant delays in verbal skills, processing speed, or attention focus, and find that the extended discussions and role plays included in the advanced elementary sessions are too difficult, it is best to use the more "hands-on" discussion exercises included in the early elementary program to increase their engagement and understanding.

Group Size and Composition

Friendship Group is developed for small groups of four to six children led by one or two staff (group leader and co-leader). However, some settings will call for alternative arrangements, including varying the group size or staff constellation. Decisions about group size, composition, staffing, and inclusion of peer partners need to be thought about carefully, as they can have a significant impact on the group process and outcome. In making these decisions, it is particularly important to consider the nature and severity of the social difficulties of the participating children. The size of the group, availability of adult support, and the characteristics of the social partner(s) all affect the degree of difficulty or social challenge associated with group participation. They also affect the capacity of the group leader to facilitate therapeutic processes during social interaction, as well as the leader's ability to manage problematic group dynamics and control negative escalation.

As groups get larger, there are more social cues to monitor, which can engender arousal and increase feelings of insecurity. Working with peer pairs or triads provides the "easiest" setting for social skill training, both in terms of the processing demands on the children and of the capacity of a single group leader to manage effectively. As the group size increases, it places greater demands on children's processing abilities and inhibitory control, as they must wait longer for their turn, and they must divide resources among more individuals. Larger groups also reduce the individual child's opportunities for social interaction, as more individuals are vying for a chance to share their opinions or participate in a task. Large intervention groups can undermine the leader's ability to implement coaching, by making it difficult to "slow down" social interaction and encourage children to reflect on the social process. For children with significant delays in verbal, attention, or processing skills, the optimal size for coaching is a *peer-pairing* or *triad* situation. For children with normative levels of verbal and processing skill, the optimal size for a therapeutic group run by two staff members is four to five children. Therapeutic groups larger than six are not recommended, although they can be effective when there are additional staff members available to assist, creating a capacity to break the larger group down into subgroups for discussions and practice activities.

The characteristics of the participating children also affect the degree to which a particular group provides a therapeutic context for social skill acquisition. Including peer partners who are socially responsive and well regulated enhances the therapeutic value of the experience for children with social skill deficits, because they create an ordered social context with predictable opportunities for social interaction and a high rate of positive contingent responding. In contrast, a group that contains multiple members with aggressive behavioral tendencies and high rates of socially domineering and intrusive behavior can be threatening and unpredictable. This kind of group provokes reactive responding and is prone to escalating conflicts, as children react to perceived threats or model rule-breaking behaviors. Research has demonstrated that, even when behavior management strategies are included to control aggressive and disruptive behavior during group sessions, children with social skill deficits benefit less when they are in groups with many aggressive partners than when they are in groups that contain partners who provide more positive role models and responses (see Lavallee, Bierman, Nix, & Conduct Problems Prevention Research Group [CPPRG], 2005). **In group interventions it is particularly important to guard against negative contagion or "deviancy training," which occurs when a child responds positively (via laughing or imitation) to another's inappropriate or rule-breaking behavior.** Regardless of adult sanctions, this type of positive peer responding increases the likelihood that children will rely on their inappropriate social habits, which in turn impedes the rate at which they adopt alternative prosocial behaviors. Although one can use behavior management techniques (e.g., rules, token systems) to maintain behavioral control within such a group, the focus of the group becomes one of managing problem behaviors with external control, which diminishes the opportunities to focus on promoting self-regulated social competence (see Chapters 3 and 4 for a more complete discussion of this issue). By avoiding the placement of highly aggressive children together in the same Friendship Group, and by including skillful peer partners, you will increase the quality of the therapeutic process and the positive impact of the intervention on the target children. As long as the group is managed well, these skillful peer partners will enjoy group sessions and may benefit from them as well.

In general, Friendship Groups are of greater benefit to children when they include children with similar social skill deficits but complementary (rather than similar) behavioral needs. That is, group members may have in common deficits in cooperative play skills or anger management, although some react with social avoidance, whereas others exhibit impulsive aggression. This kind of a group provides a common basis for skill training and may become quite cohesive, without creating a threatening or resistant social dynamic in the intervention group that impedes the coaching agenda.

In addition, you will need to make decisions regarding the gender composition of the group. Grade school friendships are typically (though not always) same-sex partnerships, and so coaching is often done in same-sex groups. However, research on the Fast Track Friendship Groups revealed that boys made greater gains in social skill acquisition and positive peer relations when their Friendship Groups contained girls and boys, rather than being composed only of other aggressive boys (Lavallee et al., 2005). The goal is to create a positive peer climate within the friendship group context, so that the sessions are enjoyable for all participants.

In some cases, it may not be possible to staff Friendship Group with two leaders (e.g., leader and co-leader). If you are running Friendship Group by yourself, it is particularly important to keep the group size small so that you are able to provide therapeutic support. If you are working alone, or if you are serving a child with severe social difficulties and behavior problems, consider starting with a small group and adding peer partners to increase group size over time. That is, begin working with dyads for initial skill training and practice; then increase the group size by adding peer partners in later sessions, when the target children are ready for the added social challenge. This strategy allows you to address the significant skill deficits or behavior problems of particular children (in dyadic sessions) first, and then work on the generalization of those skills to larger groups of nonproblematic peers later in the program.

Including Peer Partners

Helping children generalize the skills learned in the supportive Friendship Group setting to their naturally occurring peer interactions at home and school is a challenge. Natural peer interactions are often unstructured and occur in large groups that provide relatively low levels of positive peer responding. Even worse, some children face ostracism or negative reputations among their classroom or neighborhood peers, such that peers shut them out and make it particularly difficult for them to make friends or gain entry to peer activities. To the extent possible, the Friendship Group program will have a stronger impact on children if it includes efforts to create niches of social opportunity at school and home. Two kinds of coordinated programming assist with this goal.

When Friendship Group is held as a pullout program during the school day, we recommend using classroom peers as rotating peer partners in group sessions. To do so, you need to get permission from parents of other children in the classroom to attend group sessions. Once you have a list of classmates who are allowed to participate in Friendship Group, you can include them in sessions, using a rotating schedule. The unaccepted children who are the focus of the program come to every session, and other peer partners rotate every two sessions or so. This process allows the target children, who attend every session, to "demonstrate" their knowledge of social skills to classroom peers, highlighting their social skills to the peer partners. It also fosters the generalization of social skills to children's school-based peer interactions by providing practice with the same children with whom they will interact in the classroom and on the playground.

When Friendship Group is not held during the school day, it is sometimes possible to schedule peer-pairing sessions during the school day to complement the group sessions held outside of school. This strategy was used in the original Fast Track Friendship Group program. In Fast Track, the extracurricular Friendship Group sessions included only "target" children who were experiencing social adjustment difficulties. To increase the likelihood that they would use their new social skills at school and receive a positive peer response, peer-pairing sessions were conducted parallel to the friendship group program. Parent permission was acquired for classmates. Then, each week, each target child had a half-hour guided play session during the school day with a classmate. Classmate partners rotated during the course of the school year. As dyads, these children completed activities (games, art-and-crafts activities) designed to allow the target child to display improved social skills to the classroom peer and to foster mutually rewarding exchanges between the target child and a variety of classmates.

Communicating with Parents and Teachers

We recommend that Friendship Group leaders schedule periodic conferences with teachers and parents, in order to update them on children's progress in Friendship Group, and to discuss positive peer interaction opportunities that they might support outside of the group context. Each session includes a "Friendship Tips" handout that can be shared with teachers and parents to keep them informed about the focus of the group session. Supplementing these with meetings provides a chance to talk about the individual child's social needs and progress.

NUTS AND BOLTS OF SESSION ADMINISTRATION

Selecting and Preparing Space

The space available for Friendship Group will vary depending upon the setting. If you are working in a school context, your choices may be quite constrained. Some considerations to keep in mind as you identify a room follow.

Selecting a Space

The space must be large enough to include an area for a friendship circle, a tabletop for construction station activities and snack, and room for physically active games and other collaboration challenges. The optimal space will be just large enough to include these activities and no larger. Very large and open spaces, such as gyms or cafeterias, encourage running and loud voices that may disrupt the group process. The optimal space will also include few distractions. To the extent that attractive items are visible to group participants (e.g., supplies, games, books, chalkboards) or areas to explore (e.g., stairways, stage), the participants may be distracted from the task at hand and enticed into problem behaviors. The work of the coach is much greater when he or she must constantly remind children about what is "off limits" and expend energy monitoring and redirecting the children's focus. If distraction-free space of the optimal size is not available, look for a space that you can constrict by using concrete markers to identify group space. For example, in a classroom you might move desks or bookshelves around to define a well-marked group space. (Just remember to return desks or bookshelves to their original locations when you're done.) Similarly, tables or shelves may be covered with a sheet so that distracting materials are not visible during sessions. To the extent that off-limit areas must be identified, do so with clear concrete boundaries as much as possible. Avoid group locations that place children in a position where they can run away (e.g., in a room with many doors, open hallway), or where there are other people coming in and out during the session (e.g., a library). It is important to plan a setup time prior to each group session to prepare the space and thereby prevent behavior problems.

The Friendship Circle

Define the friendship circle space with a throw rug or a space marked by masking tape or a set of chairs placed in a circle or around a table. The important point is to clearly demarcate the space to which children will go routinely for the friendship circle.

Materials Storage

Consider carefully where to store materials. Children will no doubt be interested in any materials they see lying about. Power struggles over materials can be averted if initial care is taken to maintain control over these materials and to keep them out of sight until they are needed. It is important to have the presentation posters, craft supplies, snack foods, and cups carefully organized and stored, out of the reach of the children but easily and quickly accessible as they are needed.

Presession Planning

All aspects of your use of space should be planned carefully before each session. The coaches should carefully survey the preparation of the space to make sure that it is adequately "child-proofed" and clearly defined. Before you start, walk through the space together and agree upon the specific areas to be used for each part of the session.

Preparing Materials

A wide variety of materials are used in this program; the materials needed for each session are listed at the top of the session-by-session entries in the manual. We recommend stocking a supply bin for use in sessions held across the year (see Table 2.1 for suggested contents). Posters and agenda pictures that are used in multiple sessions follow Chapter 5. We recommend making colored, laminated copies of these commonly used materials. Additional materials to copy for session activities are included at the end of each unit in the Friendship Group Manual for both early and advanced elementary sessions. To keep a tight pace in the group, it is important to have the materials prepared ahead of time and well organized so that you can manage transitions effectively.

In general, you want to manage the materials so that they are available only for the period of time they are actually needed, thereby allowing you to focus your attention fully on the children. Preparedness also precludes delays and wait time for the children that might foster restlessness and disruptive

---

TABLE 2.1. Materials to Include in Friendship Group Supply Bins

General materials for supply bins

balloons; bean bags; bowls (four small); deck of cards (four); dice (six); dominoes (thick sides); glue sticks; highlighters; markers; marbles (six); masking tape (mixed colors); microphone (toilet paper roll, black duct tape, aluminum foil top); nametags; paper (white and colored); paperclips; pens and pencils; poker chips (red, white, blue); posterboard; scissors; spoons (six); stickers (star stickers and assorted) and sequins.

If opting for snack: paper plates, napkins, cups, snack foods.

Additional items for early elementary program bins

bell; blocks (40 small wooden); cars (12 small, some old, some new); cotton balls; flashlight; firefighter hats (six); funnel; hula hoops (two); jump ropes (two); pennies; playdough; plastic animals (12 small); ring; string; stuffed animals (four small); traffic cones (six small); visors (two).

Additional items for advanced elementary program

board games (junior versions of Outburst, Pictionary, Apples to Apples); clipboards (six); video recording and playback device (iPad or cellphone works fine).

behavior. Organizing activity materials into boxes is a good idea. For example, snack materials can be kept in a small box out of sight and out of reach of the children. The box can be brought down quickly when it is needed, but then easily stored back in its unobtrusive location after delivery of the snack.

Using the Manual

Read the manual carefully before conducting a session. Plan ahead with the co-leader, deciding what each coach's role will be for each part of the session, and selecting desired optional or alternative activities. Prepare and organize the materials for the session. It is not necessary to memorize the sample dialogue presented in the manual, but it is important to include some version of each of the points made. During the session itself, the coaches must rely on memory, as they will not be able to refer to the manual without losing their focus on the group. If helpful, a small, inconspicuous cue card may be brought into the session to help the coach remember the flow of the session and key presentation points.

Minor modifications in the proposed format may be necessary in response to the dynamics of a particular group. For example, a discussion should be shortened if the group is becoming restless; alternatively, an activity may be prolonged if the group is particularly engaged. When making these kinds of modifications, consider the overriding goals of the session so that the adjustments promote the program goals. For example, sometimes children will want to sustain an activity such as coloring because they enjoy it—but there is no new learning value in doing a familiar, solitary activity such as coloring, so this would not be something that is useful to sustain. In contrast, a problem-solving activity may take longer than expected, because children are actively engaged in sharing their perspectives and negotiating a solution. This kind of discussion involves the applied practice of the key skills targeted in the program, and hence it should be sustained to its conclusion, even if it means that the group will have to skip or condense some of the activities later in the session.

Roles of the Leader and Co-Leader

Small Friendship Groups can be run with one leader; larger groups should be staffed by a group leader and co-leader who remain consistent throughout the entire program. We term these leaders the Friendship Group *coaches* because their goal is to support children in the acquisition and refinement of social competencies. Children will often form strong attachments to these adults, and their interpersonal growth during the friendship group experience is fostered substantially by their ability to trust and learn from these warm, supportive, accepting, and consistent leaders. Each coach should read the manual carefully before each session. It is important that leaders and co-leaders feel confident about their ability to carry out program objectives, including the fostering of social skill acquisition, the therapeutic support strategies, and the use of noncoercive behavior management strategies (as discussed in the next chapter).

Larger groups may be run by two group leaders who are colleagues and share the role of "coach" equally, switching off in the role of leader and co-leader in different activities and sessions. In other cases, the group leader will have the primary responsibility for the organization of and preparation for each group session. This person will assure that all materials are prepared and all necessary equipment is available and ready; he or she will also serve as the liaison for communications with parents, teachers, and other program staff. This person will begin each session, providing continuity in the group routine and in the presentation of skill concepts and group rules. In this staffing configuration, the group leader has the ultimate responsibility for the group and for assuring that the group is conducted in a manner consistent with the intervention protocol.

In this latter scenario, the co-leader may have less experience or training and serve primarily to assist the leader in running Friendship Group. However, it is important for the co-leader to avoid a passive stance. In order to be an effective support, the co-leader must engage actively with the children and establish an affective connection with them in the group setting. This role is not one of an aide but one of an active co-therapist. The specific tasks to be allocated to the co-leader are not specified in the manual; individual coach pairs discuss the divisions of labor with which they are comfortable.

Individuals who vary considerably in their level of professional training have run Friendship Group effectively. Personal characteristics play a central role in determining who will enjoy and excel at the role of Friendship Group coach. For example, coaches need to enjoy interacting with children and be sensitive, responsive, and accepting of children who show problematic social behavior, including aggression. Group leaders need to feel confident in the role of instructor and feel comfortable presenting and participating in songs, activities, and games with an engaged and animated presence. The leader also needs to be well organized, able to follow the manual carefully and with fidelity, and also able to adjust the pacing and presentation of activities based upon child responses and group dynamics. Coaches themselves need to be emotionally well regulated, so that they remain unruffled in the context of behavioral challenges, able to provide calm, clear, and consistent social guidance and problem-solving support.

The Friendship Group leader role is designed for individuals with professional training in an area of social-emotional development and child mental health (special education, counseling psychology, clinical psychology, or social work), and who have work experience with children who have behavioral and developmental difficulties. With adequate training and a strong supervision model, paraprofessional staff may also become effective Friendship Group leaders. In this latter case, the regular supervisory support of a trained professional (e.g., supervision meetings, direct or video-taped session observations and reviews) is essential.

In addition to this general professional training and experience, the capacity to implement Friendship Group with fidelity requires specific training and proficiency in several key areas, including (1) a good working knowledge of the coaching model and its mechanisms of action; (2) the ability to present and discuss skill concepts in an engaging way; (3) the ability to monitor children's developmental acquisition of social skills, and to adjust skill practice opportunities in ways that maintain an optimal learning window for each child; (4) the ability to reflect, ask questions, and provide feedback during ongoing practice sessions in a way that fosters social learning; and (5) the ability to effectively implement the therapeutic processes and behavior management strategies associated with the Friendship Group program. These strategies are the discussed in depth in the next chapter.

CHAPTER 3

Therapeutic Processes

This chapter describes four therapeutic processes used in Friendship Group to promote social engagement and self-regulation skills: (1) *positive support*, (2) *emotion coaching*, (3) *induction strategies*, and (4) *social problem-solving dialogue*. These processes increase children's awareness of the positive impact of socially skillful behaviors, thereby reinforcing behavior change. They also improve understanding of cause–effect relations in peer interactions, helping children understand how their behavior affects the feelings and responses of their social partners. Finally, the strategies improve flexibility in social reasoning and behavior, giving children new options for social responding.

In addition to promoting positive social behavior, the Friendship Group program is designed to help children become more socially aware, empathic, and responsive in their social interactions. In addition, Friendship Group seeks to help children feel more comfortable socially, so that they enjoy their social interactions and feel supported by peers. To do so, Friendship Group uses a set of four core therapeutic processes: (1) positive support to increase comfort in social interaction and reduce anxiety; (2) emotion coaching to foster emotional awareness, empathy, and emotion coping; (3) induction strategies to support self-regulation; and (4) social problem-solving dialogue to enhance flexible thinking and conflict management skills.

In Friendship Group, the challenges and conflicts that emerge in the course of the session activities are considered "teachable moments." When coaches talk about feelings and focus on choices during these moments, it increases children's social awareness by slowing down the social interaction, and allowing them to clarify their own feelings and desires and to recognize the feelings and desires of others. This process gives children time to consider alternative responses and builds knowledge of cause–effect dynamics in social interaction.

How coaches deal with problem behavior is also important. Friendship Group behavior management strategies provide an important "backup" system to control aggressive, destructive, or other impulsive behaviors that disrupt the group or are harmful to others (see Chapter 4). However, the goal is not to create a classroom setting in which the adult organizes the activities and the children follow directions and comply. Instead, the goal is to prepare children for effective interactions in unstructured peer contexts, such as the playground, where they are expected to initiate and sustain their own interactions, resolving everyday social conflicts on their own. Hence, the ultimate goal of Friendship Group is to reduce adult direction and to facilitate the children's skills at self-regulation in social interactions.

The four therapeutic processes (e.g., positive support, emotion coaching, induction strategies, and social problem-solving dialogue) support self-regulation skills by improving children's understanding of how their behavior affects their own experiences and the feelings and reactions of their social partners. The strategies also strengthen children's social reasoning skills and foster flexibility and creativity in social responding. In the next sections, we describe each of the Friendship Group therapeutic strategies and their application in the group setting.

POSITIVE SUPPORT STRATEGIES

As a function of both temperament and experience, some children are insecure and anxious in peer interactions. They are unsure whether others will include them, will like them, and will care about their feelings. When children feel anxious in a social situation, they typically react in one of two ways: (1) passively, by withdrawing and avoiding social interaction, or (2) actively, by demanding attention with intrusive or strange behavior that cannot easily be ignored. Friendship Group uses positive support strategies to increase feelings of security and comfort in social interactions and to reduce anxiety, so that children are able to participate freely and can explore and practice new social behavior.

Friendly Narration

The friendly narration support strategy involves the use of frequent warm and friendly comments that describe what is going on, identify similarities (common ground) among the children, and offer opportunities for children to interact with each other. Friendly narration sends out the message that each child is personally welcome in the group, and the group is a friendly and non-threatening place to interact. Examples of this kind of social chat include:

> "Oh, here's Mike. It's good to see you Mike. We were looking for you and hoping you'd be here this week."
>
> "I see Sam chose the red paper again. Jim chose red, too, and so did I. We all like red."
>
> "Mary had an interesting idea. David, I think you might like to hear Mary's idea about snack."

Activity Options and Positive Guidance

Unstructured social situations and inactivity increase social discomfort for many children. Identifying activity options and positive roles provides guidance, directing children toward constructive social behavior (and avoiding the insecurity and "boredom" associated with unstructured waiting). For example, while you are waiting for all children to arrive, you might ask those who are early to help you set up activities, work together to color a poster to be used in the session, or fold or decorate napkins for snack. If children struggle to transition appropriately to and from their classroom to group, give them a structured role to guide transition behavior (e.g., carrying materials for you, practicing a group challenge task such as walking on tiptoes or carrying beans on a spoon as they walk). In general, monitor the pacing of group activities so that children who finish a task quickly are not kept waiting, but have something specific to do. Helpful roles, such as holding the pictures or passing out the pencils, can also aid a restless child in staying engaged in group discussions.

Making a Connection

The support strategy of making a connection involves using your body language to help children feel connected and secure in the group, especially during social situations that are stressful for some children (e.g., working out a conflict, waiting for a turn). To help children stay engaged, use nonverbal channels of communication to connect and calm the child. For example, touch the child (patting the child on the back or gently placing a hand on the child's shoulder or forearm) and use social referencing (making eye contact with the child, nodding at him or her, or giving a thumbs up) to indicate you are noticing the child and appreciative of his or her engagement. In addition, frequently use each child's name.

Specific Praise

To reinforce positive social interaction, acknowledge the specific social behavior observed and its interpersonal consequences by giving specific praise. Avoid vague praise (e.g., "Good job") or personalizing praise (e.g., "Thank you for being good for me today"). Specific praise makes the positive consequences of prosocial behavior salient, so that children see the positive impact of their behavior on others. Be particularly vigilant about praising positive behaviors when children are struggling socially. Examples include:

> "Jorge, you noticed Mary needed the glue and passed it to her. That's a nice way to take care of your friend's feelings."

> "Both of you wanted the red marker, but Nakiesha let Tamara have it this time. You were a peacemaker, Nakiesha."

Positive Support Strategies

- **Friendly narration:** Make frequent warm and friendly comments that describe what is going on, identify similarities among the children, offer opportunities for child-to-child conversation, and frequently use the children's names.

- **Activity options and positive guidance:** Avoid periods of unstructured inactivity or waiting. Monitor the pace of group activities, provide specific entry and closure transition activities, and offer restless children specific roles as helpers or assistants.

- **Make a connection:** Use your body language to help children feel connected and secure in the group setting. Use touch (gently placing a hand on the child's shoulder or forearm) and social referencing (eye contact, nodding, reassuring gesture) to support child engagement.

EMOTION COACHING

Friendship Group uses emotion coaching to increase children's emotional understanding, empathy, and emotion coping skills. The labels that children use to identify their feelings have an impact on how they evaluate situations and thereby on how they respond. Consider, for example, when a child rolls the dice to see who goes first and loses. The child could label that distress as feeling *mad*. Because feeling mad occurs when one has been wronged or mistreated, labeling the feeling *mad* increases the likelihood that the child will react against the action (e.g., feel that the game play is unfair) or against the peer (e.g., feel that the peer has done something unfair). In contrast, if the child labels the feeling as *disappointment*, the label constructs the meaning of the situation as one in which an undesired outcome occurred, but not a personal wrong. Identifying the feeling as one of *disappointment* does not set up the child for a response of retribution in the same way that labeling the feeling *mad* does. The verbal label used to define the feeling has an impact on the appraisal process and behavioral response. In Friendship Group, emotion coaching is focused on helping children develop a differentiated vocabulary of feelings so they can deescalate strong feelings. Children with peer difficulties often have an impoverished sense of their emotions; for example, they may use only two or three emotion labels (e.g., they feel either *happy* or *mad*). Emotion coaching expands their emotional understanding, helps them differentiate the feelings associated with distress, and increases their awareness of the more nuanced experiences of distress (e.g., *disappointed, frustrated, worried*).

Emotion regulation skills play a fundamental role in supporting social competence. Often children know what they should do in a social situation, but don't do it. This gap between knowledge and performance often reflects difficulties with emotion regulation. Although a child can explain the proper behavior when calm, he or she can't perform the proper behavior when feelings are running high over the child's personal stake in the outcome. To use social-emotional skills when they are upset, children need help practicing when they are emotionally engaged. Emotion coaching during "teachable moments" in Friendship Group provides an important opportunity to help children develop the capacity to regulate these feelings effectively.

Emotion coaching refers to the explicit and strategic use of "feeling talk" to promote emotional understanding and regulation. The emotion coaching strategies include (1) talking about feelings, including modeling feeling statements and asking children to describe and discuss their feelings; (2) reflecting feelings, by using feeling labels to describe a child's experience; and (3) reframing feelings, which involves the deescalation of emotional arousal in challenging situations by using less intense feeling labels.

Talking about Feelings

The strategy of talking about feelings involves increasing children's exposure to talk about feelings by making frequent statements that describe your own feelings. For example, you might comment about something that happened before the group ("I'm feeling tired today because I went to bed too late last night") or something that is happening in the group setting ("This is a difficult problem. I'm *hopeful* that you will be able to work together and solve it"). At the start of each session, children select a feeling face that fits for them and talk about how they are feeling. The goal, in this part of the session as well as when other opportunities arise, is to encourage children to describe and discuss their feelings. Examples include asking follow-up questions after your feeling statements ("Does anyone else feel tired today?"; "Are you worried about solving this problem?"), and asking children to respond to others' feeling statements ("Marcus feels frustrated by this challenge. Is anyone else feeling frustrated?").

Reflecting Feelings

The strategy of reflecting feelings involves the use of contextual and behavioral cues to identify and describe the child's feelings. For example, imagine that a child asks for the red crayon, but a peer says "No, I'm using it." Reflecting the feeling helps you set up the child for problem solving—for example: "You're disappointed that Tonya's not done with that red yet. Hmm, what could you do?" Note that it is important for the coach to refrain from jumping in and solving these small problems (e.g., by finding another red crayon or instructing Tonya to share the red crayon as soon as she is done). Instead, the coaching strategy is to reflect feelings, help the child accurately appraise the situation, and empower the child to handle situations like this one by him- or herself.

Reframing Feelings

Reframing feelings involves the selective use of nuanced feeling labels (e.g., *disappointed, frustrated, worried*) rather than more intense labels (*mad, angry*) to help children deescalate arousal and regulate emotion when they are upset. In these challenging situations, it is important to maintain a neutral and calm demeanor. Your equanimity and the use of deescalating feeling labels help children calm down, so that they are able to move forward to talk about the problem and think flexibly about possible solutions. Examples include the following:

> CHILD (*with anger*): That's my chair, Jason—get out!
>
> COACH REFRAME: You're disappointed that you did not get the chair you wanted.

> [A child goes to the front of the line out of turn, and a peer stops him or her.]
>
> CHILD: That's not fair! You always push ahead of me. You go to the end!
>
> COACH REFRAME: You're feeling impatient about the wait. You hope the line moves quickly.

> CHILD: Hers is much better than mine! Mine looks stupid.
>
> COACH REFRAME: You're feeling disappointed because your drawing didn't turn out the way you wanted this time.

In each of these examples, you are reframing a child's emotionally reactive and habitual threat appraisal with a deescalated appraisal of the problem situation, thereby fostering more adaptive social perceptions.

Emotion Coaching

- **Talking about feelings:** Make frequent use of emotion labels as you describe your own feelings and encourage children to describe and discuss their feelings.
- **Reflecting feelings:** Use feeling labels to describe a child's experience.
- **Reframing feelings:** When children are upset and angry, deescalate emotional arousal and reorient threat appraisals with a calm demeanor and the selective use of a feeling label.

INDUCTION STRATEGIES

Induction strategies encourage children to self-regulate in response to social cues by increasing the salience of prosocial opportunities (making them more explicit), and by promoting awareness of the negative social consequences of self-serving or hostile behaviors. Induction strategies are particularly useful for children who, as a function of temperament and experience, want to dominate or control social interactions and are insensitive or nonresponsive to the feelings of others. Insensitive social domination and a short-sighted focus on immediate resource control are reflected in two different types of problem behavior: (1) oppositional and rule-breaking behaviors; and (2) social inflexibility, including emotional distress in the context of a disagreement or disappointment, and a resolute resistance to negotiation.

Socially insensitive, self-serving behavior may be motivated by (1) a desire to control resources and attain rewards or (2) a reaction to perceived threat. These motivations operate at a level of automaticity below consciousness and in some children promote social interactions that are narrowly focused on immediate reward acquisition (without regard for peer displeasure or adult disapproval) and a discomfort with the "submissive" stance associated with rule compliance, peer negotiation, and reciprocal social exchange. Children may become overly vigilant to what they perceive are attempts to restrain or control them in peer interactions, and they are frequently distressed (angry, resentful) by what they feel is unfair social treatment.

Despite the social rebuke that rule-breaking behavior or sulky distress evokes, these behaviors are often reinforced socially—either positively, when others give in to the child's demands, or negatively, when others withdraw from the situation, allowing the child to "escape" from the interpersonal restriction. Often, children who display these behaviors are unaware of the negative impact on others' feelings toward them and the long-term cost of these social behaviors in relation to their peer relations. In Friendship Group, the goal is not to threaten these children into submission (e.g., "Follow these rules or you will be put out of the game") but rather to "reorient" their focus from self-serving rewards and short-term gains (e.g., getting what they want without regard for others) to a focus on the social rewards and long-term benefits of reciprocity and negotiation (e.g., maintaining fair play and winning positive peer acceptance and inclusion).

Induction strategies are designed to do several things: (1) provide support for autonomy and a nonthreatening context for change (avoid triggering negative reactivity) to allow the child to try out and experience new ways of interacting with peers; (2) make the social rewards of alternative behaviors explicit and salient for the child (e.g., the long-term rewards of friendship over the short-term rewards of immediate domination or control); and (3) foster interpersonal awareness and reinforce social responsiveness, so that socially sensitive behaviors become more automatic and easier for the child to perform.

To use induction strategies effectively, it is important to create a peer-focused group climate, rather than one focused on compliance to adults. That is, your goal is not to assure that the children are obedient and follow your directions, but rather your goal is to "coach" them in their social interactions, to help them become more effective "players" able to gain the acceptance and approval of their peers. When children behave in an insensitive, self-serving fashion, your goal is not to correct the behavior, per se, but rather to improve their awareness of its impact on other people, so that the children are now socially motivated (and able) to self-regulate. In general, you want to avoid focusing on child misbehaviors as a challenge to your authority. Instead, you want to align with the children, helping them understand how those behaviors provoke peer dislike and guiding them to consider alternatives that will support peer acceptance.

Induction strategies include (1) giving clear information about alternative desirable behaviors; (2) giving feedback regarding the negative impact of problem behaviors, using I-statements or by eliciting peer feedback; (3) focusing on consequences that matter for each child; (4) giving choices and offering constructive alternatives; and (5) responding to power struggles with deescalation strategies.

Providing Clear Information about Desired Behavior

Faced with an inappropriate or undesired behavior, this induction strategy involves providing clear information about the desired alternative and prosocial behavior. One way to provide clear information is to praise children who are displaying the behavior you would like to see—for example: "Jim has his hand up—he is showing us that he has an idea to share"; "Sue and Jill have joined the circle. They are ready to learn this new game." You can also give clear information about the desired behavior by expressing your hopes and positive expectations. For example, in the face of avoidant or inattentive behavior, you might state your hopes in this way: "I'm hoping Steve can join us for this game, because I think he will really enjoy it" (rather than "Steve, you need to join the group"); "It would be nice if Danieka could join the compliment circle; I have a compliment I'd like to share with her today" (rather than "Danieka, you need to join the circle").

Giving Feedback about the Negative Social Impact of Behaviors

This strategy provides feedback about the negative impact of a behavior. The tone is important, as the goal is not to reprimand but rather to provide nonthreatening causal information that the child can use to adjust his or her behavior. I-statements can provide this kind of neutral, direct feedback—for example: "I don't like it when you put your face against mine. It's not comfortable for me"; "I'd like to start this story for you. But it's so noisy in here, I don't think you will be able to hear me"; "I'm worried we won't have time to play if team members don't join the circle to hear the directions."

You can also give a child information about the social impact of a behavior by asking the peers involved to give feedback—for example: "I wonder how Susie feels about you leaning on her. Susie, can you tell Jason how you feel about that?" Sometimes it is important to "stop the action" in order to make sure a child registers the social feedback. For example, imagine that Jimmy pushed his way into the circle, bumping David. David looks upset but says nothing. You might comment, "Jimmy, I'd like to ask you to look at David's face. David, can you explain how you feel and why?" This method of guidance allows the child who engaged in insensitive social behavior to get immediate feedback about the effects of his or her behavior on another and to take corrective action. It is very important to maintain a neutral demeanor in these situations, so that children do not feel that you are criticizing or embarrassing them, which could trigger threat and reactive self-protective behavior (e.g., "I don't care"). Instead, your goal is to help them notice subtle peer feedback and thereby improve their friendships. You can also suggest that children elicit peer feedback directly—for example: "I wonder how Daria feels about your coloring on her paper. You might want to check it out with her to see if it's OK with her."

Focusing on Consequences That Matter for the Child

This strategy also provides feedback about the impact of a problem behavior, while focusing particularly on how that behavior will have negative consequences for the child. The goal is to make salient the loss of rewards that will occur if the child continues the problem behavior. You can point out to a child how his or her fun will be diminished—for example: "I'm afraid you won't know how to play the game if you don't listen to directions"; "I'm concerned that you will be hungry later if you don't sit down for snack." You can also point out how a behavior will have a negative impact on friendships— for example: "I'm worried that other children won't want to play with you if you push them"; "Your friends want to have fun playing this game. When you stop the game because you are upset, it stops the fun for everyone. That's why your friends want to play without you."

Giving Choices

When a behavior cannot be ignored or other induction strategies fail to elicit behavior change, you can give children choices that indicate the appropriate behavioral options. Faced with undesirable behavior, the coach might say, for example: "I'm worried that someone will get hurt if there is kicking in the circle. You can sit on the chair there and kick or stay in the circle sitting cross-legged like this"; "You can join us in the game or sit here and watch." In some cases, you may want to provide a behavioral option that diverts the child's attention from the misbehavior and restructures an opportunity for him or her to reengage with the group in a positive fashion—for example" "Erica, I'm going to set up the obstacle course now. Perhaps you would like to help"; "I could use a helper to carry these supplies so that we can start the next game." Identifying positive roles in this way can redirect a child who is behaving in an oppositional manner or has left the group.

Responding to Social Conflicts with Deescalation Strategies

Coaches can also foster self-regulation skills by helping children de-escalate when they are upset. When responding to conflicts that involve power struggles, use your voice tone, as well as words, to reduce threat and encourage self-regulation. For example, if children are getting loud (excited or angry), rather than overpowering them by raising your voice, undercut the noise by using a soft voice tone. Avoid using an angry, bossy, or critical voice tone to rebuke children for their behavior. Instead express disappointment and concern about the problem and express hope for resolution in

---

Induction Strategies

- **Give clear information about desired behaviors** by praising other children who are exhibiting those behaviors or stating positive hopes and expectations.
- **Give feedback regarding the negative impact of problem behaviors** by using I-statements or eliciting feedback from peers.
- **Focus on consequences that matter for the child** by describing the impact of the child's behavior on social rewards and peer reactions.
- **Give choices and offer constructive behavioral alternatives** by providing choices that indicate appropriate behavioral options or redirecting children into positive roles.
- **Respond to power struggles with deescalation strategies** by using a soft, neutral tone and expressing disappointment or concerns about the child's difficulties, and staying on the child's side to facilitate coping and problem-solving efforts.

the future—for example: "It took so long for you to quiet down today that I don't have time to show you this new game. That's disappointing. Next session, let's plan to get ready quickly, so you can play this game"; "Today, we could not solve the problem of dividing up the stickers. Next week, we will try again and hopefully be more successful in our problem solving." Similarly, you can express concern regarding the difficulty a particular child had coping with strong feelings, along with hope for the future—for example: "Today, you had a tough time in Friendship Group. You were so disappointed about not going first that you missed the whole game. I want to help you get more comfortable with taking turns, so that you can have more fun with your friends. Let's work on that together next week." This orientation often helps the child regain composure and puts you in a position to coach the child in coping strategies and problem-solving efforts.

SOCIAL PROBLEM-SOLVING DIALOGUE

The use of social problem-solving dialogue supports skill development in areas of anticipatory planning, interpersonal negotiation, and conflict management. Social problem-solving skills are taught in Friendship Group lessons, and many of the activities used in the program require children to use these skills to make a plan together or to solve a challenge. For example, before an activity or game, coaches often lead children in planning sessions to help them anticipate and negotiate how they will work together toward their goal—for example: "What would be a fair way to divide the snack?"; "How shall we decide which game to play?" In addition, coaches are encouraged to help children use their social-problem solving skills when the need to resolve a disagreement that emerges in the course of play.

Children are taught a three-step sequence for social problem solving, following a "traffic signals" poster: (1) stop at the red light, "Take 5" with a calming deep breath, then say the problem and how you feel; (2) go slow at the yellow light, generate ideas about how to solve the problem, check them out with your friends, and "make a deal" by saying "yes" to good ideas; and then (3) go ahead at the green light, try out your plan. In order to help children use these skills effectively in the context of emotional arousal and conflict, coaches must be active facilitators. Key steps for coaching the social problem-solving process include the following.

1. *Stop the action and encourage children to "Take 5" to calm down.* Coaches need to step in to stop the action in order to create an opportunity for problem solving. Sometimes this intervention requires gaining control of the materials the children are arguing over, restraining children from grabbing at things or pushing each other. A calm demeanor and low voice help to deescalate the situation for problem solving, and you can model and encourage children to go to the red light with you and count to 5 as they take a deep breath (three counts in, two counts out) to calm down (e.g., "Take 5" to calm down).

2. *Use active listening to help each child share feelings and explain his or her perspective on the problem.* Coaches use emotion coaching (reflecting and reframing) to help children clarify and depersonalize the problem. For example, let's say two children are grabbing at the dice: "He grabbed the dice out of my hands"; "I had them first, he grabbed them from me." You might reframe (deescalate) their feelings (e.g., "You both want to go first. You're worried that you might not get to go first this time") and clarify the problem (e.g., "Our problem is to think of a fair way to decide who goes first").

3. *Elicit solutions and support decision making to select a plan of action.* Coaches should let each child suggest a solution, with the goal of identifying at least two viable ideas. If necessary, add a suggestion yourself. If children agree on a solution, let them move ahead and try out the plan of action. If children are unwilling to agree on a solution, there are several "next steps" that you can take to facilitate their capacity to negotiate: (a) Ask another peer to suggest an alternative solution, or let another peer make a selection from the two previously generated ideas; (b) use induction strategies to point out the consequences of the stalemate and to voice hopes for resolution (e.g., "I'm worried that we won't have much time to play this game if we can't solve this problem. I'm hoping that one of you will say 'yes' to a good idea, so you have time to enjoy the game"); and (c) make an executive decision to move the process forward (e.g., "Since you can't decide right now and we're running out of time, I'll make the call this time").

4. *Recognize problem-solving efforts.* When children successfully resolve their disagreement, use specific praise to recognize their efforts and the impact (e.g., "You two did a great job of working out that problem. You listened to each other and came up with a fair plan. That was excellent teamwork"). When children are not successful, you can still praise their efforts: "Sometimes it is difficult to work through a problem with a friend. You two listened to each other and came up with some good ideas. You did not reach an agreement this time, but you put in a good effort. Next time, you may be able to solve the problem." You can also use problem-solving dialogue to discuss a problem with an individual child. To do so, frame the challenge as a problem for the child and coach to tackle together: "Eric, I've noticed that it is really challenging for you to keep your cool when you lose a game. I'd like to think of some ways to help you with that problem, so that you have more fun with your friends."

Social problem solving can be time-consuming, and coaches must decide whether to lengthen the time allotted for a particular activity in order to accommodate an extended problem-solving discussion (dropping a later activity), or alternatively, to curtail the problem-solving discussion in order to move on to the next activity. When faced with this decision, coaches need to evaluate the children's engagement to determine whether they are still actively engaged in solving the problem (such that it is useful to continue trying) or whether they are beginning to disengage and are no longer invested in the problem (such that it is best to move on, even if the problem is left unresolved). In the latter case, coaches can comment on the process and reinforce children for their efforts: "You came up with some very good ideas, even though we could not reach an agreement and solve this problem today. But we're running out of time, so we better move on to our next game."

Social Problem-Solving Steps

1. **Stop the action and encourage children to "Take 5" to calm down.**
2. **Use active listening to help each child share feelings and explain his or her perspective on the problem.**
3. **Elicit solutions and support decision making to select a plan of action.**
4. **Support implementation of the plan and recognize problem-solving efforts.**

A second challenge in using social problem-solving dialogue is that some children can "hijack" the process by refusing to consider alternative suggestions. Other children eventually tire of the conflict and give in to that child's desires, thereby reinforcing the child's inflexibility. If a child displays a recurring problem associated with resource control (e.g., the child wants the red crayon, big chair, blue cup, green marker), avoid using social problem-solving dialogue as a response. In such cases, the child's social needs are best served by helping him or her gain flexibility in accepting such small disappointments in order to have fun with a friend, rather than requiring peers to accommodate to the child's preferences. Rather than problem solving, the coach should reframe the child's emotions and encourage coping: "I know you did not get the color you wanted, but that is just a small disappointment and nothing to worry about. I hope you do not let that bother you. I don't want you to see you miss out on this fun game. I know your friends hope you will join in and have fun with them."

CHAPTER 4

Behavior Management

The chapter starts with a description of the four types of behavior problems that are most commonly observed in the Friendship Group setting and the factors that contribute to these problems. It describes a set of strategies that you can use to support positive behavior in the group by modifying the group context and strengthening the accuracy of children's social appraisals. The chapter also reviews the use of a "backup" system of token rewards to support positive behavior and manage problem behaviors in the group setting.

UNDERSTANDING COMMON BEHAVIOR PROBLEMS IN THE FRIENDSHIP GROUP SETTING

The four most common problems observed in the Friendship Group setting are:

1. *Social avoidance or disengagement.* Children hold back and appear anxious or uncertain about joining group activities. Alternatively, they join but then frequently leave the group, expressing disinterest or boredom regarding group activities.

2. *Inflexibility, inability to shift ideas, emotions, or behaviors.* Children get fixated on doing things in a particular way (their way) and are unable to consider another's ideas, opinions, or feelings. They seem unaware of or nonresponsive to others' requests or ideas. When faced with disappointment or frustration, they react with distress that immobilizes their capacity for negotiation or further social interaction, and they refuse to continue unless they can have things their way.

3. *Impulsive, intrusive, and insensitive social behavior.* Children invade others' personal space (touching, leaning on, roughhousing with others) or interrupt and intrude on conversation or play. They may try to control resources or social interaction (grabbing materials, skipping ahead in the line) or have trouble sustaining attention to a game or activity.

4. *Disruptive, rule-breaking behavior.* Children defy adult authority and transgress rules, exhibiting unacceptable behaviors (e.g., cursing, obscene gestures) or refusing to comply with defined limits (e.g., leaving the room, damaging property).

These four types of problems are listed hierarchically in terms of the seriousness of the management challenges they present for Friendship Group leaders. All reflect a lack of social competence. In addition, as one moves down the list, the problems increase in terms of the negative impact they have on other group members and the likelihood that they will undermine the integrity of the social learning experience and effectiveness of Friendship Group.

In order to make informed decisions regarding the management of these behavior problems, it is helpful to consider why some children show these behaviors in peer play contexts. That is, what motivates children to behave in these ways, and why do they continue to do so when adults and peers express disapproval and dislike? The likelihood that a child will engage in any of these behaviors is a function of the strength of the habit established to perform that behavior (vs. an alternative behavior) under a particular set of circumstances. In other words, *antecedent conditions* (A) elicit *behaviors* (B), which become established as habitual responses as a function of their *consequences* (C). Antecedents (A) include both external conditions (e.g., the social situation and group context that precede a behavior) and the child's appraisal (e.g., thoughts and feelings) about the situation. Social appraisals occur quickly, without conscious awareness, as children scan social situations for potential threats and rewards. Perceived threats trigger an emotional reaction and readiness for "fight-or-flight" behavior. Perceived rewards (anticipated pleasure) motivate approach. Over time, consequences (C) reinforce certain behaviors (making them more habitual, more likely to occur in the future) by either (1) providing a desired outcome or (2) removing or reducing threat or discomfort. In any given situation, a child's "automatic" or habitual response is the one that is most practiced, and the one that has been reinforced in the past. The important implication of this model is that there are several ways that a group leader can help a child change a problem behavior, including changing the external antecedents (situational demands), internal antecedents (the child's appraisal of the situation), or the consequences of the child's behavior.

Let's apply this model to one of the common problems seen in Friendship Group: the tendency to withdraw or avoid social interactions, rather than approach and join. Antecedents (e.g., characteristics of the Friendship Group setting and activity) affect the child's appraisal of the situation (which is also influenced by the child's temperament and past experience). This appraisal sets the stage for a behavioral response. The likelihood that a child will display one behavior (avoidance) versus another (approach) will depend upon the child's appraisal of the situation (threat vs. potential reward), past experience with the consequences of each behavior, as well as the child's level of skill (automaticity and ease of performance). For many children with peer difficulties, group interactions are threatening; it is easier to avoid social interaction than to approach, and avoidance is reinforced by reducing the anxiety associated with participation (see Figure 4.1).

In order to build a new social skill (e.g., join in rather than withdraw), coaches can take several steps. They can teach the skillful response of approaching and joining in, providing the opportunity to practice that new behavior so that it becomes more familiar and easier to do. They can influence the way that the child feels about a social entry situation and the degree to which a child appraises that social situation as a threat versus an attractive opportunity. Finally, they can heighten the degree to which the child experiences positive consequences when engaging in the new, skillful behavior by increasing the frequency and salience of positive interpersonal responding. Coaches can also increase the salience of the long-term negative consequences of the less skillful behavior, which may be less evident to the child than the immediate rewards.

This model also provides a guide to the different strategies that can be used to change a problem behavior and replace it with a desired alternative in the Friendship Group context. For problems that are less severe and that primarily affect the child who is displaying them rather than others in the group (e.g., the typical problems of social disengagement or inflexibility), it is often sufficient

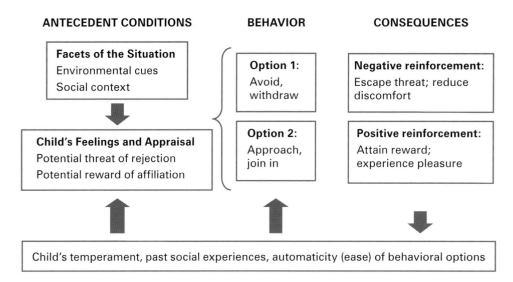

FIGURE 4.1. Factors determining social avoidance versus social approach.

to adjust the antecedent conditions that elicit the behavior in order to reduce problems and elicit alternatives. That is, you can change the situation to make it easier for the child to show the desired behavior (e.g., remove distractions from the room, decrease the group size, change the activity to make it less demanding) or change the child's appraisal of threat (e.g., by providing a secure base, positive attending, emotion coaching). For problems that are chronic and more severe, and particularly for behavior problems that affect all group members (e.g., intrusive or disruptive behaviors), it is often necessary to use a backup system of token rewards to manipulate the consequences and encourage improved behavior. Ultimately, the goal of Friendship Group is to promote self-regulated behavior, so that the child can maintain positive peer interaction without backup rewards, but sometimes the external structure is needed to foster children's engagement in the intervention—which, in turn, is necessary for them to learn alternative, desired social skills. Should you find that a child is constantly misbehaving in Friendship Group, and that you are frequently reprimanding that child during sessions, recognize these signs as a red flag indicating that you have not adjusted the situation sufficiently to create a therapeutic experience. It is important to reanalyze the situation and apply this model in order to think about what you could change to create a more therapeutic opportunity for that child to build skills.

CHANGING THE ANTECEDENT CONDITIONS THAT ELICIT PROBLEM BEHAVIOR

You can change the antecedent conditions that elicit problem behavior either by restructuring Friendship Group sessions or by influencing the way children are interpreting and feeling about events in Friendship Group. Both approaches are described in the next sections.

Reduce the Level of Social Difficulty and Self-Regulation Challenge

The most basic way to change the antecedent conditions to improve behavior in the Friendship Group context is to make the group context less challenging and provocative (e.g., less likely to elicit the problem behavior and more likely to elicit the desired behavior). There are five specific ways that you can make the Friendship Group less difficult for children.

First, *engineer the environment* to reduce distractions. For example, if a child frequently leaves the group to do something else in the space, consider how you can cover or block access to that part of the room. Consider rearranging the furniture, your materials, or other things in the room to create a less distracting space. In addition, consider making greater use of the agenda pictures and group posters and materials to highlight the desired and expected behaviors. If needed, create a separate "rules poster" to specify prohibited behaviors (e.g., "Keep your hands to yourself," "No fighting," "No put-downs").

Second, *reduce the number of transitions* and organize the group around a table to provide more structure. For some children, sitting on the floor in a circle elicits problem behaviors, such as leaning on other people or rolling on the floor. The multiple transitions within each session (e.g., moving from the circle to the table to a physical game) can also elicit disruptive outbursts or rough-house play from some children. As an alternative, children can sit around a table at the beginning of the group session, participating in friendship circle, construction station activities, and the snack without any physical transitions. When transitions are necessary, consider moving as a "transition train" or using a similarly structured process to provide behavioral support during the transition. You may choose to omit some of the active games or replace them with tabletop games if physically active games elicit disruptive behavior in the children in your group.

A third strategy for simplifying the demands of Friendship Group involves *reducing the size of the group* or breaking into pairs or triads for activities. Many children who show disruptive or disengaged behavior in larger groups find it much easier to participate effectively in a smaller group. As noted earlier, a smaller group is less threatening, more predictable, and allows children more opportunities to respond than a larger group.

A fourth and related strategy is to *reduce the level of verbal and cognitive demands* in the session. Children with less well-developed verbal skills and those who process information more slowly can be overwhelmed by the social and cognitive demands of Friendship Group sessions. By working with them in a smaller group, slowing down the presentation of new material, keeping discussions brief with supportive props and actions, children are more likely to understand and participate in the group sessions and less likely to disengage. For these children, repeating sessions is also useful, because it provides them with a second chance to hear and process the information and to consolidate their social skill learning.

Finally, you can *slow down the pace* at which you introduce new skills and new activities, and *repeat sessions* or *simplify tasks* in order to give children a chance to consolidate skill learning. The program is organized hierarchically, such that simpler social skills (imitation and parallel play) are introduced first, and more complex social skills (reciprocal, collaborative, and competitive play) follow. When the pace is too fast for some children, and the skills become too difficult, they will often disengage. Repeating sessions or simplifying the tasks (breaking them into smaller, concrete steps) gives these children a chance to feel more confident and to be more effective in skill performance.

Promote Positive Expectations and Appraisals

In addition to the actual changes in the Friendship Group context described above, you can modify the antecedents of behavior problems by promoting changes in children's expectations and appraisals (e.g., their thoughts and feelings) in the Friendship Group context. There are three ways to do this.

First, you can *provide children with advance information* about the session, so they know what to expect and can anticipate and plan for the aspects of Friendship Group that are challenging for them. For example, when possible, it is helpful to meet with a child who is struggling behaviorally before the other group participants arrive or before the formal group begins. You can review the agenda and identify the parts of the session that might be challenging for the child: "Then we will play a new game. Someone will go first, and the others will have to wait. Here is where you will wait for your turn." You can be specific about how this activity will affect the child: "I have a list that shows who will go first in each game. When we play the first game, [Name] will go first, so you will have to wait for a turn. When we play the second game, you will go first." You can also give the child a positive role to help him or her focus on the desired behavior: "I hope you will be my helper today to make sure that we take turns and everyone gets a chance to go first. I will ask you to put a check by each person's name when he or she goes first. You will be the monitor, and I will ask you to help me remember whose turn is next." You can also make *anticipatory comments* during the group session, reviewing the agenda pictures at the start of the session and referring to them during the group: "That is the end of our friendship circle. Let's look at our agenda pictures to see what comes next." For children who are impulsive, it is helpful to spell out how activities will be done before children start: "First, I will ask each one of you which animal you want for the team mascot. Second, we will count the votes for each animal. Third, the animal with the most votes will be the team mascot."

A second strategy, in addition to planning ahead with children so they know what to expect, is to *give children with challenging behaviors special roles* and jobs that help them stay focused on positive and desired behaviors at times when problem behaviors are most likely. For example, a child who is frequently distracted during friendship circle might be given jobs during circle time to keep him or her engaged (e.g., holding pictures, passing out materials, counting votes). A child who has trouble with transition might be given a role to foster transition control (e.g., leading the transition train, carrying materials over to the next activity, or checking to see if each of the team members is seated and ready to hear the directions for the next activity).

Finally, a third strategy to foster positive expectations and appraisals involves strategically responding to behavior problems to deescalate children's emotional arousal and *reframe their appraisal of the social experience.* For example, some children are extremely upset by everyday experiences with social exchange, crying or pouting when they are not first in line or it is not their turn. In this case, you do not want to comment on how disappointed or upset children feel, because that focuses their attention on their loss, amplifies their distress, and reinforces their negative appraisal of the event. Instead, a positive reframe can help them recognize the neutral, routine

---

Managing Antecedents in Friendship Group

Make the context less challenging.
- Engineer the environment to reduce distractions and cue desired behaviors.
- Reduce the number of transitions; organize around a table to add structure.
- Reduce the group size or break into pairs or triads.
- Reduce the level of verbal and cognitive demands.
- Repeat activities or simplify tasks.

Modify the child's expectations and appraisals.
- Prepare the child in advance, so he or she knows what to expect.
- Give the child a positive role to support the desired behavior.
- Deescalate and reframe the child's experience.

nature of the experience: "Our sign says that friends take turns, and you are taking turns. You are letting [Name] go first, and later [Name] will let you go first. You are being a good friend to [Name]." You can also *deescalate and reframe* their emotional reaction: "Sometimes it is your turn to be first, and sometimes it is [Name's] turn. It is a very small disappointment when it is not your turn, because you know your turn will come again later." You can also *offer a positive coping response*: "Let's go check your list to see when your turn will come."

USING A TOKEN REWARD BEHAVIOR SUPPORT SYSTEM

Some behaviors cannot be ignored in the Friendship Group setting and require immediate action by the coach to constrain the behavior, rather than (or in addition to) the use of induction strategies and the adjustment of antecedent conditions. The behaviors that require immediate limit-setting efforts are (1) aggressive or destructive behaviors that threaten or harm others in the group, or that are damaging to the materials or space used by the group; (2) rule-breaking behaviors, such as cursing, bathroom talk, or obscene language, which represent social threat and escalate arousal; and (3) behaviors that put the child or space in danger, such as standing on tables, running out of the room, or getting into materials in another part of the room.

Clear, directive rules and nonpunitive consequences are necessary when these behaviors emerge in the group setting. If these behaviors occur relatively infrequently and do not engage the reactions of other children, they may be managed effectively with simple, clear commands and follow-through action (e.g., "Bathroom talk is not allowed in Friendship Group"; "You cannot leave the room during Friendship Group"). However, if these behaviors occur with any regularity and elicit reactions from other children, it is important to establish a more systematic behavioral control plan. We recommend the use of a token reward system that allows for the provision of points when the problem behaviors are inhibited and the removal of points (response cost) when the problem behaviors are exhibited.

When determining the need for a backup behavior management system, it is important to consider how peers in the group are responding to the problematic behavior, as well as the nature of that behavior itself. Research suggests that one of the best predictors of long-term behavioral improvements following coaching interventions is the nature of partner responses during group sessions (Bierman, 1986). When peers respond favorably to positive child behaviors, these positive behaviors are likely to continue or increase in later sessions and in peer interactions outside the group context. When peers ignore negative child behaviors, these negative behaviors are likely to decrease over time. However, when peers react to negative behaviors with escalation (fighting back), encouragement (laughing, imitating), or submission (giving in), these responses increase the likelihood of repeated negative behavior in future sessions and outside of the group setting, thus essentially nullifying any positive impact of the intervention.

Problematic peer responses to negative behavior (sometimes called *deviancy training* or *peer contagion*) are most likely to emerge in groups that contain several members who are aggressive and/or highly impulsive. In such cases, the coach's attempts to provide praise for positive behavior and consequences for rule-breaking are often ineffective because the peer partners in the group are providing an alternative set of responses by laughing at, reacting to, or otherwise supporting the problematic behaviors of their peers. Under these conditions, the application of a token reinforcement system as a backup behavioral management system is necessary to establish a positive group orientation.

Token systems provide a straightforward and noncoercive method of reducing problem behaviors and enhancing compliance. Some token systems are elaborate, individualized, and detailed, explaining exactly how tokens can be earned and providing explicit guidelines linking tokens with rewards. In contrast, in Friendship Group, we use a much more general and flexible token reward system that is intentionally vague in order to allow for flexible use during and across sessions. With this system, (1) you can deliver more tokens during the parts of the group session when extra support is needed to keep children engaged, and fewer tokens during other periods. (2) The system we use is a group reward process that does not single out children. Anyone can earn or lose tokens, providing rewards to positive models as well as to children who need the behavioral support. (3) The system is nonpunitive and gives children multiple opportunities to succeed. (4) It is easy to implement and relatively easy to phase out when it is no longer needed. The steps to implementing the token reward system are as follows:

1. *Select tokens and a jar.* Any small objects can serve as tokens (e.g., poker chips, beans, buttons, pennies). The tokens should fit into a pocket, so they can be carried around during group sessions for easy access.

2. *Introduce the positive reward system to the children.* The system does not need an elaborate introduction. On the first day that you introduce the system, tell the children that today you will be awarding tokens to children when you see them following the Friendship Group rules and using the Friendship Group skills. Demonstrate how you will award tokens by pointing to one of the posters and identifying someone who is showing the skill (e.g., "Good teamwork means joining in. [Name] is joining in and paying attention"), taking a token from your pocket and putting it in the jar with emphasis. Then, point to another poster, and identify someone showing that skill (e.g., "[Name] is listening to the coaches. Nice job, [Name]"), taking another token from your pocket and putting it in the jar. Follow this step until you have pointed out skills on each of the posters (focus on the ones that are most important for children in the group), and you have rewarded each group member by noticing their positive behavior and placing a token in the jar.

3. *Explain the reward.* Decide ahead of time what you will use for a reward. It can be something tangible (e.g., pencils, stickers, erasers) or it can be a special privilege (e.g., a chance to play a favorite game at the end of the session) or a special certificate or hand stamp. Let the children know that they will get something special at the end of the group if they earn enough tokens. However, do not give explicit information about the number of tokens they need for the prize. Just explain that you will count the tokens at the end of the session to see if there are enough. (If they ask how many they need, tell them that you can't say, because it is a surprise.)

4. *Demonstrate the response cost.* Explain to the children that there is one more thing they should know about the token system—they can lose tokens if they forget to follow the Friendship Group rules. A good way to illustrate this for the children is to have the co-leader get up from the group or lay on the ground at this point in the discussion. Then, the leader can illustrate the process of token loss by commenting on the problem (e.g., "[Coach's Name] is not joining in"), while removing one of the tokens from the jar. As soon as the co-leader corrects the behavior and joins back in, the token can be placed back in the jar with specific praise (e.g., "Good work, [Coach's Name], now you are joining in and showing good teamwork").

5. *Explain the ground rules.* Explain that you will give tokens when you notice friendly behaviors during the session, but stress that tokens will not be awarded every single time you see a good behavior. The children won't know when they will get a token; you will surprise them by suddenly noticing their good behavior. Also let them know that they can't get a token by asking for one. You are the person who decides when to give tokens. These are important points because we don't want children to be overly focused on the tokens and looking to you for constant token rewards.

6. *Complete the process.* At the end of the session, count the tokens with the children and let them know if there are enough for a prize. If you feel that the children put in good effort, announce that they won the prize. If you feel that the effort was only moderate, give out part of the prize (e.g., You each won a pencil today, but not the erasers. Maybe next time, you'll earn enough for the erasers"). If you feel that the effort was poor, express your disappointment and hopes for the next session (e.g., "There are not quite enough today for the prize. I'm disappointed about that. But, we'll try again next week. I feel confident that you can earn the prize with a little more effort").

It is very important to use specific praise each time you give a token, so children know the exact behavior for which they are earning a token. In addition, use specific praise generously, even when you do not give a token. The liberal use of specific praise, coupled with the occasional use of token rewards, will make it easier to phase out the tokens over time.

One of the additional advantages of this system is that it is relatively easy to phase out over time. This token reward system often produces rapid behavior change and improved compliance in group settings in the short run by providing children with highly salient cues and contingent reinforcement to support desired behavior. However, the down side is the high visibility of the external reinforcement system. It is easy for children to rely on the external systems to guide behavior, but these systems do not necessarily foster the social awareness, emotional understanding, and self-regulation skills needed to sustain effective social interaction. In fact, providing a highly salient external reward for a social behavior can sometimes reduce children's motivation to display those behaviors, because they don't want to do the behavior unless they get an external reward. Since external rewards will not be available when children are interacting with peers in naturalistic settings, relying on this control strategy can reduce the likelihood that the behavior will be displayed outside of the group setting.

For these reasons, we recommend phasing the token reward system out gradually, once behavior problems are under control in the Friendship Group setting. To phase out the system, begin to deliver tokens less frequently, letting children know, for example, that you will use the token jar only during friendship circle this session. If this approach works, phase it out completely by leaving the tokens and jars at home. If children ask about it, explain that you are not using the token jar today, but you are still watching and noticing friendly behavior.

SUMMARY

In summary, the Friendship Group behavior management processes described in this chapter, combined with the therapeutic processes described in Chapter 3, support the development of social competencies in ways that are complementary to the skill training elements in the program. Skill training (skill presentation, practice opportunities, performance feedback) builds new skills and extends the behavioral repertoire that children have at their disposal. The therapeutic processes support the performance of new social skills by (1) fostering self-monitoring and self-regulation, (2) strengthening children's accurate appraisal of the social context, and (3) increasing awareness and understanding of social consequences. The behavior management strategies allow you to modify antecedents and consequences in the Friendship Group setting and adjust the difficulty level of the social experience to provide maximal support for positive behavior change.

CHAPTER 5

Home–School Intervention
The Fast Track Model

This chapter describes the synchronized home and school intervention components that were part of the federally funded Fast Track project, where the Friendship Group program was first developed and evaluated. First, we describe the multiple intervention components that were included in Fast Track and highlight the school-based and family-focused intervention components that were used with Friendship Group. Fast Track research findings are described briefly, providing evidence that validates the intervention approach. We offer suggestions for extending the impact of the Friendship Group program with the use of parent training and school-based programming.

The original Friendship Group program was part of Fast Track, a federally funded prevention project for children who entered kindergarten showing high rates of aggressive-disruptive behaviors. Such behaviors can trigger a cascade of negative school experiences (e.g., peer rejection, conflict with teachers, academic difficulties) that increase the likelihood of long-term poor outcomes for children. Early aggression, combined with social rejection and learning difficulties, fuels school disengagement, putting children at risk for school failure. In turn, school disengagement increases the likelihood that children will initiate risky behaviors in adolescence, ranging from alcohol/drug use and early sexual activity to antisocial behavior, including criminal activity.

The goal of the Fast Track project was to develop and evaluate a prevention program for children with early starting aggressive-disruptive behavior problems, in order to disrupt the negative cascade and promote positive adjustment. Fast Track focused on building child competencies to promote the social-emotional and academic skills needed for self-regulation, positive peer relations, and school success. The long-term goal was to help children control their aggression, establish positive peer relations, reduce risky adolescent behavior, and ultimately reduce negative adult outcomes, including criminal activity and substance use. Fast Track had two phases. The Friendship Group program was delivered during the elementary school years, which is described below. In addition, an individualized case management program extended into midadolescence.

THE FAST TRACK PROJECT DESIGN

The Fast Track project design was based on the assumption that prevention efforts to reduce child aggression are most effective when they focus on the promotion of child competencies, and when they link services across home and school contexts (CPPRG, 1992). In Fast Track, children with high levels of aggressive-disruptive behavior problems were identified at school entry based upon parent and teacher ratings. The elementary school intervention began in first grade and continued through the fifth grade. In the classroom, teachers taught the Promoting Alternative Thinking Strategies (PATHS) curriculum (Kusche & Greenberg, 1994). In addition, families with aggressive-disruptive kindergarten children were invited to attend extracurricular groups held after school or on the weekend when Friendship Groups, parent groups, and parent–child sharing activities took place. In addition, peer pairing and academic tutoring services were delivered by an educational consultant at school, and home visits were conducted by a family consultant. Three of these components (PATHS, Friendship Groups, and peer pairing) were focused specifically on the promotion of social competence, self-regulation skills, and positive peer relations. Parent groups, parent–child sharing sessions, and home visiting were designed to promote positive parenting, high-quality parent–child relationships, and home–school communication. (For more detail on program implementation design, see CPPRG, 2002a; Bierman & CPPRG, 1997.)

The PATHS Curriculum

The PATHS curriculum (Kusche & Greenberg, 1994) was taught by classroom teachers during twice-weekly 20- to 30-minute lessons in grades 1–5. PATHS targets multiple skills, including emotional understanding, self regulation, communication skills, friendship skills, and problem-solving skills. Skill concepts are presented via instruction, discussion, modeling stories, or video presentations, and discussion and role-playing activities follow to support skill practice. In addition to these formal lessons, teachers were instructed in how to generalize their use of PATHS concepts across the school day. For example, teachers were encouraged to help children identify their feelings, communicate clearly with others, and, as interpersonal problems emerged, to use self-control strategies and problem-solving steps to resolve conflicts. Each classroom had a mailbox in which students could write down problems or concerns for discussion in classroom problem-solving meetings. In Fast Track, an intervention staff member, the Educational Consultant, met regularly with teachers to answer questions about PATHS and to provide suggestions and consultation in the area of effective classroom management of disruptive behavior (e.g., establishing clear rules and directions; providing positive and corrective feedback for appropriate behavior; applying reprimands, time out, or response cost procedures contingent upon the occurrence of problematic behavior). PATHS was designed to promote a positive peer climate at the classroom level. Fast Track staff also consulted with the school principal to bring the philosophy of PATHS to the entire school, resulting in various efforts (on a school-by-school basis), such as placing PATHS posters in school hallways, implementing new school behavior guidelines, and painting problem-solving "stoplights" on school playgrounds. The goal was to create a positive school climate and reduce peer conflict and victimization.

Family Sessions: Friendship Group, Parent Group, and Parent–Child Sharing Activities

Kindergarten children at high risk for negative school experiences and problem outcomes were identified on the basis of parent and teacher ratings (see the "Fast Track Project Research Findings" section later in this chapter). These children and their families were invited to attend extracurricular sessions, which were 2-hour sessions held at the school building during an after-school, evening, or weekend time period. The intervention model involved intensive support for children and families in grade 1 (22 weekly extracurricular sessions) and grade 2 (14 biweekly sessions), with maintenance support in grades 3–5 (8 monthly sessions each year). Each extracurricular session included 90 minutes in which children met in Friendship Group and parents attended parent groups. It also included 30 minutes for joint parent–child sharing activities. Educational consultants led the Friendship Groups, and Family consultants led the parent groups. The early elementary Friendship Group sessions included in this manual represent a combination of sessions used in Fast Track grades 1 and 2, as well as sessions developed more recently for kindergarten children. The advanced elementary Friendship Group sessions represent a combination of sessions used in Fast Track grades 3–5, with some revisions based upon staff feedback and subsequent clinical experience with the intervention. The Friendship Group program is designed to coordinate with the PATHS curriculum. The two programs focus on promoting skills in the same domains, with the classroom program providing an introduction to the skills, and the Friendship Group providing at-risk children with additional coaching and practice to remediate skill deficits. Friendship Group can be run effectively as a "stand-alone" intervention program, without PATHS. However, when it is possible to deliver both PATHS (at the classroom level) and Friendship Group (for children who need additional support to develop social-emotional skills), the combination is optimal. If PATHS is being used in concordance with Friendship Group, we advise coaches to use PATHS feeling faces and social problem-solving posters in the Friendship Group context, in order to maximize cross-setting consistency and support for skill development (see Bierman, Greenberg, & CPPRG, 1996).

The parent groups that were held in parallel to Friendship Group focused on promoting positive family–school relationships and effective communication and discipline skills (including praise and ignoring, clear instructions and rules, and time out) (McMahon, Slough, & CPPRG, 1996). The skill topics addressed in the parent group followed a developmental sequence, with an increasing emphasis over time on communication skills, homework study skills, goal setting, and negotiating parent–child conflicts (see McMahon et al., 1996, for more detail). The last 30 minutes of each family session included a parent–child sharing session, in which parents and children participated in joint activities to promote positive relationships and provide parents an opportunity to practice new parenting skills with staff guidance.

Individualized Components: Peer Pairing and Home Visiting

In the Fast Track project, Friendship Groups were held outside of the school setting and included only children who exhibited high rates of aggressive-disruptive behavior. Although these extracurricular groups provided a context for intensive social skill training, they were limited in two ways: (1) All group members had similar skill deficits, limiting children's exposure to normative peer interactions; and (2) there was no direct opportunity to practice skills with classmates and thereby to promote the generalization of skills to the school setting. To address these limitations, Fast Track included a peer-pairing program that ran parallel to Friendship Group, designed specifically to increase exposure to normative peer interactions and to enhance generalization of friendship skills to interactions with classmates. Peer-pairing sessions were held once per week in the school setting. Each peer-pairing session included a 30-minute supervised indoor play opportunity, in which each target child (the Friendship Group participants) met with a classmate and engaged in games and activities designed to provide practice in the Friendship Group skills. Any classmate with parental permission participated as a partner, rotating over the course of the year. The topics covered during weekly Friendship Groups were repeated and reinforced during these weekly peer-pairing sessions. These sessions provided children with additional practice in the social skills and also showcased their improved behavior to peers. Peer-pairing sessions were conducted by trained paraprofessionals, who worked under the supervision of the educational consultants. In the Fast Track model, children also received academic tutoring in reading skills during the early elementary years, conducted by the same paraprofessional and supervised by the Educational Consultant.

Complementing the parent group, family consultants visited the participating parents in their homes. The goal was to provide individual support, helping parents to apply the program skills in their family context and to problem-solve challenges to effective parenting. Many of the parents who participated in Fast Track faced multiple stressors, including poverty, maternal depression, limited educational attainment, marital conflict, and single parenting, among others. These stressors often fuel demoralization and feelings of helplessness, impeding effective parenting. The home visiting program focused on providing individual support to primary caregivers, and helping them address personal and parenting challenges with the use of problem-solving strategies. On average, home visits occurred every other week, although some families were visited weekly and others were visited monthly, depending upon family needs.

FAST TRACK PROJECT RESEARCH FINDINGS

Fast Track was evaluated using a randomized controlled design. In January 1991, 55 schools in four geographic sites across the United States (Durham, North Carolina; Nashville, Tennessee; Seattle, Washington; rural central Pennsylvania) were selected as high risk. Within each site, the schools were divided into multiple paired sets matched for demographics (school size, student poverty, ethnic composition), and one of each pair was randomly assigned to intervention or "usual practice" conditions. For each of the following 3 years, all of the kindergarten children in those schools were screened for aggressive-disruptive behavior problems by teachers. If the kindergarten teacher reported elevated behavior problems at school entry (e.g., the child scored in the top 30–40% on teacher ratings), the parents were interviewed and invited to rate the child's aggressive-disruptive behavior problems at home. Teacher and parent ratings were combined into a sum score, which served as the basis for child selection into the Fast Track project (for more information about the screening process, see Lochman & the CPPRG, 1995; Hill, Lochman, Coie, Greenberg, & CPPRG, 2004). Overall, 891 children and their parents participated in the study, with 445 receiving the Fast Track intervention and 446 experiencing the "usual practice" supports available in their schools and communities. Two-thirds of the participating children were boys. Approximately half of the participating children were European American and the others were primarily African American. During the course of the program, annual assessments were conducted to track child progress. Each year, teachers and parents provided ratings of child competencies and behavior problems. In addition, in the early years of the program, peer ratings and observations were collected.

Elementary School Findings

Significant benefits to children and parents were evident by the end of first grade. Compared with the high-risk children receiving "usual practice," the high-risk children in the intervention schools showed improvements in social, emotional, and academic skills. Specifically, direct assessments with the children revealed improved emotion recognition, emotion coping, and social problem-solving skills, reflecting the focus of the Friendship Group and PATHS curriculum (CPPRG, 1999a, 2002b). In addition, these intervention children showed higher rates of positive peer interaction at school. They were nominated more often as "most liked" by their classmates and less often as "least liked," demonstrating that the social competence training reduced their peer rejection and improved their acceptance by peers. Parents and teachers reported reductions in child aggression. Because Fast Track is a comprehensive program, the gains in children's social competence and peer relations are not necessarily due to single components, but rather to the fully integrated intervention program. Thus, the parent groups, through their focus on helping parents to facilitate their children's developmentally appropriate academic and social skills, may well have facilitated these outcomes as well. Indeed, Fast Track improved parenting, reducing parents' reliance on physical punishment and increasing parent–child warmth and appropriate, consistent discipline. Teachers reported that parents who received Fast Track were more positively involved with their children's schools.

At the end of grade 3, we calculated a "clinical caseness" index to determine the overall impact of Fast Track on child behavior adjustment. We considered a child to be "problem free" if he or she showed none of the following indicators of risk: (1) was not diagnosed with an oppositional defiant disorder or conduct disorder in structured interviews with parents, (2) did not have an individualized education plan (IEP) reflecting a need for special education, and (3) was not rated by teachers or parents as having significant aggressive-disruptive behavior problems (e.g., scores in the top 15% of the sample). Using these criteria, 37% of the children receiving Fast Track services emerged as "problem free" at the end of grade 3, in contrast to only 27% of the children receiving "usual practice." This represents a powerful one-third increase in the rate of "problem-free" status by the end of grade 3 among children who entered school at high risk (CPPRG, 2002b).

Late Adolescent and Early Adult Outcomes

Children who participated in the Fast Track Project were followed through age 25. Children who received Fast Track services were less likely than the children in the comparison group to be arrested as juveniles (CPPRG, 2010). Among those with juvenile arrests, children who received Fast Track were 24% less likely to commit serious juvenile crimes. Among the children exhibiting the highest rates of challenging behavior in kindergarten, Fast Track also reduced the likelihood of receiving a diagnosis of conduct disorder, ADHD, or any externalizing disorder through the end of high school (i.e., grade 12; CPPRG, 2011). Significant benefits remained evident at age 25, when those who had received Fast Track as children showed lower levels of internalizing and externalizing behaviors and lower rates of substance abuse (CPPRG, 2015).

IMPLICATIONS FOR PRACTICE

The ability to coordinate school-based or family-focused intervention components with Friendship Group will vary, depending upon the context of Friendship Group implementation. However, when it is possible to create connections with parents and teachers, it is highly recommended and likely to extend the impact of Friendship Group.

Connecting with Teachers

If you are located within a school context and have the capacity to explore the PATHS curriculum as a complement to Friendship Group, it is highly recommended. PATHS has benefits for all students in the classroom (CPPRG, 1999b, 2010a). In addition, the social-emotional skills targeted in Friendship Group are reinforced by the PATHS program and by classroom teachers who are using PATHS. PATHS utilizes support processes in the classroom that are parallel to those used in Friendship Group, including emotion coaching, induction strategies, and social problem-solving dialogue. Hence, the use of PATHS in the classroom (as a "universal" prevention program) with pullout Friendship Groups to provide intensive, remedial support to children with social skills deficits (as an "indicated" prevention program for children at risk) is a powerful combination. Even if you are not able to use PATHS in the classroom, connecting with classroom teachers is important for (1) planning Friendship Group, (2) eliciting teacher support to promote the generalization of program gains to classroom peer interactions, and (3) evaluating children's response to Friendship Group and assessing their progress in gaining peer integration.

Connecting with Parents

The Fast Track project included a parent group program that was held at the same time as Friendship Group. This organization enabled us to provide intensive support to parents, and also to hold parent–child sharing sessions when parents and children could practice new interactions with staff support. The intensive parent group experience was particularly important in the Fast Track project because children were selected for inclusion based upon high levels of aggressive-disruptive behaviors. Children who are highly impulsive and/or aggressive are quite challenging to parent effectively. Hence, if this is the population you are focused on serving, we recommend using the Fast Track Parent Group in conjunction with the Friendship Group. Even if you are not able to use the parent group program, connecting with parents is still important for (1) planning Friendship Group, (2) addressing relationship problems at home that may be related to peer difficulties, and (3) giving parents feedback about children's peer challenges and progress, and helping them consider how they might support their children's positive peer integration at home.

Commonly Used Materials in Friendship Group

The session posters, agenda pictures, and award pictures
on the following pages are used throughout the Friendship Group sessions.
Session-specific activity sheets appear at the ends of units.

Friendship Group Guidelines

In Friendship Group, we:

Listen to each other.
Support each other.
Respect each other.

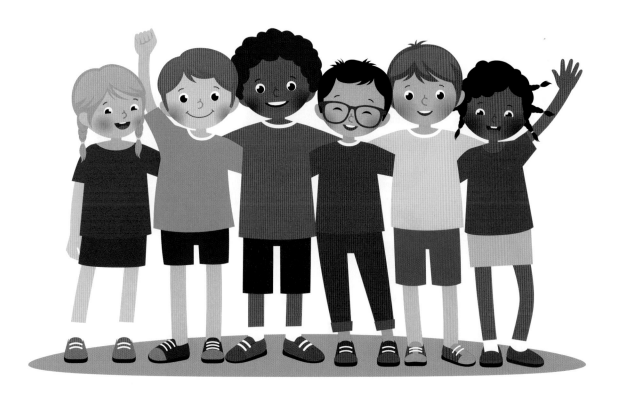

Good Teamwork

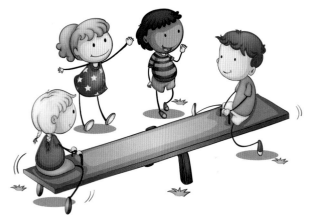

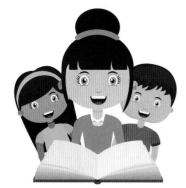

Pay attention.

Join in.

Support your friends.

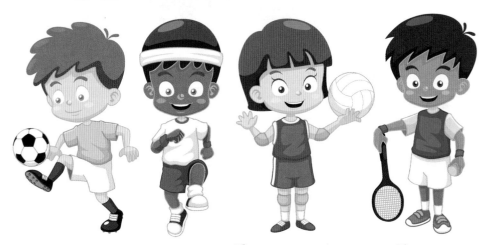

Listen to the coaches.

Care for Your Friends

Help each other.

Share.

Think before
you act.

No fighting.

Take care of our place.

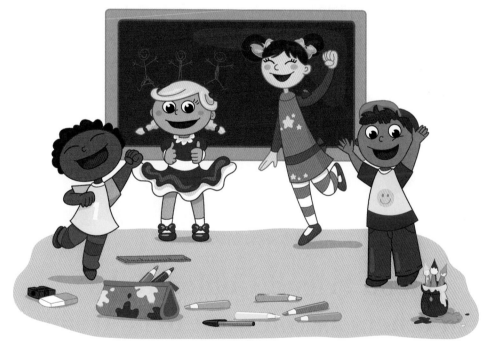

Fair Play is Fun Play

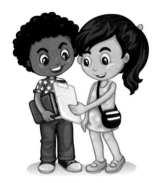

Take turns.

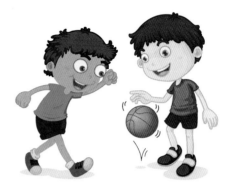

Follow rules.

Treat your friends
with respect.

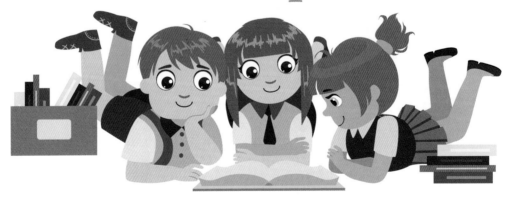

Good Friend Golden Rule:
"Treat others as you want to be treated."

Make a Deal

Give an idea.

Check it out.

Okay?

YES!

Say "yes" to good ideas.

Traffic Light Poster

When You Have a Problem, Work It Out

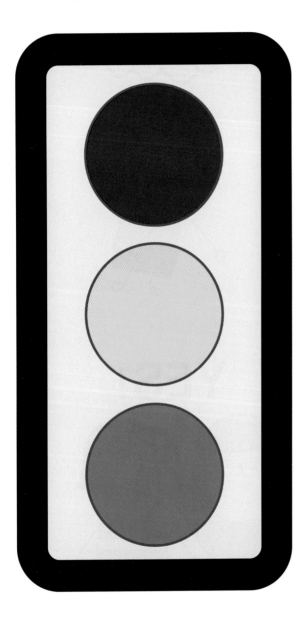

- Stop, calm down, Take 5.
- Tell what the problem is and how you feel.

- Give an idea.
- Listen to others' ideas.
- Say "yes" to good ideas.

- Give it a try.
- Did it work?

Communication

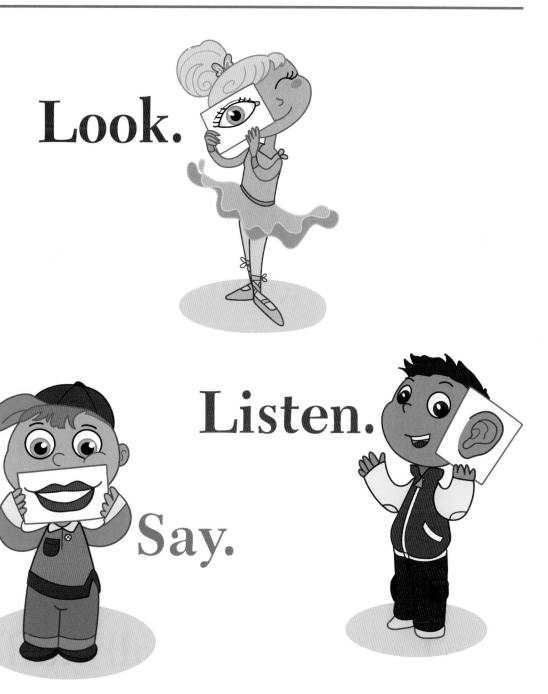

Look.

Listen.

Say.

Positive Thinking

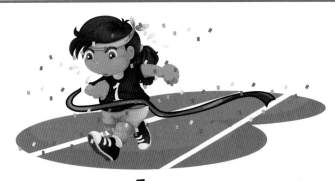

Focus on the <u>positive</u>.

Make a good effort.

Tell yourself that you can do this.

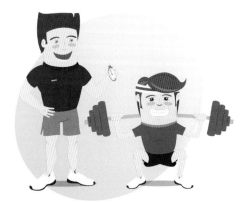

Don't sweat the small stuff.

Snack Jobs

Plates _____

Napkins _____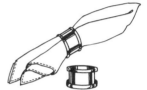

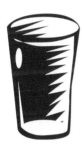

Drinks _____

Food _____

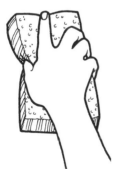

Clean-Up _____

Baxter's Feeling Faces

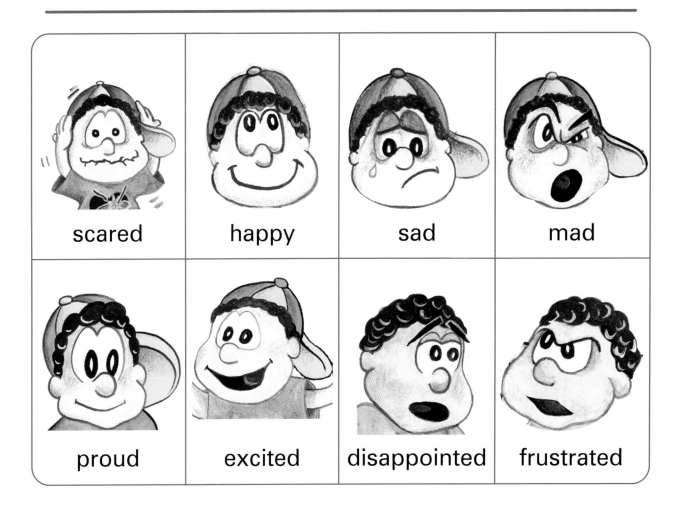

| scared | happy | sad | mad |
| proud | excited | disappointed | frustrated |

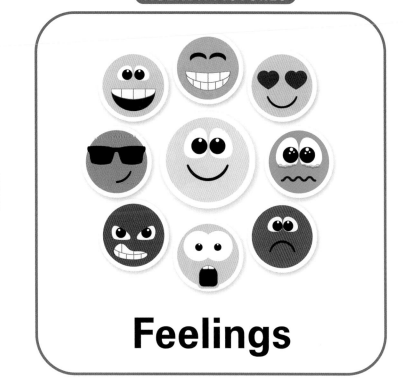

1

Feelings

2

Friendship Circle

3

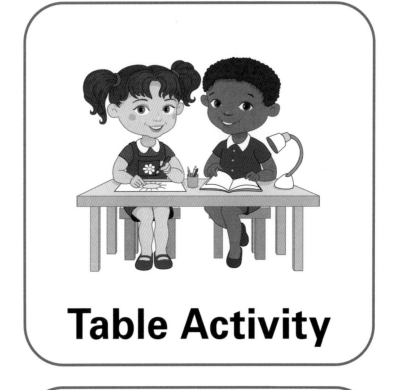

Table Activity

4

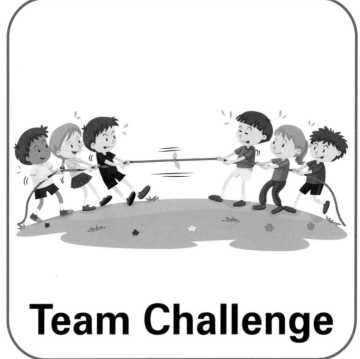

Team Challenge

5

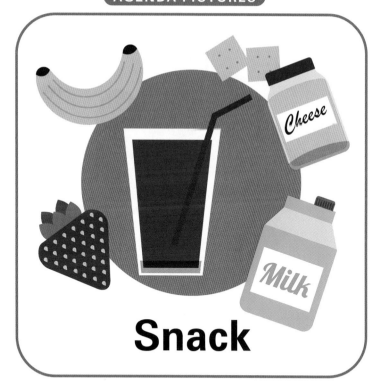

Snack

6

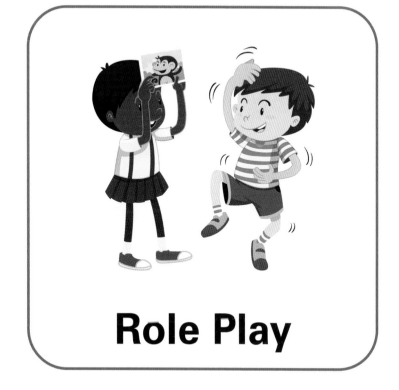

Role Play

7

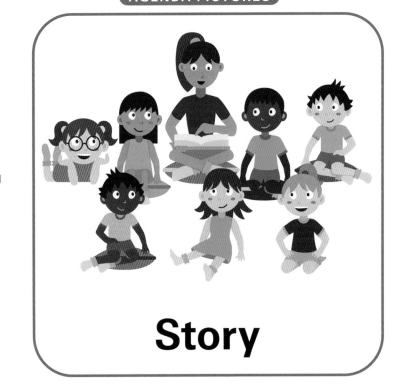

Story

8

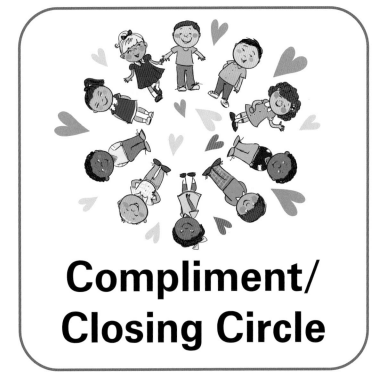

Compliment/ Closing Circle

Friendship Star Medals

Cut out, add children's names, fasten on with tape.

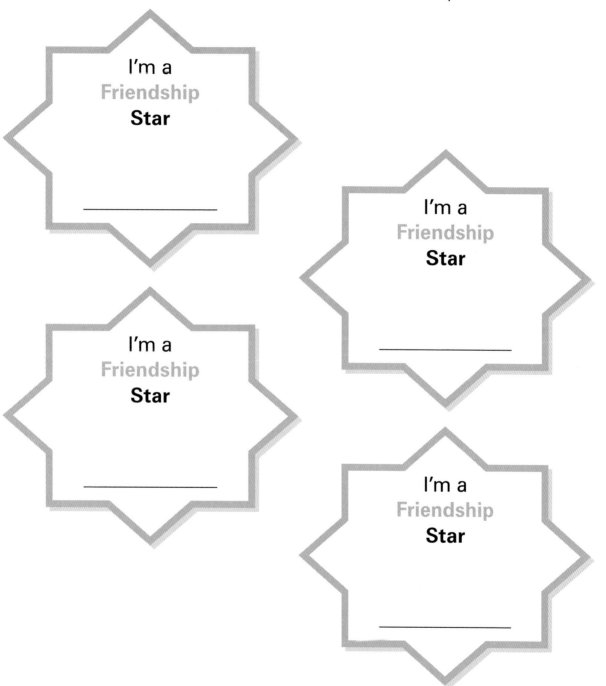

FAIR PLAYER AWARD

Presented to

_____

FOR FAIR PLAY IN FRIENDSHIP TEAM

Friendship Award

To:

For:

PEACEMAKER AWARD

To: _____

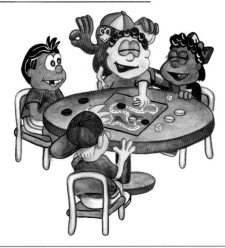

For: _____

_____

_____

_____

Friendship Group Manual
EARLY ELEMENTARY SESSIONS

Establishing Common Ground

SESSION 1. Joining In and Getting Acquainted

GOALS

1. Introduce the purpose of the group.
2. Present the concept of participation (Good Teamwork) and group rules.
3. Help children become familiar and comfortable with each other.

MATERIALS NEEDED

- Agenda Pictures: 2, 3, 4, 5, 6, and 8
- Posters: Good Teamwork and Snack Jobs
- My Friendship Team (Activity Page 1.1, see p. 90; one per child)
- A set of stickers for each child with group members' names, star stickers, markers
- Pictures of (1) firehouse, (2) firetruck, (3) house on fire (Activity Page 1.2, see p. 91; one per group)
- Props for the Firefighters' Show (hats, rope to use as the fire hose)
- Friendship Tips Handout for Session 1 (Activity Page 1.3, see p. 92; one per child)

SESSION OUTLINE

- *Friendship Circle:* Introductions, Good Teamwork skills, name game (15 minutes)
- *Construction Station:* Decorate Activity Pages, My Friendship Team (10 minutes)
- *Snack* (optional, 15 minutes)

- *Collaborative Challenges:* Firefighters' Show (10 minutes)
- *Closing Circle:* Play the Describing Game and share compliments (10 minutes).

ADVANCE PREPARATION

- Hang agenda pictures, Good Teamwork poster, and Firefighters' Show pictures.
- If you are having snack, assign children snack jobs and hang poster.

DETAILED SESSION CONTENT

Friendship Circle: Introductions, Good Teamwork Skills, Name Game (15 Minutes)

Invite the children to sit together, forming a "friendship circle." Introduce yourself and provide a brief description of the group schedule and purpose.

> "Hello, everyone, my name is _____ and I'm going to be the coach of this Friendship Group. I'm glad to see you all here today. We are going to meet in our Friendship Group every week. We'll get to know each other and have fun together."

Explain that the children will make friends, try out new activities and games, and learn how to solve problems and work together. Have the children introduce themselves, then ask the children what they know about teamwork. Encourage the children to think about different kinds of teams (sports teams, dance teams, etc.) and how the people on a team work together to help each other and get things done. Reinforce the idea that team members like each other and have fun together. Ask the children to think about things they like to do with friends, and why it is more fun to play with friends than to play alone.

> "In Friendship Group, we are a team. Has anyone been on a team? What does it mean to be on a team? What do team members do? Why do people like to be on a team?"

Summarize the discussion by reviewing the Good Teamwork poster, as follows:

> "For good teamwork, there are four things that you need to do [point to poster]:
> 'Join in,' 'Pay attention,' 'Support your friends,' and 'Listen to the coaches.'"

As you read the items on the poster, point out children who are showing the skill and describe what they are doing—for example: "I notice that [Name] and [Name] are joining in; they are sitting with the group and sharing good ideas in our discussion"; "I notice that [Name] and [Name] are paying attention; they have their eyes on me and they are listening." When you read the last two items, include counterexamples that are prohibited in the group.

> "When you're part of a team, you need to support your friends. So, we don't yell at each other or say mean things, and we don't push or hit. That would be breaking our Friendship Group rules. We notice the good things our friends do and cheer them on. The last teamwork idea is

to "Listen to the coaches." Our job is to help you get along with each other, make friends, and play safely. It's important to listen to us so that you know what to do in the group. Right now, I'd like to give our whole team a hand for your great teamwork—joining in, paying attention, and listening to the coaches. Great job!" [Lead children in clapping for themselves.]

Next, select and play a game to help the children learn each others' names. A popular choice among young children is Friend, Friend, Chase. This game is played like Duck, Duck, Goose. Children sit in a circle. The person who is "it" walks around the outside of the circle tapping each person lightly on the head and saying his or her name. (Coaches and other group members can also say the names aloud to aid memory.) At some point, the person who is "it" will add the word *chase* after someone's name. That person then stands up and chases "it" around the circle. When "it" reaches the chaser's seat, he or she sits down and the chaser becomes "it." Explain the rules of the game and choose a child from the group to go first. Let each child have a turn. As the children play, point out and praise good teamwork.

An alternative name game is Group Juggle. Children sit in a circle with their hands in front of them. The coach introduces a soft object, such as a beanbag or small stuffed animal (something that will not bounce away), calls out the name of a child sitting across the circle and tosses the object gently to that child ("Hi, [Name], here you go"). The coach instructs that child to say "Thank you, Coach" and then call out the name of another child in the circle and toss the object to that person. That person says "Thank you, [Name]," and then calls out the name of another child who has not yet had a turn. This process continues until each person has had a turn. Then the coach introduces the challenge, which is to repeat the same pattern (greeting by name, tossing the object, thanking by name) in the same order. If desired, two additional challenges can be attempted: (1) seeing how quickly the group can remember and complete the tossing sequence; and/or (2) adding a second object around the circle in the same sequence midway through the first sequence, so that two objects are circling around the circle, one after the other. At the end of the activity, comment on positive skill performance.

"WOW! That was really great! I noticed a lot of good teamwork during that game—everyone was joining in and paying attention! I think we should give ourselves a hand for joining in together so well." [Lead the children in clapping for themselves.]

Construction Station: My Friendship Team Activity Page (10 Minutes)

Have children sit around a table and show Activity Page 1.1. Explain that each child will have a chance to complete a team page to take home and show to his or her parent(s). Demonstrate how the children will put on stickers to show each team member's name, and then decorate the page with stars and markers. Ask the children how they will be able to show Good Teamwork when they are working on their pages. As children work, engage them in a discussion about firefighters and teamwork, as this will set the stage for the later group activity.

"Did you notice the firefighter picture on your team page? What does a firefighter do? Right, and also firefighters work as a team, just like our Friendship Group. They help each other out and work together to put out fires and save people."

During the art activity, coaches can ask about firefighter experiences—for example: "Have you been to a firehouse? What was it like? Have you climbed on a firetruck?" They can also ask about the activity—for example: "What colors are you going to use on your page?" To help establish common ground, comment on the similarities you notice among the children—for example: Both [Name] and [Name] have seen firetrucks in a parade"; "[Name] and [Name] are coloring their firefighters red." In addition, praise examples of Good Teamwork behaviors.

Snack (Optional, 15 Minutes)

Lead children to the snack table and show them the completed Snack Jobs chart. Explain that each child has a job to do for the team: distributing plates, napkins, drinks, food, or helping with cleanup. Jobs will change each week. During snack, support conversation that helps the children get to know each other, and point out examples of good teamwork.

Collaborative Challenges: Firefighters' Show (10 Minutes)

Before the show, post the three pictures at different locations marked by chairs and/or colored tape to represent the (1) firehouse, (2) firetruck, and (3) house on fire. Introduce the play.

> "Now it's time to put on a play about firefighters and show how well you can work as a team. You will be firefighters, and this is your firehouse. When our show starts, you will be in the firehouse. What can you do when you are in the firehouse? [Encourage the children to generate a few ideas, such as playing cards, polishing their boots, drinking soda or coffee, taking a nap.] Then you will hear the alarm ring. [Make the sound of a bell ringing.] What do you do then? Yes, it means there is a fire. You have to get on your helmet, grab the ladder, get onto your firetruck and drive to the fire. [Indicate the picture and location of the hats and truck.] What can you do on the truck? [Help the children generate a few ideas, such as driving the truck, making the siren go, keeping a lookout for cars or people who are in the way.] You get to a burning house [indicate picture], and then what do you do? You will need to work as a team. You will each take a turn holding the hose to put water on the fire."

The coach should serve as the "director," reminding the children of the actions as they move through the play. Remind children to act out their roles at each station (e.g., playing cards, polishing their boots in the firehouse). At the burning building, remind them to help carry the hose and take turns being in the front to spray water on the fire. Praise children for their good teamwork—paying attention, joining in, and supporting their friends. If time allows, have the children put the play on a second time.

Closing Circle: Compliments (10 Minutes)

Join in a friendship circle for the closing activity, the Describing Game, and compliments.

> "Have you had a good time in our Friendship Group today? I really enjoyed spending time with you today and seeing all of your good teamwork. I can tell you are going to be a very special team! We end each Friendship Group with compliments, noticing positive things about each other. I am going to give each one of you a compliment about your good teamwork. You will have to guess who I am thinking of."

Start the Describing Game with general clues ("The person I'm thinking of has two eyes"). Allow one guess after each clue. Proceed to give more specific clues ("The person I'm thinking of has brown hair") until children make a correct guess. Then, give that child a compliment, describing positive behavior observed during the session. Proceed until each child has received a compliment. Then distribute Friendship Tips Handout for Session 1 for parents and teachers.

SPECIAL ISSUES

1. Children who are anxious during the first session may resist joining in initially. Provide encouragement and reassurance, but do not pressure children. Allow them to watch for a while if they need time to feel comfortable in the group setting.

2. Children who feel insecure may engage in intrusive, attention-getting behavior. Ignore as much inappropriate behavior as you can, and put effort into forging a positive connection. Use your attention and proximity to reinforce appropriate behaviors, and give these children specific positive roles when possible (e.g., holding materials, helping to distribute papers).

3. To establish a sense of comfort and security in the group context, use extensive praise to support appropriate behavior, and focus on positive expectations (e.g., telling children what you would like them to do). However, do not allow children to engage in behavior that is harmful to others in the group (e.g., aggression or put-downs) or that is damaging to property. Immediately explain that these behaviors are against the Friendship Group rules, and redirect children to appropriate behaviors. Significant problem behaviors in the first session indicate that you will need to put in special efforts to manage the environment, focus your attention, and use behavior management supports (e.g., token reward system) to maintain a positive group context.

4. In general, Friendship Group emphasizes positive behaviors (e.g., Good Teamwork) rather than rule prohibitions (e.g., No Fighting). Children who show minor infractions can be reminded to "Listen to the Coaches." However, if needed, specific rule prohibitions can be added (e.g., No Fighting, No Put-Downs, Take Care of Our Place, Keep Your Hands to Yourself), along with response cost consequences (see Chapter 4).

5. For very impulsive children, consider using a "Team Train" to move from one activity to another. Have children follow the coach in a line and copy actions (e.g., clap high, clap low, walk on tiptoes) as they move to the new activity.

SESSION 2. Initiating Friendships: Tell about Yourself and Listen to Your Friend

GOALS

1. Review the purpose of the group, Good Teamwork skills, and group rules.

2. Introduce the concept of self-expression (Tell about Yourself) as a way to make friends.

3. Provide opportunities to practice skills with supportive feedback.

MATERIALS NEEDED

- Agenda Pictures: 2, 3, 4, 5, 6, and 8
- Posters: Good Teamwork and Snack Jobs
- Pretend microphone, cards for Pass the Mike (Activity Page 2.1, see p. 93; one set per group)
- Cards for You and Me card sort (Activity Page 2.2, see p. 94; one set per dyad/triad)
- Markers, glue sticks, tape, note cards labeled *None*, *Some*, and *All*
- Three pictures and props (helmets, rope) for the Firefighters' Show (see Session 1)
- Friendship Tips Handout for Session 2 (Activity Page 2.3, see p. 95; one per child)

SESSION OUTLINE

- *Friendship Circle:* Review teamwork and self-expression, play Pass the Mike (15 minutes)
- *Construction Station:* You and Me card sort activity (15 minutes)
- *Snack* (optional, 15 minutes)
- *Collaborative Challenges:* Replay the Firefighters' Show (10 minutes)
- *Closing Circle:* Play the Describing Game with compliments (5 minutes)

ADVANCE PREPARATION

- Hang agenda pictures and posters and a new Snack Jobs poster (if needed).
- Cut out the cards for Pass the Mike and You and Me activities.
- Create a pretend microphone with a toilet paper roll, black paper, and aluminum foil.
- For the You and Me card sort, write *None*, *Some*, and *All* on note cards.

DETAILED SESSION CONTENT

Friendship Circle: Review Teamwork and Self-Expression, Play Pass the Mike (15 Minutes)

Review everyone's names. Use choral responding to read through the Good Teamwork poster—for example: "Let's read through our Good Teamwork ideas together. I'll read it first, and then we'll all say it together." Ask children for a favorite memory from the prior session, and note how the activities they remember illustrate the goals of the group (e.g., making friends and learning to have fun working and playing together). Review the session agenda. Then introduce the idea of telling about yourself and listening to your friends, as follows.

> "I'm so glad to see you again for our Friendship Group. We had fun getting to know each other last week and learning to be a friendship team. Today, I'd like to tell you about a good way to make friends, and that is to talk with them—tell about yourself and listen to your friend. What could you tell someone about yourself, so he or she could get to know you better? [Restate their

ideas.] How could you learn about them? Right, listen to what they say. We are going to play a game that will help you learn more about your friends in this group by talking with them."

Put the Pass the Mike cards face down in the middle of the circle. Explain that you will turn on music (or hum some music) as the children pass a (pretend) microphone around the circle. When the music stops, the child with the mike picks up a card from the center and turns it over to see what the category is. (You will need to read the card for children who do not yet read.) That child tells about him- or herself by responding to the category (e.g., for the category of favorite foods, the child might say, "My favorite food is pizza"). Then the child asks the others in the group to raise their hands if they also like pizza. Play the music and pass the mike again; let each child have one or two turns picking a category, giving a response, and seeing who shares his or her interest or feeling. As children play, praise their good teamwork (joining in, paying attention, supporting their friends) and conversation skills (telling about themselves and listening to their friends). Foster common ground with your comments—for example: "Everyone in our group likes pizza! Both [Name] and [Name] have cats—isn't that neat to find out?"

Construction Station: You and Me Card Sort Activity (15 Minutes)

The You and Me activity provides an opportunity to practice basic conversation skills in a structured context and facilitates the establishment of common ground. Have the children split up into pairs or triads, and create some distance between the groups. Tape note cards saying *None, Some,* and *All* onto the tabletops. Place the picture cards from Activity Page 2.2 face down. Children take turns choosing cards and sorting them into these piles, indicating things that no friends like, some friends like, or all friends like.

"We just learned that a good way to make friends is to talk with others—tell about yourself and listen to your friend. We are going to learn more about our friends by talking with them. First, one of you will draw a card from this pile. Show the picture and tell your partner[s] if it is something that you like. Then ask your partner[s] to raise a hand if it is something that he or she [or they] like. Now you have to put it into one of these piles."

Let the children take turns choosing a picture, telling about their likes, asking how the other(s) feels, and putting it into the pile indicating how many liked it. As they play, praise good teamwork and conversation skills (telling about you, listening to your friend).

Snack (Optional, 15 Minutes)

Remind children of the snack routine and Snack Jobs.

"I'm so pleased to see how you all remembered to come over to the table, take a seat, and quiet down; you remembered just how we get ready for snack in our Friendship Group. Let's look at the jobs for today. Review assigned jobs. We'll have new jobs each week, so you will get a chance to do each job. That's how we work together as a team."

During snack, encourage the children to discuss what they learned about each other during the activities. Facilitate general conversation and socializing among the children.

Collaboration Challenges: Replay the Firefighters' Show (10 Minutes)

The goal of this activity is to provide children with an opportunity to practice teamwork in the context of a large group and active game. Begin by asking the children to remember the three things that happen in the show and what they do at each station, using the pictures as a guide. After this review, the children can put on the show, with the coach providing support as needed. Be sure to remind the children to elaborate their actions at each point in the play, pretending to do different things while they are waiting at the station, getting on their uniforms and riding the truck, and taking turns putting out the fire. Praise instances of good teamwork and encourage the children to clap for themselves at the end of their show.

Closing Circle Compliments (5 Minutes)

Join in a friendship circle for the Describing Game and compliments.

> "What a great job you did today! We learned about Good Teamwork, and also how to talk with friends to get to know them better. I have some compliments to share, but first you will need to guess who I am thinking of."

As in Session 1, give clues and let children guess about whom you are thinking. Give that child a compliment, focusing on the good teamwork or good conversation skills demonstrated during the session. Then ask the group whether anyone else has a compliment for that child, and let a peer give a compliment. Continue until each child has had a turn. Distribute Friendship Tips Handout for Session 2.

SPECIAL ISSUES

1. If the active games and transitions disorganize the children, consider different strategies for providing more support. Holding the entire session around a table with children seated in chairs can be helpful. Strategic staff attention to children who need more positive support can also be helpful. If impulsive or emotional behavior is disrupting the session, initiate a token reward system to establish behavioral control and increase children's positive engagement.

2. If an individual child is showing difficulty engaging with the group (exhibiting withdrawal or intrusive behavior), focus on providing a "secure base" for him or her. To provide secure support, attend carefully to that child, maintain positive eye contact, and provide frequent physical or verbal support (e.g., pat on the back) and extensive specific praise for appropriate behavior. In addition, this child can be given "helper" roles, such as passing out materials.

3. If desired, Friend, Friend, Chase can be replayed at the start of the session to review children's names, or at the end if there is extra time. In a variation, this game can also be used to review the Good Teamwork ideas. As children go around the circle, they repeat a teamwork idea as they tap each child's head (e.g., "Join in, join in, join in, chase").

4. The goal of the conversation activities is to identify common ground, rather than celebrate individual preferences. It's important to recognize and accept an individual child's preferences, and no child should be compelled to agree with others. At the same time, many children who struggle

with friendship issues do so because they are self-focused and have trouble finding common ground with others. These activities are designed to encourage children to listen to others, exploring and seeking areas of common ground. Hence, it is important to maintain a focus on finding common ground, rather than simply expressing individual opinions.

SESSION 3. Talking about Feelings

GOALS

1. Review the teamwork skills and Tell about You as a way to make friends.

2. Introduce and discuss the "core four" basic feelings (happy, sad, mad, scared).

3. Practice expressing feelings in a game, fostering teamwork and empathy.

MATERIALS NEEDED

- Agenda Pictures: 1, 7, 5, 6, 2, and 8
- Posters: Good Teamwork, Snack Jobs, and Baxter's Feeling Faces
- Four feeling faces cards for circle activity (Activity Page 3.1, see p. 96)
- Baxter Story 1, "Baxter's Feelings" (pp. 97–102)
- Leader Hat for Follow the Leader game
- Award certificates and Friendship Tips Handout for Session 3 (Activity Page 3.2, see p. 103; one per child)

SESSION OUTLINE

- *Friendship Circle:* Review skills, play Guess My Feelings (15 minutes)
- *Construction Station:* Read and discuss the story "Baxter's Feelings" (15 minutes)
- *Snack* (optional, 15 minutes)
- *Collaborative Challenges*: Follow the Leader game (10 minutes)
- *Closing Circle:* Distribute awards and share compliments (5 minutes)

ADVANCE PREPARATION

- Hang agenda pictures, posters, and (if needed) a new Snack Jobs poster.
- Cut out the core four feeling faces cards (Activity Page 3.1).
- Choose and complete an awards certificate for each child (in the Commonly Used Materials that follow Chapter 5).

DETAILED SESSION CONTENT

Friendship Circle: Review Skills, Play Guess My Feelings (15 Minutes)

If needed, review children's names. Ask children for their memories of prior Friendship Group activities and reinforce the skills on which they worked.

> "It's great to see all of our friendship team members here again today! I really had fun with you last time. Who can remember something we did last time? What did you like the best? Yes, that was fun! What friendship ideas did we talk about?"

Review the Good Teamwork poster and ideas with the children, and the value of getting to know each other by telling about yourself and listening to your friend. Review the agenda pictures and the activities planned for the session. Begin the discussion of feelings by pointing to Baxter's Feeling Faces poster (with just the top row showing), starting with the happy face and then moving to the sad, scared, and mad faces, and letting children identify each one. Make sure all are labeled correctly. Introduce the Guess My Feelings game by saying something like this:

> "Now we're going to play a game. I'm going to put pictures of these faces down in the middle and mix them up. I'm going to pass this ball around the circle and turn on some music. When I stop the music, you stop passing the ball. OK, the ball stopped at me. So, I pick up a feeling face and peek at it, but I'm not going to show it to anyone. I am just going to show you that feeling on my own face and tell you something that makes me feel that way. Your job is to guess which feeling I chose—happy, sad, mad, or scared. Pay attention, Team, and we will see if you can guess my feeling."

Model the process of making a feeling face and giving an example, and let the children guess. Then play the music and pass the ball around again, giving someone else a turn to pick a feeling card, make a feeling face and give an example, and let the group guess his or her feeling. Give each child a turn, and if children are interested, give them each a second turn.

Construction Station: Baxter's Feelings Story and Discussion (15 Minutes)

Introduce the idea that feelings are something you can talk about with friends. Use an interactive reading style to read and discuss the story about Baxter's Feelings, encouraging responses from the children as indicated. Questions to encourage discussion are embedded within the story; feel free to add questions or comments to support discussion within the group. The goal is to introduce each of the four core feelings (happy, sad, mad, scared) and discuss how each feeling looks on the outside and feels on the inside. In addition, children can be helped to discuss the kinds of events or experiences that make them feel each feeling.

Snack (Optional, 15 Minutes)

Following the usual snack routine, review the Snack Jobs poster and then distribute the snack. As they eat, support conversation among the children. Following the theme of the session, coaches can ask children about experiences they had that made them feel happy, sad, scared, or mad, and note shared experiences—for example: "Sounds scary. Has that happened to anyone else?" Encourage peer-to-peer conversation as much as possible.

Collaborative Challenge: Follow the Leader Game (10 Minutes)

Sit or stand in a circle and put on a visor (the Leader Hat). Tell the children that you will do something with your hands and they must try to copy your motion. Start with a simple action, such as clapping hands, and keep up the action until the children copy it. Then switch to a different action, such as slapping hands on knees, and continue the action until all of the children copy it. Lead a few additional hand motions so that children get some ideas (e.g., hand rolls, fist bounces), and then pass the Leader Hat to the child sitting next to you. Give each child a chance to lead two or three hand motions, before passing the hat on to the next child.

Then, try a Follow the Leader challenge in which you add feeling faces into the mix. Add a different feeling expression to each motion. For example, start by clapping hands and smiling, with a happy expression. Once all are copying you, ask the children, "What feeling are you showing?" and praise them for figuring it out and copying you. Then switch to a different action, such as hot potato fists, with a sad and crying expression. Continue until all of the children copy your motion, let them name the feeling, and then switch to air punches with a mad expression. Finally, try jazz hands with a scared expression. See if other children want a turn to lead actions with feelings.

For an even more difficult challenge, show the children an action and then stop. Explain that their challenge is to remember what you did and then copy it after you are done. Start with a single hand motion, such as three claps, and then stop and let the children copy it. Next do a sequence of two hand motions, such as three claps followed by a hand roll. If the children can do that well, try a sequence of three hand motions, such as three claps followed by a hand roll, followed by hitchhiker thumbs. Throughout this activity, praise children for their attention and effort at mastering the challenge, and for good teamwork in joining in, paying attention, and supporting their friends. At the end of the game, encourage the children to clap for themselves.

Closing Circle Compliments (5 Minutes)

Call the children into a friendship circle and review the highlights of the session.

> "That was really wonderful! I saw a lot of good teamwork I especially liked. [Provide examples of particular observed instances of good teamwork and the children's discussion of feelings.] I'd like to talk about feelings some more next time—how about you? Today, I'd like to recognize each person's good work with an award certificate and compliment."

One by one, hold up an award certificate with a child's name on it. Give that child a compliment about his or her behavior during the session, and ask if someone else has a compliment for that child. Set a limit of one additional compliment per child in order to keep the pace moving along and to make sure that each child has a turn to receive an award. Distribute Friendship Tips Handout for Session 3.

SPECIAL ISSUES

1. If some children find it difficult to talk about their feelings or to respond to the prompts in the Baxter story (e.g., "How about you?"), add some suggestions for nonverbal responses instead (e.g., "Show me how you'd look if that happened to you").

2. At this point in the program, some children will find it difficult to negotiate basic social decisions (e.g., "Who would like to go first?"). Later in the program, negotiation skills become a

focus. However, at this point, avoid conflicts by assigning roles (e.g., tell the children who will go first each time).

3. Several adjustments can be used to simplify the Follow the Leader game if it is difficult for a group. You can try doing it as a "parade" rather than a static circle game. Children may be more familiar with the parade idea, and it may be easier for them to start as a parade, and then try it in a circle. If the Leader Hat is a problem in your group, it is not necessary to use it. The third level of imitation (in which the children have to copy the actions from memory) may be too difficult for some groups at this point in the program. Stick with the first level (direct imitation) and do not overstress the children if you see that it is too difficult for them.

SESSION 4. Talking More about Feelings

GOALS

1. Review the unit skills (Good Teamwork, Tell about You, Talk about Feelings).

2. Practice emotional expression using the feeling cards and by sharing feelings.

3. Provide opportunities to role-play feelings and practice emotion regulation and teamwork.

MATERIALS NEEDED

- Agenda Pictures: 1, 4, 3, 5, 6, 2, and 8
- Posters: Good Teamwork, Snack Jobs
- A laminated Baxter's Feeling Faces poster or set of face cards for each child
- Pictures for feelings card sort (Activity Page 4.1, see p. 104; one set per group)
- Friendship Tips Handout for Session 4 (Activity Page 4.2, see p. 105; one per child)

SESSION OUTLINE

- *Friendship Circle:* Introduce individual feeling faces, feelings song (15 minutes)
- *Construction Station:* Feelings Card Sort and Feelings in Motion games (15 minutes)
- *Snack* (optional, 15 minutes)
- *Collaborative Challenges:* Rock Around the Clock (10 minutes)
- *Closing Circle:* Distribute feeling faces armbands and share compliments (5 minutes)

ADVANCE PREPARATION

- Hang agenda pictures and Good Teamwork and (if needed) Snack Jobs posters.
- For each child, hang a laminated Baxter's Feeling Faces poster or provide a set of feeling cards.

- For the feelings card sort, cut a set of four core feeling faces and tape them on the table.
- For the clock game, place tape with numbers on the ground to represent a clock face.

DETAILED SESSION OUTLINE

Friendship Circle: Introduce Individual Feeling Faces, Feelings Song (15 Minutes)

The friendship circle starts by sharing feelings, using individual posters or feeling faces cards. One option is to hang up a laminated feelings face poster for each child. Children place an indicator on their chosen feeling face, for example, by using a pushpin (if the posters are on a bulletin board), a small magnet (if the posters are on a metal background), or a dry erase marker (if the posters are on the wall). A second option is to give children their own sets of laminated feeling faces cards on a ring, letting them display their current feeling on top. Children will use their feelings poster or feeling faces cards to show how they are feeling at the start of each group, and to note changes in their feelings during the session.

> "Hi everyone. I'm so pleased to see all of you here today! I have so much fun with you when I come here each week; I always look forward to it. Today I brought feeling faces for each of you. Every time you come to Friendship Group, you will get to place a marker on the picture [or choose the card] that shows how you are feeling that day."

Let each child take a turn putting the marker on a feeling face (or selecting a feeling face card) and telling the group why he or she feels that way. After each person has shared his or her feelings, review the session agenda. Then ask who can tell you one of the Good Teamwork ideas and help children review the four ideas on the teamwork poster. Continue by noting that it also helps friendships when you talk with each other and when you pay attention to your feelings and your friend's feelings. Explain that you brought a feeling song for the group today, as follows.

> "First, think of something that makes you happy. I'm thinking of a sunny day—that makes me happy. [Name], what are you thinking of? OK, is everyone thinking of something that makes them happy? I think so—I see a lot of smiling faces. Sing the song.] 'If you're happy and you know it, clap your hands; if you're happy and you know it, clap your hands; if you're happy and you know it then your face will surely show it; if you're happy and you know it, clap your hands.'"

Next ask a child to think of something that makes him or her sad. Note that this game will extend too long if the entire group generates ideas for each feeling, so to keep it moving at a good pace—just ask one child to generate an idea for each feeling, and rotate who you ask. If the child has trouble thinking of something, offer a suggestion or see if a friend in the group has an idea to offer. With each emotion, comment that you will be looking for facial expressions and body language that shows the feeling—for example: "This time, I'll be looking for sad-looking faces and droopy heads, because we are thinking of sad things." The additional verses are "If you're sad and you know it, hang your head"; "If you're mad and you know it, shake your fist"; "If you're scared and you know it, shiver and shake." At the end of the song, praise the children for joining in and paying attention, and for sharing their feelings. Let them know you enjoyed learning about their feelings.

Construction Station: Feelings Card Sort and Feelings in Motion Game (15 Minutes)

Have children sit around the table. There should be feeling faces taped down on the table, so that children can "sort" their cards by placing them in a pile under a feeling face. Note that this activity can be done in pairs if it is difficult in the large group. Explain as follows:

> "Today, we are going to play a card game. I will give you each a card. First, you turn it over and we will talk about what is happening in the picture. Then, decide how you would feel if that happened to you, and put the picture under the feeling face that shows how you'd feel."

If you think the children need a model, take a card and model the process. Then deal the cards out to the children. For restless groups, deal out the same card to each child on each turn, so that they are all involved and they are each thinking about the same event, and comparing how it would make them feel. At the end of the activity, comment on how behaviors affect others' feelings, and when friends show good teamwork and support each other, it makes everyone feel happy. Then explain the Feelings in Motion game.

> "Before we go to snack, I want to show you a funny game. I am going to call a feeling word and show you a movement that goes with that feeling. Your job is to remember the motion, and do it when I call the word. Here is the motion that goes with *Happy*. [The coach should smile and wave jazz hands, looking happy.] Let's see everyone try it. Great job, Team. Everyone is making the Happy motion."

Proceed to show the children the motion for sad—frown and use your hands to wipe away pretend tears, looking sad. Have the children try that motion, and praise them for their efforts. Then call out *Happy* and lead children in changing their facial expression and motion, smiling and waving jazz hands. Encourage the children to make the matching feeling face along with the hand motion. Go back and forth, calling *Sad* and *Happy* again. This emotion switching should be fun and funny for the children, so encourage them to enjoy it. Once children have the hang of it, add a motion for *Mad*, such as making a mad face and shaking fists in the air. Mix up the calls for children to show the motions for happy, sad, and mad. In most groups, three motions will be all children can do, but if your group accomplishes these three with ease, add a fourth motion for *Scared*, forming your mouth in an "O" shape, with your hands on either side of it. Let the children try switching between all four motions as you call different feeling words.

Snack (Optional, 15 Minutes)

Guide the children through their usual snack time routine. Be sure to foster socialization by modeling and encouraging conversation among the children.

Collaboration Challenge: Rock Around the Clock (15 Minutes)

To set up for this game, Rock Around the Clock, use small pieces of numbered tape to mark 12 spots on the ground in the shape of a circle, corresponding to the 12 locations of numbers on a clock. (The children will be moving around these spots, so use small pieces of numbered tape rather than taping down paper on which children might slip.) The game is played like this: You tell the children what kind of motion they must use to move around the clock numbers, going from each number to the next, in order (e.g., march forward, tiptoe, hop on one foot, walk backwards use "twirl-around" steps). Periodically, make the clock "chime" (e.g., by saying "*ding-dong.*") At that point, the children must freeze. Then give them another type of motion to use in moving around the clock. As you explain the game, demonstrate the actions.

> "This is a really fun game. To play it, you will need to listen carefully, because I will be telling you what kind of steps you need to use to move around the clock. First, you will need to walk on tiptoes. [Start walking around the clock on tiptoes.] After a while, you will hear the clock chime, like this: '*ding-dong.*' When you hear that sound, you have to freeze. [Freeze.] Then, I will tell you a new way to rock around the clock. Now you must hop on one foot around the clock. Come try it!"

After the children have tried a few different kinds of movements around the clock, add in new challenges. Ask them to move together (e.g., "Now find a partner and tiptoe"; "Now, switch partners and skip"), or add a "no talking" rule, so that they have to figure out the new motion by watching carefully. You can also ask them for ideas about how to "rock around the clock." Praise them for their teamwork, listening skills, and following directions.

Closing Circle: Compliments (5 Minutes)

Following usual procedures, give each child a compliment by recognizing a positive friendship behavior, and allow a teammate to offer a compliment as well. Distribute Friendship Tips Handout for Session 4.

SPECIAL ISSUES

1. Often there is an increase in behavior management problems between Sessions 3 and 6. As the novelty of the group wears off, the social difficulties that brought children into the group become more apparent. This is a good time to reread Chapter 4 "Behavior Management." Children need to be positively engaged in order to benefit. Use as much positive induction as possible, but add a positive token reward system if needed to control negative group contagion or increase engagement. Low engagement may also occur if the group setting is too difficult for the participants. If children have low verbal skills or significant attention difficulties, consider working in a smaller group and repeating parts of sessions to give the children extra skill practice.

2. If a particular child is struggling to engage effectively in group, provide a "secure base" by maintaining close physical proximity, frequently looking at this child, whispering positive praise, using his or her name, and giving pats of encouragement.

3. As program activities become more collaborative, some children will show inflexibility and a desire for dominance (e.g., doing it their way, controlling the materials). Avoid a power struggle with these children. Instead, use active listening to reflect their concerns, and remind them of the benefits of Good Teamwork skills—for example: "I can see that you would like to do this yourself, but taking turns with your team members is also fun. It is a good way to make friends and have fun playing with others"; "I see that you are very excited about getting your turn, and I know it is hard for you to wait. The other kids really enjoy playing with you when you let them have their turn. They want to be your friend when you do that."

SESSION 5. Good Teamwork Review

GOALS

1. Discuss and consolidate the friendship skill concepts presented in this unit.

2. Practice coordinated play with planning and group problem solving.

3. Practice emotion regulation and impulse control in the context of coordinated play.

MATERIALS NEEDED

- Agenda Pictures: 1, 4, 3, 5, 2, and 8
- Posters: Good Teamwork, Snack Jobs
- Individual feeling faces
- Hula Hoop™ for team challenge
- Two Hey Friends, Let's Talk game pages (Activity Page 5.1, see p. 106; one for each dyad/triad)
- Two sets of Hey Friends, Let's Talk game cards (Activity Page 5.2, see pp. 107–108; one per dyad/triad)
- A penny marker for each child, and two dice for each pair of children
- For toy play: 50 dominoes/blocks (large enough to stand up on edge), eight plastic animals, poker chips for animal food dishes, folded tissue for beds, a few plastic/wooden trees
- Helping Hands certificates (Activity Page 5.3, see p. 109; one per child)
- Star stickers (cut strips, four stickers of the same color, one strip/color per child)
- Friendship Tips Handout for Session 5 (Activity Page 5.4, see p. 110; one per child)

SESSION OUTLINE

- *Friendship Circle:* Review skills, group Hula Hoop, group cookie chant (15 minutes)
- *Construction Station:* Hey Friends, Let's Talk game (10 minutes)
- *Snack* (optional, 15 minutes)
- *Collaborative Challenges:* Collaborative toy play (15 minutes)
- *Closing Circle:* Helping Hands certificate creation and compliments (5 minutes)

ADVANCE PREPARATION

- Hang agenda pictures, posters, and (if needed) a refreshed Snack Jobs poster.
- Cut out the cards for the Hey Friends, Let's Talk game.
- Write children's names on the Helping Hands certificates and cut stickers into strips.

DETAILED SESSION CONTENT

Friendship Circle: Review Skills, Group Hula Hoop, Group Cookie Chant (15 Minutes)

Greet children and invite them to display a feeling face and share their feelings.

> "It's good to see everyone! Go ahead and show us how you're feeling today. Let your friends know why you feel that way today."

After reviewing the agenda, then proceed to review the unit skills.

> "Today, I thought we'd go around the circle and let each person tell one good idea for making friends and having fun together. If you'd like to, you can pick an idea from our posters or you can add your own. [Let children voice their ideas, and highlight the target skills in your summary.]"

Next, explain that you brought a challenging activity to test their skills at Good Teamwork. You are curious to see how well they will manage this challenge.

> "We have to stand up for this challenge. I brought a Hula Hoop, and we are going to see if we can pass it all around our circle. Sounds easy, but here is the challenge. We can't touch it with our hands. We need to hold hands in a circle the whole time, and pass the Hula Hoop using other parts of our body—we can't let go of each other's hands. How important is it for us to work together to win this challenge? Right, we are really going to need to help our friends. Let's give it a try and see if we can do it."

As the group works on this challenge, praise children for their cooperative behaviors. If they have difficulty, ask them to think about what they can do to help their teammates. Don't worry if some children have difficulty with this task and can't manage it without some use of their hands. This is a challenge that gets easier with more practice. Praise them for their effort. Have them talk about what they did and try a second time.

> "I saw a lot of friendly teamwork during that challenge. You were really joining in, working as a team and supporting your friends! It was hard not to use your hands to pull the Hula Hoop. We're going to try it one more time. Who has an idea about how we can do this challenge without breaking our handholds in the circle?"

The next team challenge is the "Who ate the cookies?" group chant. The group sits in a circle and starts by chanting together "Who ate the cookies in the cookie jar?" The person who is "it" will name someone. They say "[Name] ate the cookies in the cookie jar." Then the person whose name was called answers "Who, me?" and the group replies, "Yes, you." The named person says "Not me" and the group replies "Then who?" The named person names someone else, saying, "[Name] ate the cookies in the cookie jar," and the whole sequence is repeated. What makes this activity challenging is that the chanting is done to a repetitive clapping beat (two slaps on knees and two claps of hands), and the children must try to join in with their part in time to the clapping beat. The beat can start very slow and then speed up.

> "Great! How did you like that funny game? I saw a lot of great teamwork in that game! You really have to pay attention to keep the beat going. I noticed how well you were joining in!"

Construction Station: Hey Friends, Let's Talk Game (15 Minutes)

The Hey Friends, Let's Talk game provides children with opportunities to practice good teamwork, identify feelings, and talk with each other, thus fostering consolidation of the skills introduced thus far in the program. If there are two coaches, have children divide into pairs or groups of three, each getting a game board, a pair of dice, and two pennies to use as markers. If children do not yet read, coaches will need to read the cards. Explain as follows:

> "Here is how you play this game. First, you each shake and roll the dice, and the highest score goes first. When it is your turn, you shake and roll the dice and move forward that many spaces. When you land on a smiling space, you pick a card. If you can answer the question on the card, you can stay on the space. If you need help to answer, you can ask your friend."

Guide the children as they play, liberally praising good teamwork and positive behaviors. If a child has difficulty thinking of an answer, suggest that he or she ask a friend for help.

> "Wow, that was really great. By joining in, paying attention, and talking with your friends, you made this game a lot of fun. What a team!"

Snack (Optional, 15 Minutes)

Follow the usual routine to support conversation.

Collaboration Challenge: Collaborative Toy Play (15 Minutes)

Have children sit around a table and show them a plastic zipper storage bag full of dominoes/blocks, and another bag of plastic animals. Explain the task as follows.

> "Today, we are going to build an animal pen together as a team. First, you'll need to share the blocks and work together to build a large fenced area to mark the animals' living space. Does anyone have ideas about how to share the blocks and make a large fence together?"

Encourage children to share ideas, and if needed, provide a "multiple-choice" array of options and ask children which ones they like. The goal is to come up with a simple plan, such as passing the bag of blocks around and letting everyone take some, or putting the blocks in the middle and letting everyone share them. Next ask the children for ideas about how they can work together to make one large fenced-in area for the animals. In some cases, particularly with younger children, coaches may need to show the children how to put the dominoes on their sides and connect them so that they make an enclosure, because some children may have a habit of stacking the blocks into a pile. Once the animal pen is made, give the children the materials they can use to set up a home for the animals inside the enclosure—food dishes (e.g., poker chips), animal beds (e.g., folded tissue), and trees. Give some to each child and ask everyone to work together to set up the materials. When the children are ready, hold up the bag with the animals and let each child pick one. Once everyone has one animal, let each child pick a second animal. If conflicts arise at any point, ask the children to think about how they could share the animals (or materials). Get ideas from the children who are in conflict, and from their peers. If possible, let the children come up with ideas about how to share, rather than directing them in this task. A key goal is to build their capacity to make plans with peers and gain agreement before they start the activity. At the end, give the children a few minutes to play with the animals, pointing out and praising the children's cooperative behaviors. Comment on and encourage pretend activities, such as helping the animals play together, eat, and sleep. Then ask children to help place the materials back in the bags so you can move on to the next game.

Closing Compliment Circle with Helping Hands Certificates (5 Minutes)

> "You showed terrific teamwork today—you all participated and supported your friends. I am going to give you each a compliment and a Helping Hands award, because you were such good helpers."

Make sure that you have written children's names on the certificates in advance. Pass out a strip of four stickers (all one color) to each child. Hold up a certificate, announce the child's name, give that child a compliment, and elicit a compliment from a teammate. Then pass the certificate around the circle, asking each child to put one star sticker on one of the fingers of the helping hand. Explain that, after it has gone around the circle, the will have all four colored stickers, and can go back to the child who will take it home. Proceed in a similar manner for each child in the group. To keep the pace up, you can start with the next child's compliments as the group finishes putting stickers on for the first child. Praise good teamwork.

SPECIAL ISSUES

1. Team Hula Hoop will be challenging for some groups. Don't worry it if it is. Praise effort, and do not be a stickler for complete mastery of the task, but keep the session moving along. These challenges repeat later in the program, so children will have a chance to try them again.

2. The game Hey Friends, Let's Talk is well liked by some children, but less appealing to others. To help the game start off well, you can "stack the deck" so that some of the more engaging cards are on the top of the deck. Use two die to keep the game moving. If you anticipate that competition between children may be a problem in your group, you may want to have the children share a marker so they move together, or just use the cards but not the game board.

3. This is the first session in which children are encouraged to use toys for pretend play. Some children will find it challenging to coordinate play (e.g., making a large animal pen as a team). They may revert to established play habits (e.g., stacking blocks, playing by themselves). In addition, some children will find it difficult to talk about and plan because they want to start playing. The goal of this activity is to encourage collaborative play, which is more developmentally advanced than parallel or cooperative play. This first activity will give you a chance to see where children are developmentally, and how much support they need to engage in this level of play. It is important to "stretch" the children's capacities to inhibit impulsive activity, make a plan, and work together in their play. At the same time, it is important to monitor the difficulty level and provide support if needed, so that the task does not become so effortful that the children disengage.

My Friendship Team

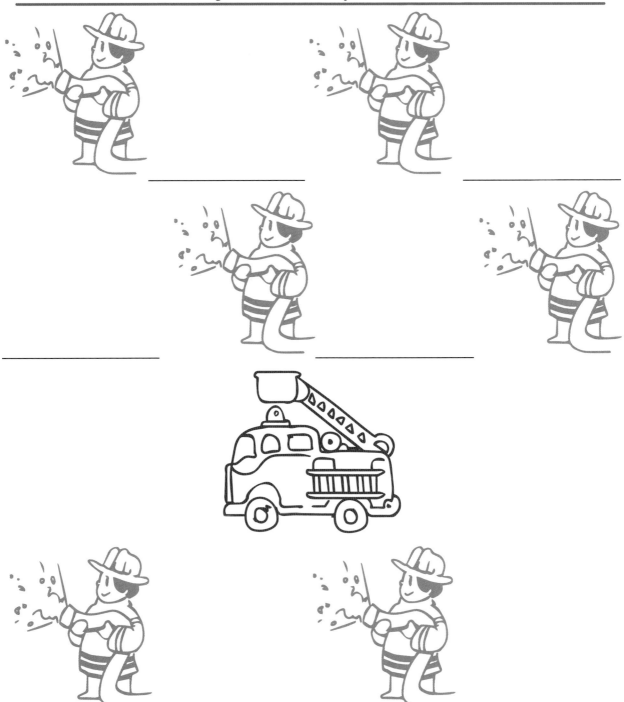

Pictures for the Firefighters' Show

FIRETRUCK

FIREHOUSE

FIRE!

Friendship Tips Handout for Session 1

In Friendship Group, children learn how to make friends and get along with others. They try out new activities and games, and learn how to solve problems and work together. These **Friendship Tips** are to share with teachers and parents who can support friendship skills at school and home.

Remember

To be a good friend and good teammate:

Join in.

Pay attention.

Support your friends.

Try It Out

Give a compliment.

Notice the positive things around you!

You can compliment others on:

    The way they look and things they have.

    The nice things they do.

School and Home Check

- *At school:*
  Did you join in, pay attention, support your friends? Share a compliment with your teacher?

- *At home:*
  Did you join in, pay attention, support your friends? Share a compliment with your family?

Cards for the Pass the Mike Activity

Favorite Food	Pets You Have	Favorite TV Show
Animals You Like	Favorite Color	Your Birthday Month
Food You Don't Like	Toppings You Like on Pizza	Favorite Game to Play

Cards for the You and Me Card Sort

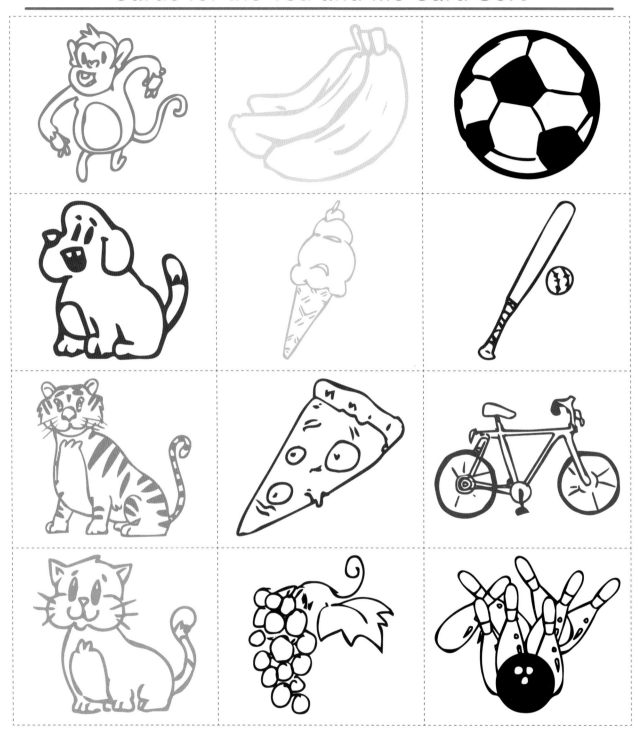

Friendship Tips Handout for Session 2

Share these **Friendship Tips** with teachers and parents who can support friendship skills at school and home. This week, Friendship Group focused on talking with friends and listening skills.

Remember

Talk with a friend:

Tell about you.
Listen to your friend.

Be a good friend:

Join in.
Pay attention.
Support your friends.

Try It Out

Play Pass the Mike with a friend.

Find out what you both like.

School and Home Check

- *At school:*
  Did you talk with a friend?
  What did you learn about your friend?

- *At home:*
  Did you tell your friend about you? Listen to your friend?
  What do you both like?

Feeling Cards for the Feelings Card Sort

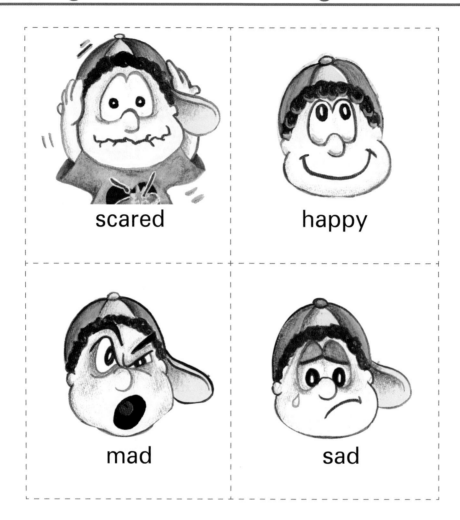

scared

happy

mad

sad

Baxter's Feelings

Text by Karen L. Bierman   Illustrations by Andrew Heckathorne

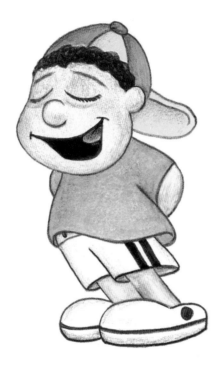

This is Baxter. Baxter is a boy about your age. He likes to ride his bike and play with friends. I think you would like Baxter if you got a chance to meet him, and I think he would like you.

(page 1 of 6)

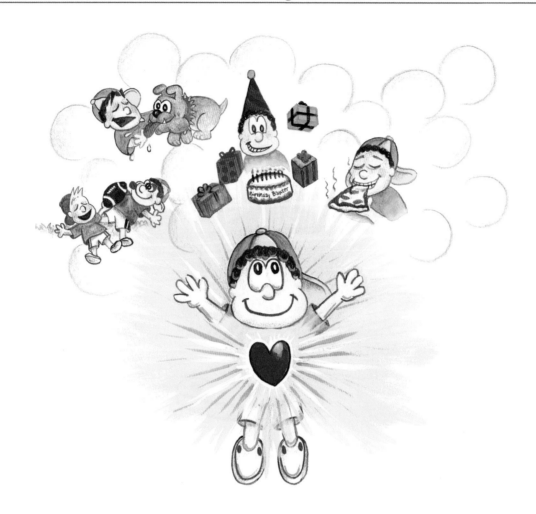

Just like you, Baxter has all kinds of feelings. Sometimes he feels happy.

Can you guess what makes Baxter happy?

Baxter feels happy when he plays with his friends and when his dog gives him a kiss. He feels happy when it's his birthday and when he gets pizza.

What makes you feel happy?

When Baxter is happy, he feels warm and light inside, with his heart shining like the sun.

How do you feel inside when you're happy?

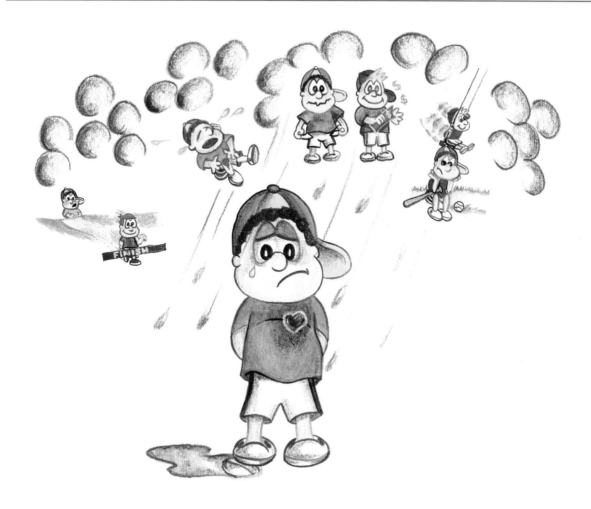

Sometimes Baxter feels sad.

Can you guess what makes him sad?

He feels sad when he's last in a race, and when he scrapes his knee. He's sad when he loses his lunch money, and when his friends can't play.

What makes you feel sad?

When he is sad, Baxter feels heavy and cold and empty inside.

How do you feel inside when you're sad?

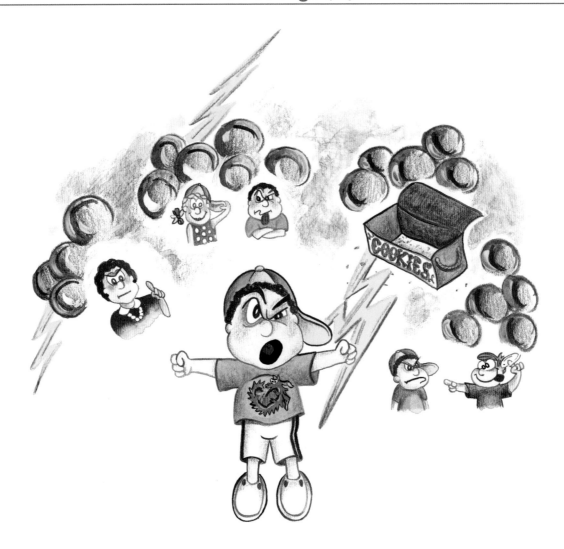

Sometimes Baxter feels mad.

Can you guess what makes him mad?

He feels mad when his mom tells him "No!" or when his sister takes his hat or eats all the cookies. Baxter feels mad when someone makes fun of him.

What makes you feel mad?

When he is mad, Baxter feels red and hot like a volcano inside, like a fire-breathing dragon.

How do you feel inside when you're mad?

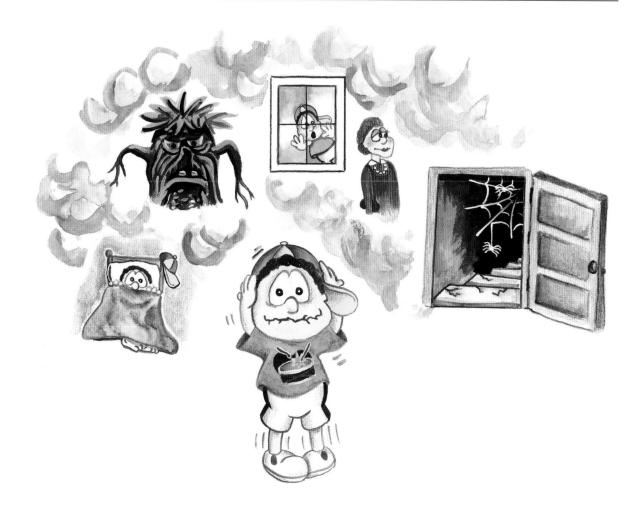

Sometimes Baxter feels scared.

Can you guess what makes him scared?

He's scared when he hears strange noises at night and when he dreams of monsters. Baxter feels scared when his mom is gone or when he goes into the basement and sees spiders on the wall.

What makes you feel scared?

When he is scared, Baxter feels his skin tingle and his chest feels tight. He can hear his heart beating like a drum—"Watch out, watch out, watch out."

How do you feel inside when you're scared?

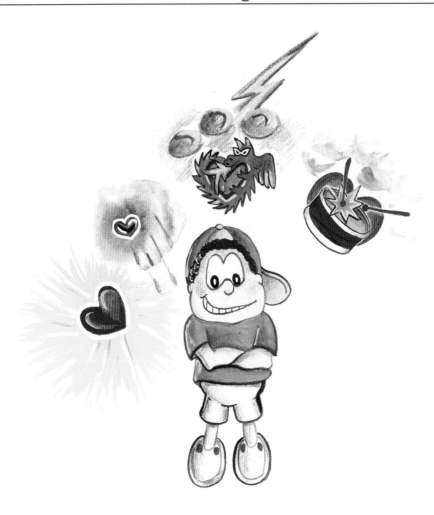

Baxter has all kinds of feelings and they change all through the day. His feelings tell him if everything's fine or if something is wrong. When he pays attention to his feelings, they help him figure out what is wrong and what he can do to feel better.

How do your feelings help you?

Friendship Tips Handout for Session 3

Share these **Friendship Tips** with teachers and parents who can support friendship skills at school and home. This week, Friendship Group focused on talking with friends about feelings.

Remember

Feelings are important:

Share your feelings.

Pay attention to others' feelings.

Good ways to make friends:

Join in. Pay attention. Support your friends.

Talk with your friends.

Try It Out

Play Follow the Leader with a friend.

Find out what makes your friend feel:

Happy

Sad

Mad

Scared

School and Home Check

- *At school:*
  What makes you feel happy?
  What makes you feel sad or scared or mad?

- *At home:*
  Share your feelings. What makes you feel happy?
  What makes you feel sad or scared or mad?

Cards for the Feelings Card Sort

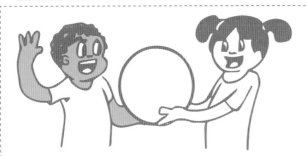

Someone shares with you.

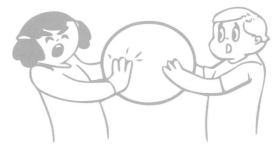

Someone takes your things.

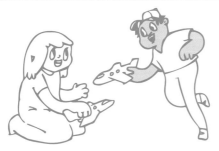

Someone plays with you.

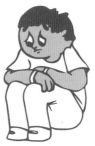

Someone says "You can't play."

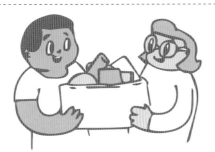

Someone helps you.

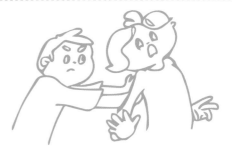

Someone pushes you.

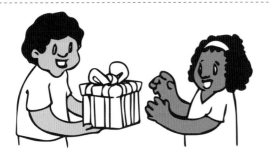

Someone gives you a present.

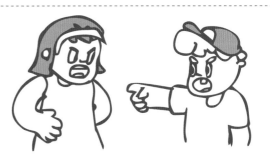

Someone yells at you.

Friendship Tips Handout for Session 4

Share these **Friendship Tips** with teachers and parents who can support friendship skills at school and home. This week, Friendship Group focused on sharing feelings and cooperating during group games.

Remember

Things you can do to make friends:

Join in and cheer for your friends.

Tell about yourself, listen to your friends.

Share your feelings.

Everyone has feelings:

The way someone treats you affects your feelings.

The way you treat others affects their feelings.

Try It Out

Join in and play with a friend. Talk with your friend.

Notice your feelings. How do you feel?

Notice your friend's feelings. How does your friend feel?

School and Home Check

- *At school:*
  How is your teamwork? Talk to a new friend this week.
  How do you feel when you make a friend?
  See what you can do to make a friend feel happy.

- *At home:*
  How is your teamwork?
  Share your feelings and give a compliment.
  See what you can do to make a family member feel happy.

Game Board for Hey Friends, Let's Talk

Hey Friends, Let's Talk

SCHOOL START

☺

☺

Heavy Traffic

STOP

Go Back 1

☺

☺

☺

Skateboard Ride

Go Ahead 1

☺ ☺

Stop for Ice Cream

Go Back 1

☺

☺

Green Light

Go Ahead 2

☺

☺

☺

Windy

Go Ahead 1

☺

☺

☺

☺

Train Coming

Go Back 1

HOME

FINISH

☺

☺

☺

☺

Smell the Flowers

Go Back 1

☺

☺

☺

Chase the Ball

Go Ahead 1

☺

Game Cards for Hey Friends, Let's Talk

Tell about a game you like to play.	Tell about something you are good at.	What is your favorite TV show?
If you could turn into an animal, which one would you choose?	What makes someone sad?	What makes someone happy?
A boy did something nice for his friend. What was it?	Show a mad face and tell what you are thinking of.	A child is crying. What is she crying about?
What makes someone mad?	Show a happy face and tell what you are thinking of.	What sport or outdoor game do you like to play?
A boy fell down and cut his knee. How did he feel? How did he look?	Say something scary.	Hop on one foot 10 times.

(page 1 of 2)

How can you make a friend feel happy?	What does someone do that hurts your feelings?	See if you can touch your nose with your tongue.
Make a silly face.	What makes someone scared?	Pretend tomorrow is your birthday. What will you do?
Show a scared face and tell what you are thinking of.	Tell about something that made you feel proud.	A child did not have a friend to play with. How did she feel?
Tell a knock-knock joke. See if anyone in your group knows another.	What hurts your feelings?	See if you can say "Toy Boat" very fast five times in a row.
Show how you would look if you were a space alien.	Show a sad face and tell what you are thinking of.	Try to pat your head and rub your tummy at the same time.
A boy did something nice for his mother. What did he do?	If you got into a fight with a friend, how could you make up?	Samantha is sad. She said, "BJ hurt my feelings." What did BJ do?

Helping Hands

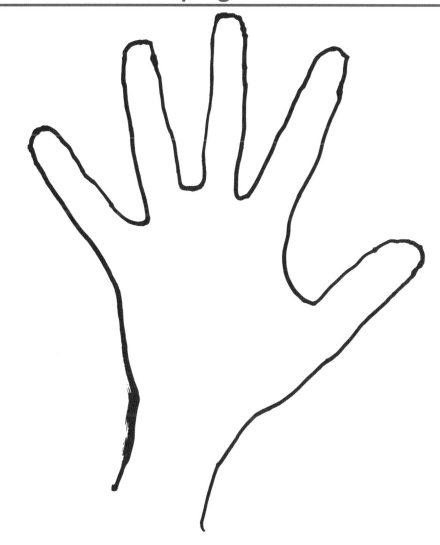

_____ helped friends today!

Friendship Tips Handout for Session 5

Share these **Friendship Tips** with teachers and parents who can support friendship skills at school and home. This week, Friendship Group included a review of the Good Teamwork skills in Unit I. Children worked together to plan a way to succeed at group challenges.

Remember

Tips for Good Teamwork:

Join in.

Pay attention.

Support your friends.

Try It Out

In a group:

Give an idea about how you can play.

Listen to your friends.

Work together and have fun.

School and Home Check

- *At school:*
  Join in to make friends and have fun together.
  Practice good teamwork.
  Talk with your friends about what they want to do.

- *At home:*
  Try a team challenge with your friends and family.
  Try the Hula Hoop challenge or make an animal pen together.

UNIT II

Caring and Controlled Behavior

SESSION 6. Caring for Your Friends: Help and Share

GOALS

1. Recognize the importance of thinking about other people's feelings.

2. Identify behaviors that are "OK" and "not OK" in friendship.

3. Practice cooperation skills—sharing and taking turns.

MATERIALS NEEDED

- Agenda Pictures: 1, 3, 4, 5, 2, and 8

- Posters: Good Teamwork, Baxter's Feeling Faces, and Care for Your Friends

- Pictures for OK or Not OK game (Activity Page 6.1, see p. 129; one set per group)

- Poster board or large sheet of paper to decorate with markers, stencils, and stickers

- OR materials for toy play: 50 dominoes or blocks, plastic animals (two per child), poker chips, tissue, plastic/wooden trees, 3″ × 5″ cards (one each per child)

- Colored tape for the Beetles and Ants game

- Friendship Tips Handout for Session 6 (Activity Page 6.2, see p. 130; one per child)

SESSION OUTLINE

- *Friendship Circle:* Care for Your Friends skills; OK or Not OK game (10 minutes)

- *Construction Station:* Decorate a banner or make an animal pen together (15 minutes)

- *Snack* (optional, 15 minutes)

- *Collaboration Challenges:* Beetles and Ants group game (15 minutes)
- *Closing Circle:* Pass the Mike and share compliments (5 minutes)

ADVANCE PREPARATION

- Hang agenda pictures and posters in the room.
- Cut apart the pictures for OK or Not OK game (Activity Page 6.1).
- Prepare poster board for banner; place markers and stencils/stickers in separate bags.
- For toy play option, put dominoes/blocks and plastic animals in separate plastic bags.
- Use colored tape to make "safety squares" and a skipping route for Beetles and Ants.

DETAILED SESSION CONTENT

Friendship Circle: Care for Your Friends Skills, OK or Not OK Game (10 Minutes)

As children enter, invite them to share their feelings and then review the agenda so they know what is going to take place. Introduce four new feelings: *proud, excited, disappointed,* and *frustrated.* Explain each feeling, discuss when someone feels that way, and describe what it feels like inside. Ask children to show you the way their faces look for each feeling. Then show children the new "Care for Your Friends" poster:

> "I brought a new idea about friendship today. At the top, it says 'Care for Your Friends.' Who can tell me what it means to care for something or to take care of something? [Ask for examples of things they care for, and of things they have taken care of.] When something is important to us, we want to keep it safe and help it grow. This poster has three ideas about how you can keep your friendships safe and help them grow."

Review the first two statements on the poster ("Help each other," "Share") and ask the children for examples of how they do those two things in Friendship Group and with their friends at school and home. Then read the last statement ("Think before you act"). Ask the children why that idea is on the poster. What could happen to end a friendship or make a friend sad and upset? Encourage the children to think of examples when a friend made them sad or upset. Usually, these examples will involve some kind of insensitive or aggressive behavior. Summarize the discussion by saying something like this:

> "That's why 'Think before you act' is on this poster. It's a reminder to think about how your friend will feel before you do something that could hurt your friendship."

To play the OK or Not OK game, you will pass a ball around the circle to music (or humming). The person holding the ball when the music stops draws a card from the center. That person describes what is happening in the picture (Activity Page 6.1) and then explains why the behavior is "OK" or "Not OK." If a child gives a simple answer such as "Hitting is bad," ask questions so children discuss how the behavior affects a friend's feelings and hurts a friendship (or makes it stronger). Pass the ball until everyone has had one or two turns.

Construction Station: Toy Play or Art Activity (15 Minutes)

The purpose of the next activity is to give children practice in cooperation: that is, in helping, sharing, and taking turns. If children enjoyed making the animal pen during the last session and could use more practice in cooperative toy play, that activity can be repeated and extended. Alternatively, children can create a banner cooperatively. Each activity is described briefly.

For the animal pen activity, present the dominoes/blocks and animals in plastic bags, and ask children for ideas about how they might share the materials in order to build a pen in which the animals could live. This task should be easier for them the second time through. Encourage children to explain their ideas about how to divide the blocks evenly and work together. Let the children make a plan and carry it out as independently as they can. After the pen is ready, present the additional materials (e.g., poker chips for food, tissue for beds, and wooden trees) and ask the children for ideas about sharing those materials. If the group is ready for an extra challenge, demonstrate how $3'' \times 5''$ cards can be folded slightly to make roofs for animal houses. When the pen is done, let the children choose animals and play a little.

The alternative group activity involves cooperatively decorating a banner. A large poster board or sheet of long paper is needed, with the words "We Care for Our Friends" written on it. There should be two bags of materials in plastic bags to decorate the banner (one containing the markers, and one containing the stickers and stencils). Start by explaining the task and asking children to develop a plan—for example: "We're going to decorate this poster together. I'd like your ideas about how you can share these markers and stickers, so that everyone has some. Who has an idea about that?" After one child gives an idea, praise the effort and ask if anyone else has an idea. If the group is having trouble deciding which idea to use, go around the table to let each child say which idea he or she would like to try today (and note that the group can try the other idea on another day). If conflicts arise at any point, use them as opportunities for discussion and problem solving. If possible, let the children generate ideas about how to share and solve the problem rather than directing them in this task. Praise their positive behaviors and efforts.

Snack (Optional, 15 Minutes)

Follow the usual snack time routine.

Collaboration Challenges: Beetles and Ants Game (15 Minutes)

In the game of Beetles and Ants, children wear colored wristbands (colored tape or construction paper loops) to identify them as beetles or ants. As you give out the wristbands, explain the basic rules. To stay safe, beetles and ants must work together and arrange themselves on safety squares (taped squares on the ground) in different ways. When an elephant is coming, they must get in a square with the partner who is like them (i.e., ants on one square, beetles on the other). When a hippopotamus is coming, however, they must get in a square with a partner that is different (i.e., an ant and a beetle on each square). It is a good idea to mark off the area where the children are allowed to skip around during the time when the "coast is clear," including a pathway they can follow as they skip around. The coach should do a few practice rounds, before starting the game, asking the children to demonstrate what they will do when they hear that an elephant or hippopotamus is coming. Ask the children how they can help each other succeed at this game, and get their ideas. When children are ready, start to alternate calls of "The coast is clear," "An elephant is coming," and "A hippopotamus is coming." Be prepared to support the children with problem solving if needed. For example, if children fail to arrange themselves correctly on the safe spots, note that "Someone is about to get squished. What can you do to make sure everyone is safe from the hippopotamus [elephant]?" Encourage children to help each other in moving around so that everyone is safe. Praise good teamwork and communication skills. To add challenge, keep score by giving the first two who land safely on a square a point (planning your "stops" to give children an equal chance to earn points). At the end, ask the children, "How did you help each other in that game?"

Closing Circle (5 Minutes)

Play "Pass the Mike" to music. When the music stops, let the mike holder share his or her favorite part of the session and receive compliments from the coach and a peer. Distribute tips.

SPECIAL ISSUES

1. Setting the right level of difficulty is important for the planning tasks. To decrease the challenge level, reduce the number of problem-solving discussions. For example, if children struggle, provide a plan for sharing the markers and then let them generate a plan for sharing stickers.

2. Consider carefully the amount of supplies you provide. If there are too many, it removes the challenge of sharing because there is more than enough for everyone. However, if there are too few, the challenge of sharing may become too difficult for the children to master.

3. If there is a group problem with physical crowding or roughhousing, avoid the Beetles and Ants game, and add this item to the Care for Your Friends poster: "Respect personal space." Discuss what it means to give people personal space (e.g., "Keep your hands to yourself, and do not lean on or push others"). Praise and compliment children when they successfully behave in a way that indicates a respect personal space.

SESSION 7. Think before You Act: Calming Down

GOALS

1. Introduce the distinction between "what you feel" and "what you do."
2. Discuss the value of calming down when excited or upset.
3. Introduce "Take 5" to calm down, then say the problem and how you feel.
4. Practice cooperation, social awareness, and self-control.

MATERIALS NEEDED

- Agenda Pictures: 1, 4, 7, 5, 6, 2, and 8
- Posters: Good Teamwork, Baxter's Feeling Faces, Care for Your Friends
- Feelings and Behavior game cards (Activity Page 7.1, see p. 131; one set per group)
- A bell for the Pass the Bell game

- Baxter Story 2, "Baxter's Temper" (pp. 133–142), What My Temper Looks Like coloring page (Activity Page 7.2, see p. 132; one per child)
- Snack components for shared group snack activity (optional)
- Pictures and props for the Baxter and His Temper role-play show (Activity Page 7.3, see p. 143; one per group)
- Materials for choice of games, if desired
- Friendship Tips Handout for Session 7 (Activity Page 7.4, see p. 144; one per child)

SESSION OUTLINE

- *Friendship Circle:* Skill review, Feelings and Behavior game, "Take 5," team challenge (15 minutes)
- *Construction Station:* Baxter's Temper story; What My Temper Looks Like activity (15 minutes)
- *Snack* (optional, 15 minutes)
- *Collaboration Challenges:* Baxter's Temper role play (10 minutes)
- *Closing Circle:* Circle game and round robin compliments (5 minutes)

ADVANCE PREPARATION

- Hang agenda pictures, posters, and (if needed) a refreshed Snack Jobs poster.
- Cut up pictures for the Feelings and Behavior game and put them in a basket.
- For snack (optional), have ingredients in separate packages for children to share.

DETAILED SESSION CONTENT

Friendship Circle: Skill Review, Feelings and Behavior Game, "Take 5," Team Challenge (15 Minutes)

As children enter, greet them warmly and invite them to share their feelings. Review the agenda so they know what to expect. Next review the Care for Your Friends poster by asking children what they remember about it, and then taking children through it using choral reading. Ask children why it is a good idea to care for their friends and what happens if they don't. Then introduce the Feelings and Behavior game:

> "This game is about the difference between how you feel on the inside and what you do on the outside. Sometimes that is tricky to figure out. The game works like this. First, we'll pass this basket of pictures around the circle with music. When the music stops, the person holding the basket will draw a card. That person will have to decide what the character in the picture is doing—the *behavior*—and what the character in the picture is feeling on the inside—the *feeling*. If anyone is not sure, just ask friends for help."

Before you start, pick out a card and do one as an example. Note that the distinction between feelings and behaviors is quite difficult for children at this age. The purpose of this activity is to get them to start thinking about this distinction. There is no single "right" answer for these pictures. Be liberal in accepting descriptions of feelings, and encourage children to ask their friends or coach for ideas, if needed. Praise positive behavior, emphasizing good teamwork, attention, and communication skills. After the game is done, ask these questions.

> "Raise your hand if this is true for you: Have you ever felt so mad that you wanted to hit someone or yell at him or her? [Allow a show of hands and raise your own hand.] I have felt that mad before—I wanted to yell at someone, but I didn't do it. Who has felt so mad that they wanted to yell or hit someone—but didn't? [Allow a show of hands and raise yours.] How did you keep yourself from yelling or hitting when you felt like doing it?"

Allow children to talk about this kind of experience for a little bit, and then sum up the discussion by noting that feelings are different from behaviors: "You can feel like doing something, but you don't have to do it. If you are able to calm yourself down, you can take control of your behavior." Now explain that you'd like to share a little trick that they can use to calm down when they are upset:

> "Here's something I have noticed. When I have a very strong feeling—for example, if I am very scared or very angry—I can feel my heart beating faster. It pounds in my chest. Have you noticed that? So, I put my hand right here over my heart to steady it. I take a deep breath, and I count to 5 to calm myself down. I 'Take 5' and tell myself quietly to calm down. I want to give you a chance to try that trick today and see how it works for you."

Explain that you have a new challenge that will require everyone to be very calm, so you'd like to "Take 5" as a group, and see if everyone can get calm and ready to hear the challenge. Ask the children to copy you in placing their hand over their heart, taking a deep breath while counting quietly—breathing in through their noses for a count of 3 and out through their mouths for a count of 2, blowing out the stress to feel calm inside. Now, using a quiet, calm voice, explain the "Pass the Bell" challenge.

> "Nice job, everyone. You look calm and ready now. This game is called 'Pass the Bell' and that is our challenge—to pass the bell around the circle. That sounds pretty easy—but here is the hitch. We need to pass it *without* letting it ring. That means we'll have to stay calm and help each other. Do you think we can do it? OK, let's try it."

Praise good teamwork and self-control, as the children try this challenge. If the bell rings, the group must start again. Be sure to choose a bell that will ring easily to provide a challenge.

Construction Station: Baxter's Temper Story and Coloring Page (15 minutes)

The illustrated story of "Baxter and His Temper" provides a model of how one boy learned to recognize his angry feelings, calm himself down, and talk about his feelings in order to control his behavior. The coloring page of Baxter allows the children to draw what their own temper looks like as they listen to the story, which will help them sit and focus on the story more effectively.

> "Today I have a new story about our friend Baxter. Do you remember him? This story is called 'Baxter and His Temper.' Do you know what a temper is? Right, your temper is your mood, the way you feel inside. Some people, like Baxter, get mad very easily, so we say they have a hot

temper. In this story, Baxter is going to find out what his temper looks like on the *inside*. Here is a picture for you that says 'My Temper' at the top. While you listen, you can color to show what your temper looks like inside of you."

Read through the story using an interactive, conversational style. The story includes questions (*in italics*) to ask as you read the story to keep children engaged and to help them think about their own angry feelings. Recognizing their feelings and being able to describe them in words provides children with the first step in being able to manage those feelings effectively.

Sharing Snack (Optional, 15 Minutes)

Explain that today's snack time will differ from the usual routine. This time, each child will be responsible for one part of the snack (e.g., crackers, peanuts, raisins). Each child will need to go around the table and ask whether or not each friend wants the snack ingredient he or she is serving. This activity prompts children to communicate with their friends as they ask for each friend's preferences, tell their friends what they'd like, listen to their friends, and share.

Collaborative Challenges: Baxter's Temper Role Play (15 Minutes)

Explain that the group will put on a play of the story "Baxter's Temper." First ask the children to re-tell the story using the story pictures. Then let them choose to play either the part of Baxter or the bird (multiple children can play each part), and act out the play by following the pictures and show-ing the actions and feelings of the characters. If time allows, let them enact the play twice, switching roles the second time. Encourage children to ad lib dialogue as well as actions, as they act out this story. If you have additional time left in the session, replay a cooperation game from an earlier ses-sion, such as Friend, Friend, Chase; Group Juggle; Follow the Leader; Who Ate Cookies?; or Team Hula Hoop. Praise positive behaviors.

Closing Circle (5 Minutes)

For closure, start a round robin compliment circle. Give the child next to you a compliment about a positive in-session behavior. Then ask that child to give the next compliment by turning to the child sitting next to him or her and giving a compliment about a positive in-session behavior. If children have trouble thinking of compliments, provide suggestions.

SPECIAL ISSUES

1. Be sure to familiarize yourself completely with the story before the session so you can tell the story in an animated, interactive, and child-focused way.

2. For some children, having the picture to color makes it easier to pay attention to the story. For others, the coloring is distracting. Options include using that coloring page after the story rather than during it, or not using it at all.

3. Now that you have introduced "Take 5," remind children to use it whenever it might be helpful—at least several times each session. For example, suggest that the group "Take 5" to quiet down for circle time or compliments, or if a conflict arises or a child is upset about something.

SESSION 8. Sharing Toys

GOALS

1. Focus on social awareness: on how your behavior affects your friend's feelings.

2. Demonstrate the importance of self-control, helping, and sharing for good teamwork.

3. Practice self-control, social awareness, and cooperation in collaborative team activities.

MATERIALS NEEDED

- Agenda Pictures: 1, 4, 3, 5, 2, and 8
- Posters: Good Teamwork, Baxter's Feeling Faces, and Care for Your Friends
- 12 matchbox cars, ramp (binder), signs to sort cars
- Poster board, paper towel rolls, dominoes, markers, tape for Test Track
- Props, as needed, for Game Choice
- Friendship Tips Handout for Session 8 (Activity Page 8.1, see p. 145; one per child)

SESSION OUTLINE

- *Friendship Circle:* Review skills, Coach's Problem, Battle of the Beat (15 minutes)
- *Construction Station:* Test and select cars, cooperatively create a Test Track (15 minutes)
- *Snack* (optional, 15 minutes)
- *Collaboration Challenges:* Choose from a list of Friendship Group games (10 minutes)
- *Closing Circle:* Round robin compliments circle (5 minutes)

ADVANCE PREPARATION

- Hang agenda pictures and posters.
- Put 12 cars in a bag, set up ramp, make signs: "Cars That Can Race" and "Cars That Need Repair."
- Prepare a list of the games from which children can choose.

DETAILED SESSION CONTENT

Friendship Circle: Review Skills, Coach's Problem, Battle of the Beat (15 Minutes)

Greet children and invite them to share their feelings. Coaches should put up "sad" and "mad" feeling faces. Let the children know that you have a problem and that you hope they can help you solve it today. Briefly review the agenda pictures and use choral responding to review the Care for Your Friends poster. Ask who remembers how to "Take 5" to calm down. Have them demonstrate and lead the group in the "Take 5" practice. Then explain the coach's problem. (Note that the problem dialogue is written for two coaches. If you have just one coach, you will need to explain both perspectives, describing what you said and also what your coworker said.)

> "Today I need your help. I put up my 'mad' face today, and Coach put up his 'sad' face. We want to explain our problem. Will you help us solve it? Yesterday, I went to Coach's house to get cars for our Friendship Group game. We had to divide up the cars so we each had some. He had some really shiny, new cars and some old, crummy cars. He said that I could play with the old, crummy cars, and he was going to keep all the shiny new cars for himself. I did not think that was fair and I felt mad." [Now give the other coach's point of view. If there is just one coach, explain what the other said.] "Well, I had some brand new cars, and I didn't want them to get scratched or dirty. So, I told Coach that she could use the old ones, and I would keep the new ones for myself. But she got mad. It made me sad to see that my friend was upset. How can we solve this problem?"

Ask the children for their ideas about this situation. Use active listening to summarize their comments and highlight these points: (1) It is not fair for one person to have all of the good cars, even if there is a good reason; and (2) friends have fun together when they share in a fair way. In addition, point out that you could have "Taken 5" to calm down and find a fair way to share the cars. Thank the children for their helpful advice. Let them know they will have a chance to divide up cars today, and you want to see how they give everyone a fair share.

Next introduce the Battle of the Beat challenge. Begin by slapping a slow, steady rhythm on your knees with your hands, asking the children to join in and clap with you. When all are slapping their knees, tell them you are going to change the beat; they should listen and join in the new beat. Choose a new position (clapping hands together) and clap at exactly twice the speed (two claps for every one slap on the knee you did before). Continue until all are clapping double-time in unison. Explain that when you call "Slow beat," everyone needs to switch back to the original slow beat. Then call "Slow beat" and switch back to the first tempo and position. Explain the challenge:

> "I think you are ready for the Battle of the Beat challenge. When I call out either 'slow beat' or 'fast beat,' your challenge is to change your beat and get into beat with the group as fast as you can. Let's see how we do."

Try this several times, calling out "Slow beat" or "Fast beat." As children master this skill, a variation is to change leaders so that a child is in the lead. You can increase the challenge by having some children do slow beat while others do fast beat at the same time, and then switch. After playing a few rounds, compliment the group on teamwork, cooperation, and listening skills.

Construction Station: Test and Select Cars, Cooperatively Create a Test Track (15 Minutes)

For this activity, you will need a ramp to test out the cars. Any ramp will work. One option is to prop one side of a notebook binder up on a book to make a raised flat area on which to set cards, with the other side tilting down to the floor, creating the ramp. Explain the children's task as follows:

> "I have 12 cars in this bag. Some of these cars will be good for racing—they can go down this ramp fast and coast for a long time. Some are not good for racing—they won't go very fast or

coast very long—they are in need of repair. To make our game fair, we need to work together to find the good racing cars. Later you can pick a car to race. To find the good racing cars [demonstrate as you explain], you will each take a turn, pick a car out of this bag, and send it down the ramp. You will talk with your friends and decide if you should put it in this pile [indicate the pile marked 'Cars That Can Race'] or here [indicate the pile marked 'Cars That Need Repair']. After we have tested all of the cars, then we will be ready to play our racing game, and you can pick the car you want to race."

This is a challenge for young children, because they want to pick a car and keep it. However, the purpose of the activity is to help them control the impulse to act for themselves (e.g., get a car they want) and work instead to create a fair situation for the team (e.g., find the good cars and then divide them up). Before they start, ask the children to review what they are going to do. Check for understanding: that they are not picking cars for themselves, but finding the good cars so that everyone on the team will have a good racing car. If children are not attending to others' cars, remind them that the whole team is trying to find the best racing cars.

Once the good cars have been identified, the racing game starts. The goal of the racing game is to see how far the cars can go. Children take turns picking a car and sending it down the ramp, marking where it ends with a piece of tape or other marker. Use a coin flip or dice throw to determine the order in which children will go. Each time they take a turn, they can keep the same car or trade it in for another car from the "good car" pile. If two children want to race the same car, suggest they "Take 5" with you to calm down. Using induction, suggest that it would be more fun if they selected different cars, so the team can see how far different cars go. If they cannot agree to try different cars, let them take turns with the same car. After each child has had a few turns, celebrate how well the cars did, and move on to create the Test Track.

Creating the Test Track provides practice in sharing and helping. The goal is to use the poster board and create a Test Track that has (1) a road for the cars to travel on (children draw this road with markers), (2) tunnels for the cars to go through (children cut up paper towel rolls and tape them on to make the tunnels), and (3) pit-stop areas where the cars can rest and get gas (built with the dominoes). It is ideal when children can plan and enact this cooperative task themselves, but some groups may need additional support. *If needed*, provide structure to assist the children at each step of the construction. If the planning becomes difficult and children start to disengage, lead the group in "taking 5" to calm down, and provide some direct suggestions—for example: "Now I will give each one of you a tunnel to tape onto the track." Throughout the activity, praise teamwork, helping, and sharing. Save time to let children take cars through the Test Track.

Snack (Optional, 15 Minutes)

Usual snack procedures are followed in this session.

Collaborative Challenges: Choice of Games (10 Minutes)

Show children a list of the games they can choose from and let them indicate their preferences, including any of the following: Friend, Friend, Chase; Group Juggle; Follow the Leader; Who Ate Cookies; Feelings in Motion; Team Hula Hoop; Rock Around the Clock; and Beetles and Ants. Once a game is selected, ask them to review the way the game is played, and praise good teamwork and positive behaviors observed during the game.

Closing Circle (5 Minutes)

Conduct a round robin compliments circle, giving the child sitting next to you a compliment focused on teamwork and caring for friends. Then ask that child to compliment the child sitting next to him or her. Provide suggestions if needed. Distribute Friendship Tips Handout for Session 8.

SPECIAL ISSUES

1. Cooperative activities typically go more smoothly when an adult directs them by stating rules about sharing and taking turns. However, in the "real world" of the playground and neighborhood, children need to be able to regulate and monitor their own behavior. So, rather than tell children what to do, we encourage coaches to boost child self-regulation skills by using induction strategies to focus attention on the interpersonal rewards of positive social behavior, restating the friendship ideas on the poster, and using ample praise to support these behaviors.

2. Some children will have difficulty managing disappointment; if they don't get the car they want, they may refuse to play. Provide feedback with a nonjudgmental, neutral tone—for example: "I see you are disappointed that you did not get a turn with the red car. You are so upset, you don't want to join the group and have fun with everyone." Then state positive expectations about their ability to cope—for example: "I'd like to help you learn how to cope with this kind of disappointment, so that you can enjoy playing with your friends. It might help to 'Take 5' with me." Model the "Take 5" practice and praise the child if he or she joins in the exercise. If the child still refuses to participate, praise the children who are joining in, commenting on the fun they are having. Do not show distress or become overly solicitous of the child's feelings (remain affectively neutral) and do not try to negotiate or fix things for the disappointed child. Periodically express your hopes—for example: "You had a small disappointment with the car. I hope you can calm down, because I hate to see you miss all the fun. I'd love to see you join in and have fun with the others." When the child eventually rejoins the group, praise the coping effort—for example: "I'm so glad you were able to manage your disappointment and did not let it keep you from having fun with your friends." If the child is not able to reengage and misses out on the activity, note your supportive hopes for the future—for example: "You had a disappointment today and were not able to calm down in time to join the fun. But you will have another chance soon. It will get easier for you to calm yourself the more you practice." If children act out and kick the track, calmly state that the feeling is OK, but not the behavior: "I see you are disappointed you did not get the red car. It is OK to feel disappointed, but it is not OK to kick the track."

3. If induction and praise are not sufficient, add a short-term token system or a Fair Player Award to give extra support for coping skill development. Plan to fade out the external rewards as children become more skillful at sharing and negotiation.

SESSION 9. Expressing Concerns: Say the Problem and How You Feel

GOALS

1. Introduce the Traffic Light poster; practice the steps of the red light.

2. Discuss positive problem solving: Explain the problem and how you feel.

3. Practice social awareness, cooperation, and self-control skills in collaborative activities.

MATERIALS NEEDED

- Agenda Pictures: 1, 4, 5, 6, 2, and 8

- Posters: Good Teamwork, Baxter's Feeling Faces, Care for Your Friends, and Traffic Light

- Puppets, paper, crayons, and cars for problem role plays

- For partner challenges: three rings, string, a hook, a bunny picture, cotton balls, tape

- Props for the Three Little Pigs Show, storyboard cards (Activity Page 9.1, see pp. 146–148; one per group)

- Friendship Star Medals (in the Commonly Used Materials that follow Chapter 5) and Friendship Tips Handout for Session 9 (Activity Page 9.2, see p. 149; one per child)

SESSION OUTLINE

- *Friendship Circle:* Traffic Light introduction and puppet problem solving (15 minutes)
- *Construction Station:* Partner challenges (10 minutes)
- *Snack* (optional, 15 minutes)
- *Collaboration Challenges:* Three Little Pigs Show (15 minutes)
- *Closing Circle:* Friendship Star Medals (5 minutes)

ADVANCE PREPARATION

- Organize the puppets and puppet show props in a box for hidden storage and easy access.

- Identify stations for the partner challenges and have materials ready for use.

- Use signs and chairs for pig houses and tape for the road. Cut out the storyboard pictures.

DETAILED SESSION CONTENT

Friendship Circle: Traffic Light Introduction and Puppet Problem Solving (15 Minutes)

Greet the children and invite them to share their feelings. Briefly review the agenda pictures. Ask for a model of how to "Take 5" and lead a discussion to review the skill, as follows:

> "Last time we talked about how to 'Take 5' to calm down when you get excited or upset. Who can show me how to 'Take 5'? Let's all do it together. Who had a problem and used 'Take 5' to calm down this week? Tell us what happened and what you did."

If a child has an example, let him or her explain how he or she used "Take 5." If no one volunteers, give an example of how you "Took 5" to calm down when you were frustrated with a friend, and how you explained the problem. Summarize the key ideas and introduce the Traffic Light poster:

> "When you feel upset, you can 'Take 5' to calm down. This new friendship poster shows what you can do next. What do you do at a red light? [Let children respond.] When you have a problem with a friend, you can go to the red light in your head and tell yourself to stop and calm down. What can you do to calm down? [Let children respond.] That's right, 'Take 5.' Then, you can tell your friend what the problem is and how you feel."

Read through the poster with the children, and then introduce the puppets. Explain that the children have a special job to do at the puppet show. They must watch the puppets carefully and raise their hand when they see a friendship problem. They will need to show the puppets how to go to the red light when they have a problem. In the first show, the happy puppets decide to color. Puppet one (a girl) gets the crayons and picks the nicest colors, saying: "I need the blue, red, green, and yellow crayons, because I am going to make a beautiful rainbow. You can have the black and white crayons." Puppet two (a boy) has just two crayons and complains: "Hey, that's not fair. I don't even want to be your friend anymore. I'm going home." Children will notice there is a problem and raise their hands. Have the children explain what is wrong. They will note that the puppet needs to share. Praise them for paying attention and giving the puppet good advice. Then ask them to think about the second puppet—how he felt, why he said he was going home. Ask them what the second puppet could do to calm down and explain his feelings in order to solve the problem and have fun with his friend. Have them show the puppet how to go to the red light, "Take 5" to calm down, tell what the problem is, and describe how he feels. Replay the scene using the children's advice. Ask the children to evaluate the replay and praise them for good ideas.

Next, move on to the second puppet show. Remind the children to raise their hands when they see a problem. Have puppet two (the boy) set the scene: "I got all my cars out. I set up a car track and some blocks to make a city. It was really neat." Then puppet one should explain: "Now I want to show you what happened when I came over to his house, because we were going to play together." Puppet one requests the opportunity to play several times—for example: "This looks neat. I would like to play with you. Can I have some cars?" But puppet two asks her to wait each time—for example: "Just a minute. I'm still setting this up. You need to wait. I'm still playing with this part." After making three polite requests, puppet one grabs a couple of cars. Puppet two is upset: "Hey, stop it! Those are my cars. You can't take them. Give them back!" Children will raise their hands and note two problems (not sharing and grabbing the cars). Ask questions to explore each problem more fully, and summarize their comments on the importance of sharing to have fun with friends. Ask what puppet one could have done when puppet two did not share. Reinforce the suggestion that she could have gone to the red light, used "Take 5" to calm down, and explained the problem and how she felt—for example: "I'm frustrated because I am waiting and waiting, but you are not giving me any cars to use." Replay the scene following the children's advice. Ask them to evaluate the replay and praise them for their good ideas.

Construction Station: Partner Challenges (10 Minutes)

Children do these challenges in pairs, standing together arm-in-arm or holding hands. If needed, a coach can serve as a partner. Explain that these challenges will test how well the children can help and share with their friends:

> "Today's challenge requires helping and sharing and working as a team. Do you think you can do it? Let's 'Take 5' together so we are calm and ready to hear the directions. ['Take 5.'] Each one of you will stand next to your partner and put your hand behind his or her back. [Demonstrate.] You will pretend you are glued together, and you can use only your one free hand to do the challenges. How does that sound? You really have to work as a team for this game. [Demonstrate as you explain.] First, you need to put this ring on a string. One person can't do this alone; you have to work together! Then you coil this string and put it on this hook. Next, you put tape on a cotton ball and put it on the bunny. To work as a team, you will have to talk to each other and work out who is going to do what. Ready to try it? OK, great, I'll be watching for good teamwork!"

> Provide support as needed and praise good teamwork and communication. After they finish, ask children to reflect: "What made the challenge difficult?"; "How were you able to do it?"; "How did you help each other?" Then let them switch sides and try the challenges again.

Snack (Optional, 15 Minutes)

Follow the usual snack process.

Collaboration Challenges: Three Little Pigs Show (15 Minutes)

This show gives the children the opportunity to work as a team, controlling their expression of happy, scared, and mad feelings. The coach serves as the director, providing guidance and supporting children in their roles. Children can choose to be pigs or wolf (they will have a chance to be both). It is fine to have more than three children play pigs or more than one play the wolf. Review the storyboard pictures with the children in an interactive manner, asking them to guess what happens next and how the characters feel. Show children where the pigs will build their houses, and the road they will run down as they move from house to house. It works well to have a chair represent each house, so the "pig" can hide behind it as the wolf tries to blow it down. Before starting the action, have the children talk with each other and decide who will build the straw house, stick house, and brick house. As director, guide the action by showing the storyboard pieces (Activity Page 9.1) one at a time to remind the children what happens next. Model emotional displays and remind the children to show how the characters feel as they act out the story. Praise children for positive behaviors and tell them to give themselves a hand.

Closing Circle (5 Minutes)

During the closing circle, present each child with a Friendship Star Medal. Display them one by one, giving a compliment and soliciting a peer compliment. Distribute Friendship Tips Handout for Session 9.

SPECIAL ISSUES

1. Puppets can be exciting and stimulating. If you have concerns, use plain paper stick puppets or coach a role play without puppets. Children may want to play with the puppets, so decide ahead of time how you will handle this issue. Avoid wild puppet play.

2. The problem-solving challenges place demands on children's attention and verbal skills. Some groups may disengage if the discussion tasks are too difficult or go on too long. Adjust the pace accordingly to maintain interest. For example, if children appear fatigued or disinterested after one puppet role play, move onto the game rather than continuing with the second role play.

3. If children in your group wrestle or roughhouse, do not have them put their arms around each other for the partner challenge. Have them hold hands or place one hand behind their back.

4. If a conflict emerges, point out the red light poster and have children walk through the steps.

SESSION 10. Finding a Fair Solution

GOALS

1. Foster consolidation of the unit skills (cooperation and self-control).
2. Review and practice the steps of the red light.
3. Practice using unit skills during collaborative play.

MATERIALS NEEDED

- Agenda Pictures: 1, 4, 3, 5, 2, and 8
- Posters: Good Teamwork, Baxter's Feeling Faces, Care for Your Friends, and Traffic Light
- Basket of problem cards (Activity Page 10.1, see p. 150; one set per group), music
- For circle challenges, spoons (one per child), beans, penny, cotton ball, button
- For awards, varied stickers and markers (Activity Page 10.2, see p. 151; one per child)
- Picture storyboard and props for the Three Little Pigs Show
- Three unusual objects for "It's a WHAT?" game
- Friendship Tips Handout for Session 10 (Activity Page 10.3, see p. 152; one per child)

SESSION OUTLINE

- *Friendship Circle:* Review, problem discussions, and team challenges (15 minutes)
- *Construction Station:* Cooperative award decoration (10 minutes)
- *Snack* (optional, 15 minutes)
- *Collaboration Challenges:* Three Little Pigs replay (10 minutes)
- *Closing Circle:* Compliments and "It's a WHAT?" game (10 minutes)

ADVANCE PREPARATION

- Cut up and fold the problem cards and put them in a basket (Activity Page 10.1).
- Select sets of stickers for award decoration negotiation.
- Arrange props and tape road for the Three Little Pigs replay.

DETAILED SESSION CONTENT

Friendship Circle: Review, Fair Play Problems, and Team Challenges (15 Minutes)

Greet children warmly as they enter and invite them to share their feelings. Review the session agenda and the Traffic Light poster. Then let the children know that you are going to act out one of the friendship ideas from one of the friendship posters (point to the "Good Teamwork" and "Care for Your Friends" posters), and their job is to raise their hand when they guess which idea you are acting out. Step away from the group, and then come back into the circle with spoons, pretending to greet everyone and handing out a spoon to each child. Let the children guess which friendship ideas you acted out (e.g., in this case, joining in and sharing with your friends). Tell them that they will need the spoons for an activity, but first you are going to act out another friendship idea. Remind them to raise their hands when they know what it is. Look around and show that you just realized that you don't have a spoon, and reach over and start to grab one from one of the children. Pull at it, looking frustrated, saying, "I need one to play the game." Suddenly remember to go to the red light, "Take 5" to calm down, and then say the problem and how you feel —for example, "There's not enough spoons, and we each need one. I better look for another." Let the children explain which friendship idea you were acting out (e.g., in this case, red light and "Take 5").

Explain that you have some challenges for the team, and that you will pass a basket around the circle to music. When the music stops, the child holding the basket will pick a card, choose a partner, and solve the friendship problem shown on the card. Explain that, to solve the poster, you want them to follow the steps of the red light. Next, you will give the team a physical challenge. Pass the basket while you hum a tune or play music; when the music stops, let the child with the basket pick a card and a friend to help solve the problem. Ask the children what they see happening in the picture and how the children in the picture feel. Help them read the problem. Find out if they have experienced a similar problem, and ask them for ideas on how to solve the problem. Praise them for good teamwork ideas and ask them to role-play the solution, showing the use of the red light. Let other children in the group add additional ideas.

After each problem card is discussed, instruct the group to try a physical challenge. Have everyone "Take 5" to get calm and focused and ready for the physical challenge. The challenge is to pass an object all the way around the circle using the spoons, passing it from one spoon to another. After each problem card, have the group try to pass a new kind of object—a cotton ball, a penny, a bean, a small button (or similar objects). Praise the children for good teamwork, staying calm, and supporting each other.

Construction Station: Patchwork Medal Decoration and Problem Solving (10 Minutes)

Give each child a Friendship Patchwork Medal (Activity Page 10.2) to color and provide the group with markers to share. Explain that they will each get to color a page for themselves, and in addition, they will be able to choose four stickers to put in the four squares of their medal. While they color, show them the set of stickers and ask for ideas about fair ways to divide them for the medals. It is important to provide a varied set of stickers, so that children have to plan and negotiate in order to share them. Once children share ideas and reach a consensus on a plan, follow the plan to divide the stickers and finish the medals.

Snack (Optional, 15 Minutes)

Follow the usual snack routine, encouraging group conversation. Ask the children how they have used Friendship Group ideas at school or at home, and praise their efforts.

Collaboration Challenges: Replay of the Three Little Pigs Show (15 Minutes)

Divide the group into two teams; let each team retell the story using the storyboard cards, explaining the story events, actions, and feelings. Let children choose roles and enact the play; then reverse roles (pigs become wolves and vice versa) and let them enact the play again. The coach can again serve as director, reading through the storyboard cards, or a child can serve as director. At the end, praise the children's teamwork and tell them to give themselves a hand.

Closing Circle: It's a WHAT? Game (10 Minutes)

During the closing circle, hold up each child's Friendship Patchwork Medal. As you display each one, give that child a compliment and ask for a compliment from a friend that is focused on the child's friendly efforts and behaviors during the session. If time allows, play "It's a WHAT?" before distributing Friendship Tips Handout for Session 10.

The coach begins to pass objects around the circle, one at a time.

"I am going to pass an object to [Name], right next to me. I'll say, '[Name], this is a pretty pickle.' [Name] will say 'A what?' I will say 'A pretty pickle.' Then [Name] is going to pass it to the next person in the circle, and say, '[Name], this is a pretty pickle.' [Name], you say 'A what?' and [Name] will say, 'A pretty pickle.' [Let this object go all the way around the circle, with all participants going through the correct motions with your help.] Now, that wasn't too difficult, was it? Are you ready for another challenge? Do you think you can do two?"

Now have the group pass the "pretty pickle" in one direction and introduce a "red hot pepper" going in the other direction (following the same procedure of neighbor asking neighbor about the object each time it changes hands). When finished, ask the children what they needed to do to accomplish the task—for example, pay attention, remember which direction, and listen. For an additional challenge, try three objects going around the circle. At the end, pass out Friendship Tips Handout for Session 10.

SPECIAL ISSUES

1. Decision-making activities (e.g., suggesting ideas for how to solve the problems presented in the session) can be quite effortful for young children. These tasks are demanding because children have to think ahead about a possible action (anticipatory planning), and they have to put their strategies into words (rather than just taking action). Many children would prefer to play rather than talk, but these kinds of thinking exercises play a very important role in building self-control and problem-solving skills—core elements of social competence. Monitor the pace of the session, allowing children some time to struggle with these problems and put their ideas into words, but keeping the pace moving so that children do not become disengaged. Use active listening to support the children in expressing their ideas. Stop after the first two or three problem-solving challenges if children become restless and disengaged.

2. If children have difficulty negotiating, use the opportunity as a "teachable moment" for the application of the program skills. Encourage the children to go to the red light, "Take 5" with you, calm down, and tell what the problem is and how they feel. Using an inductive approach, remind them that joining in and sharing is a good way to take care of friendships and enjoy spending time with each other. If the process reaches an impasse, flip a coin to choose one of the ideas for a solution in order to move forward.

Cards for the OK or Not OK Game

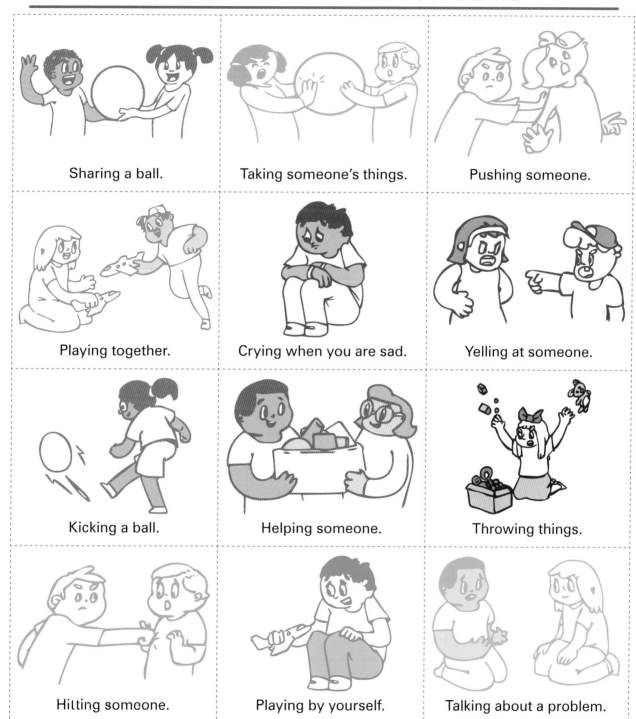

Sharing a ball.	Taking someone's things.	Pushing someone.
Playing together.	Crying when you are sad.	Yelling at someone.
Kicking a ball.	Helping someone.	Throwing things.
Hitting someone.	Playing by yourself.	Talking about a problem.

Friendship Tips Handout for Session 6

Share these **Friendship Tips** with teachers and parents who can support friendship skills at school and home. This week, Friendship Group focused on the importance of caring for your friends—helping, sharing feelings, and cooperating during group games.

Remember

Take care of your friendships:

Help others.

Share with others.

Think before you act.

Try It Out

Join in and play with a friend.

Talk with your friend.

Share your feelings.

Have fun together.

School and Home Check

- *At school:*
  How is your teamwork?
  Talk to a new friend this week.

- *At home:*
  How is your teamwork?
  Share your feelings and give a compliment.

Cards for the Feelings and Behavior Game

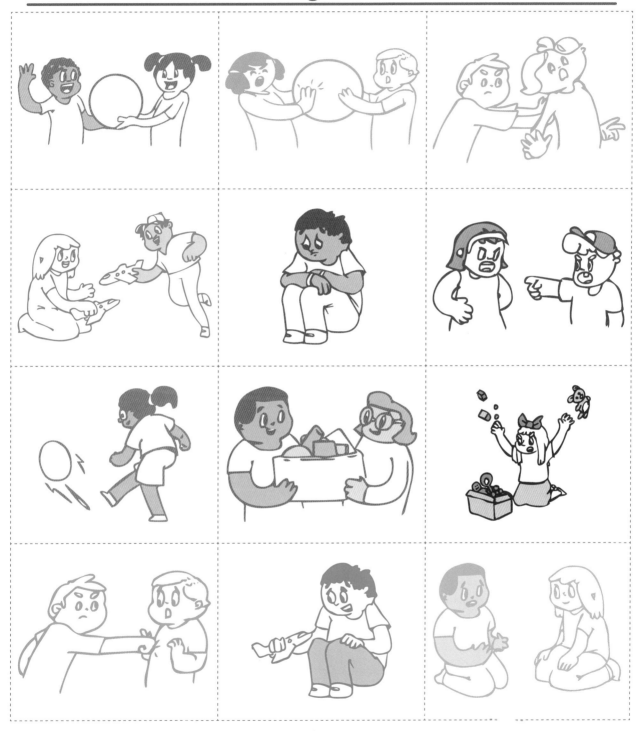

What My Temper Looks Like

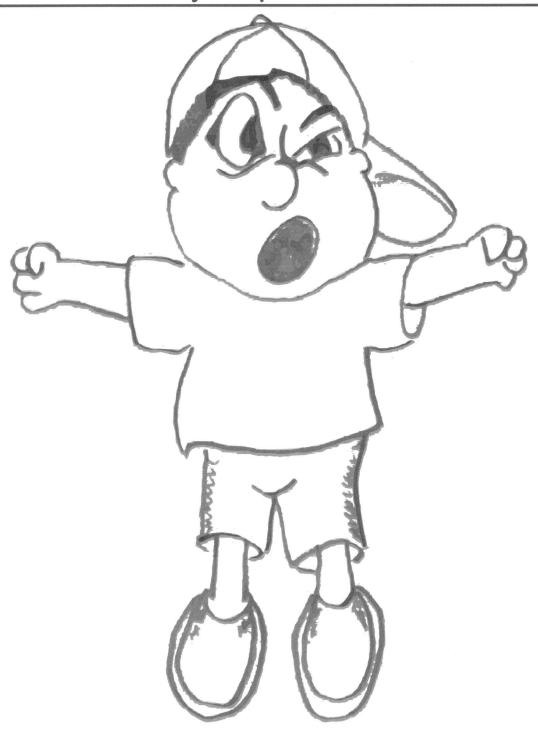

Baxter's Temper

Text by Karen L. Bierman   Illustrations by Andrew Heckathorne

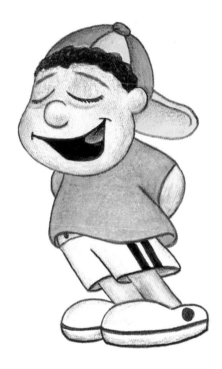

This is Baxter. *Do you remember him?*

Baxter is a boy your age. Baxter likes school, especially recess.

He loves to play with his friends. Baxter is a lot like you.

(page 1 of 10)

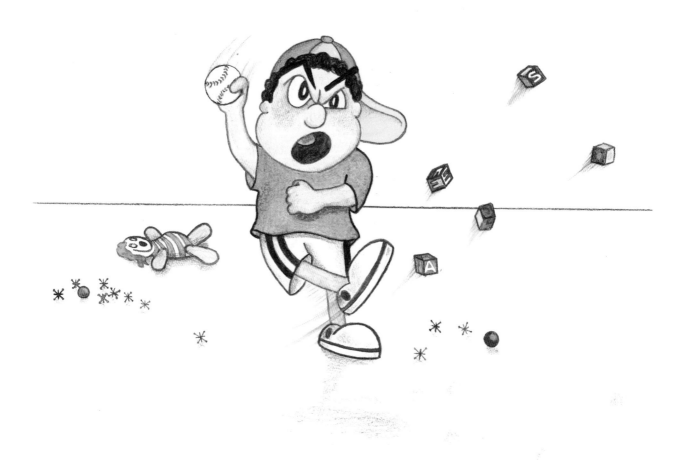

Baxter had a terrible problem. When he felt really mad, he lost control.

Look at the picture. What did he do when he felt mad?

When he felt really mad, Baxter's face would turn red. He would stomp his feet and yell and sometimes even throw things.

What happened then?

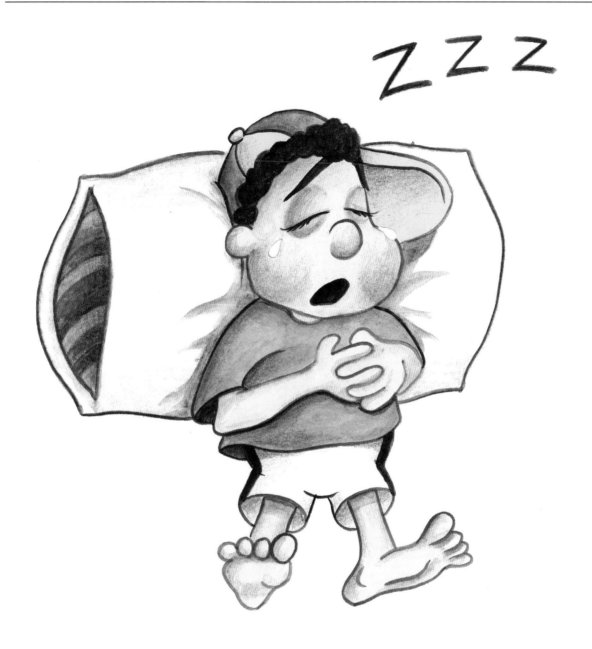

Poor Baxter—he was sent to his room, and he lost his allowance. It made his mother cry. "Oh, Baxter," she'd say in a very sad voice, "you'll lose all your friends if you act that way."

Baxter didn't like to feel so out of control. But how could he stop his temper? He didn't know how. One day, Baxter was sent to his room. He was so sad and so mad that he began to cry, and he cried so hard he fell asleep.

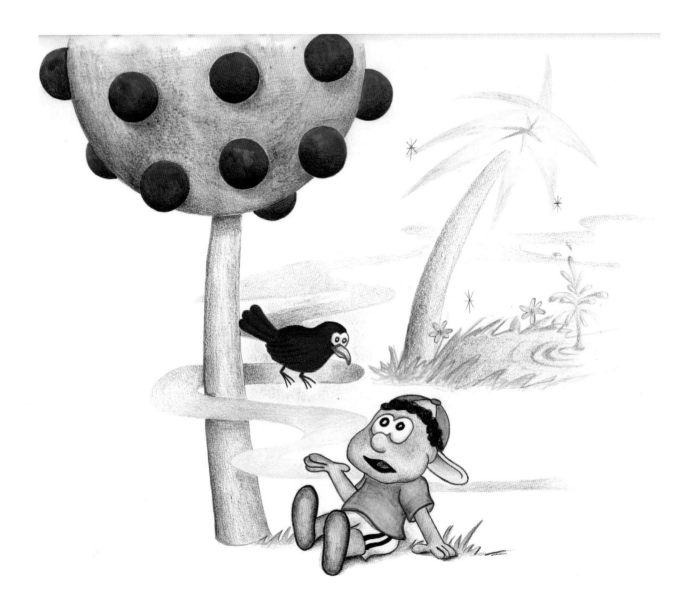

Baxter woke up in a dream. He was in an enchanted forest, and a beautiful red bird was looking down at him. "I can help you," said the bird. *Look at Baxter's face. How does he feel now?*

"How can you help?" asked Baxter. "I can show you your temper," said the bird, and she spread her wings and started through the forest. *What will Baxter do next?*

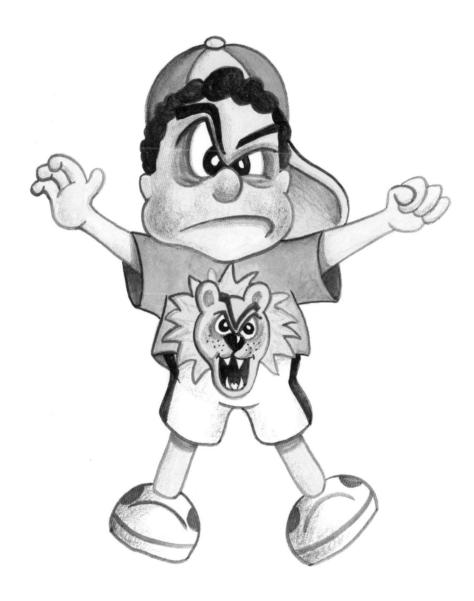

Baxter ran after the bird. "What is my temper?" asked Baxter. "A roaring lion? A screaming wild beast?" "No," said the bird. "It's no beast."

"A monster, then?" asked Baxter, "An ugly, screeching monster?" "No," said the bird. "It's no monster. But here, you can see for yourself." *What do you think Baxter's temper looks like?*

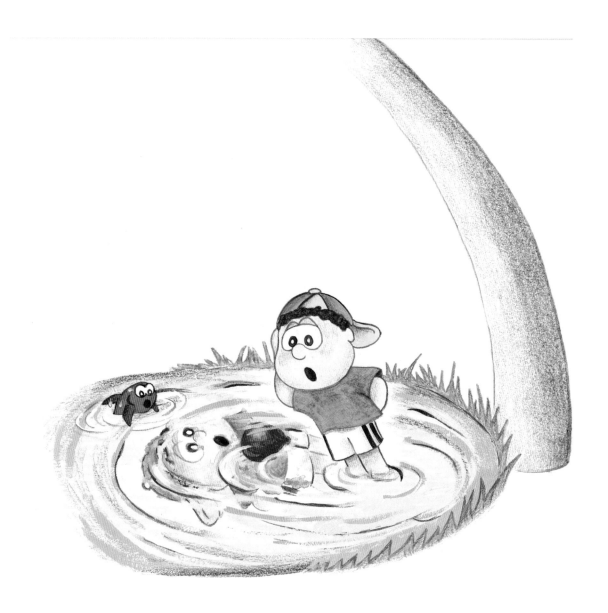

"Look down into the waters of the enchanted forest," said the bird, "and you will see your temper for what it really is."

What does Baxter see?

"I don't understand," said Baxter. "All I see is a balloon."

"It's a special kind of balloon," said the bird. "It holds your uncomfortable feelings—your sad and scared and mad feelings."

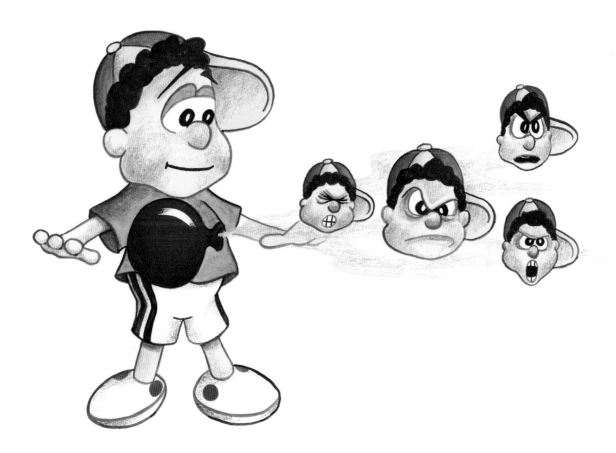

"When things happen that upset you, uncomfortable feelings fill the balloon," explained the bird. "What happens when the balloon gets so full of uncomfortable feelings that it can't hold anymore?"

What do you think happens then?

"It bursts?" wondered Baxter. "Exactly," said the bird, "and that is your temper." "But then how do I stop it?" asked Baxter.

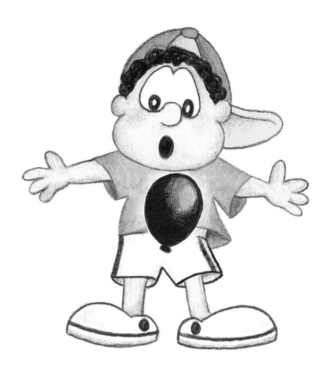

"Well," said the bird, "you must let the feelings out slowly."

How can Baxter do that?

"Pay attention to how you feel," said the bird. "If you feel upset and tight inside, your balloon is filling up. Better let your feelings out."

"I can take a deep breath and blow some of the mad feelings out," suggested Baxter.

"Good idea," said the bird, "and talk with someone, a friend or your teacher or your mom. Tell someone how you feel."

How will this help Baxter control his temper?

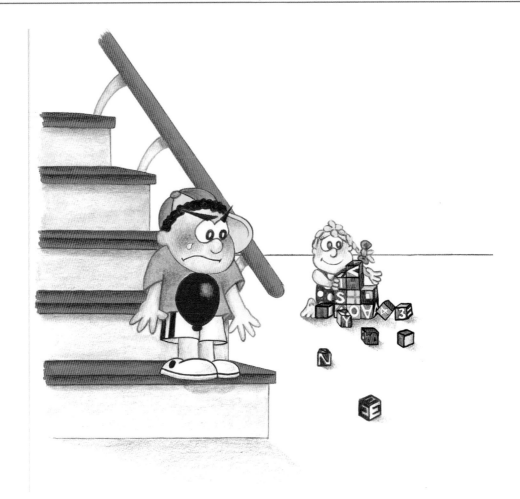

Suddenly, Baxter woke up. He felt happy inside. He had seen his temper and he knew just what to do.

Baxter headed downstairs to play with his favorite blocks. But when Baxter reached the bottom stair, he saw his sister playing with his blocks. Baxter felt himself getting red and hot. He was about to roar when he heard the voice of the bird inside his head.

"Remember your balloon, Baxter. Take a deep breath and let some mad out." So, Baxter took a deep breath and felt better.

"Now," said the voice, "tell her how you feel."

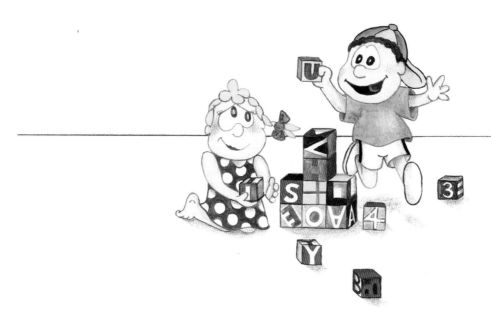

Baxter told his sister how he felt—and he stayed calm!

After that day, Baxter found it easier to control his temper. When he got mad, he thought of his friend, the bird, took a deep breath, and talked about his feelings instead of yelling.

Storyboard Steps
for the Baxter and His Temper Role-Play Show

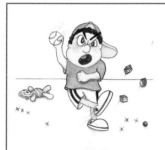 When Baxter got mad, he felt hot. He turned red, stomped his feet, and he yelled.

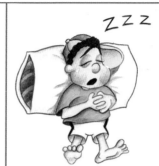 He was sent to his room. He felt mad and sad, and he fell fast asleep.

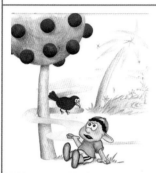 He saw a beautiful red bird in his dream. The bird said it could show Baxter his temper.

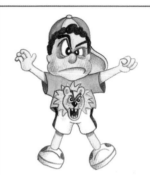 Baxter wondered what his temper looked like—a monster or a lion?

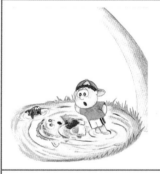 In a magic pond, Baxter saw a balloon inside him holding all his feelings.

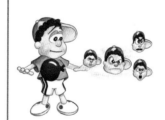 The bird said to take a deep breath and talk about his feelings, so his balloon would not burst.

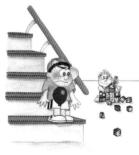 When Baxter saw his sister, he knew what to do. He took a deep breath and talked about his feelings.

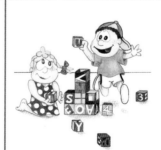 It worked! Baxter learned to stop, calm down, and talk about his feelings instead of yelling.

Friendship Tips Handout for Session 7

Share these **Friendship Tips** with teachers and parents who can support friendship skills at school and home. This week, Friendship Group focused on the difference between feelings and behaviors. When you have strong feelings, like anger, it is important to "Take 5" to calm down and talk about your feelings before you act.

Remember

Feelings are inside:

Sometimes you feel angry, scared, or sad. All feelings are OK. You can't help how you feel.

Behaviors are what you do and how you treat others:

Some behaviors are OK. Some behaviors are not OK. When you have a strong feeling, "Take 5."

Calm down, then say the problem and how you feel.

Try It Out

Pay attention to your feelings.

"Take 5" if you feel angry, sad, or scared.

Calm down and talk about your feelings before you act.

School and Home Check

- *At school:*
  When is a good time to "Take 5"?
  Who can you talk to about your feelings when you have a problem?

- *At home:*
  When is a good time to "Take 5"?
  Who can you talk to about your feelings when you have a problem?

Friendship Tips Handout for Session 8

Share these **Friendship Tips** with teachers and parents who can support friendship skills at school and home. This week, Friendship Group focused on fair play and making sure that everyone in the group is included and has a fair share of the toys and a fair part in the game. We noticed that making it fair and fun for everyone can be hard; you have to watch out for everyone's feelings and not just your own.

Remember

Caring for your friends means:

Making sure the game is fair for everyone.

Watching out for your friends and not just yourself.

Sharing your feelings and listening to your friends.

Try It Out

When you play with a friend:

Give your ideas *and* ask what your friend thinks.

Check it out: Is the game fair and fun for everyone?

When you make an effort to share with a friend:

You and your friend will have fun.

It will build a stronger friendship.

School and Home Check

- *At school:*
  Share with a friend and see how your friend feels.

- *At home:*
  Share with someone in your family, and see how he or she feels.
  How do you feel when you share?

Picture Cards for the "Three Little Pigs" Story

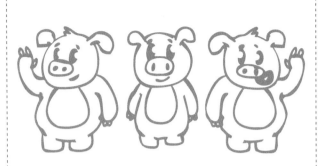

1. One day, three little pigs left home to explore the world.

   (The pigs walk down the road. The wolf follows, spying on them.)

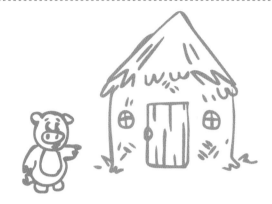

2. One pig was in a hurry. He built a house very quickly using straw. He stayed to rest.

   (The first pig builds a straw house. The others walk on. The wolf spies from a distance.)

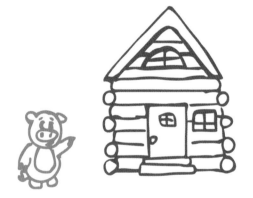

3. Another pig was also in a hurry. He built his house of sticks, and he stayed to rest.

   (The second pig builds a stick house and stays there. The other pig walks on. The wolf spies from a distance.)

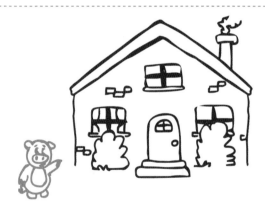

4. The last pig took his time. He worked very hard and built a very strong house with bricks.

   (The third pig builds a house and stays there. The pigs rest in their houses. The wolf watches)

(page 1 of 3)

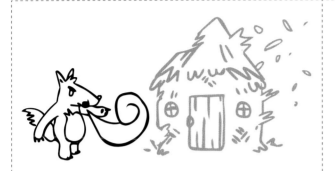

5. At the straw house, wolf says: "Little pig, little pig, Let me in!" Pig: "Not by the hair of my chinny, chin, chin." Wolf: "Then I'll huff, and I'll puff and I'll blow your house down."

   (The wolf threatens the straw house. The pig hides behind the chair and answers).

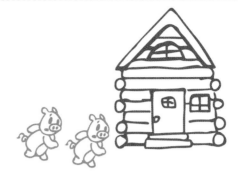

6. The wolf blows down the straw house. The pig runs to stay with his brother in the stick house.

   (After the wolf blows the house down, the pig climbs up and jumps off the chair and runs to hide with the pig in the straw house.)

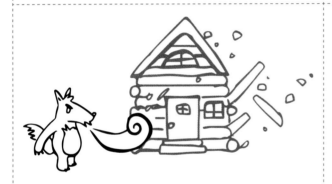

7. At the stick house, the wolf says: "Little pigs, little pigs, let me in!" Pigs: "Not by the hair of our chinny, chin, chins." Wolf: "Then I'll huff, and I'll puff and I'll blow your house down."

   (The wolf threatens and blows the stick house. The two pigs hide behind the chair and answer.)

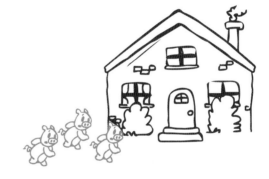

8. The wolf blew down the stick house, and the little pigs ran to stay with their friend in the brick house.

   (Both pigs jump off the chair as the wolf blows down the house, and they run into the brick house.)

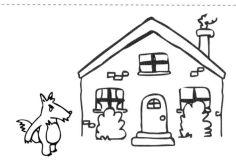

9. At the brick house, the wolf says: "Little pigs, little pigs, let me in!" Pigs: "Not by the hair of our chinny, chin, chins." Wolf: "Then I'll huff, and I'll puff and I'll blow your house down."

   (The three pigs hide behind the chair. The wolf tries to blow the house down three times, but he cannot blow the house down.)

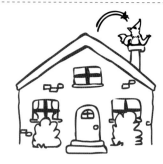

10. So, the wolf snuck up on top of the house and jumped down the chimney.

    (The wolf climbs up on the chair and jumps off.)

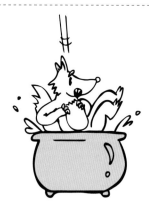

11. The pigs were too smart for the wolf. He landed in the pot. He got up and ran away, and was never seen again. The pigs lived happily ever after.

    (The wolf runs away; the pigs dance in celebration.)

Friendship Tips Handout for Session 9

Share these **Friendship Tips** with teachers and parents who can support friendship skills at school and home. This week, Friendship Group focused on managing strong feelings during a conflict. Children learned to "go to the red light," "Take 5" to calm down, and explain the problem and how they feel.

Remember

If there is a problem and you are upset:

Go to the red light

 Stop, calm down, "Take 5."
Explain the problem and how you feel.

Try It Out

If you have a problem, tell yourself to stop.

Think of the red light. "Take 5" to calm down.

When you are calm, you can talk about the problem.

School and Home Check

- *At school:*
  If you feel upset with a friend, go to the red light, "Take 5," and calm down. See if it helps you talk about the problem.

- *At home:*
  If you feel upset at home, go to the red light, "Take 5," and calm down. See if it helps you talk about your feelings.

Problem Cards

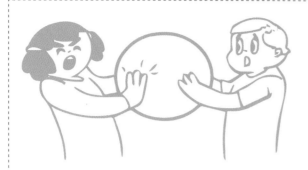

These children are fighting over the toys.

Can you solve this friendship problem?

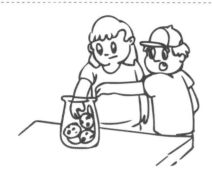

Each child wants a cookie, but the other one is in the way.

Can you solve this friendship problem?

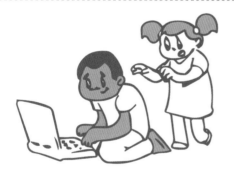

The boy is using the computer. The girl wants to use the computer too.

Can you solve this friendship problem?

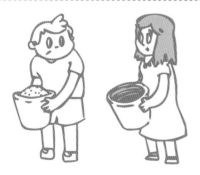

The girl wants some sand in her bucket, but the boy wants to keep the sand for himself.

Can you solve this friendship problem?

Friendship Patchwork Medal

Name _____

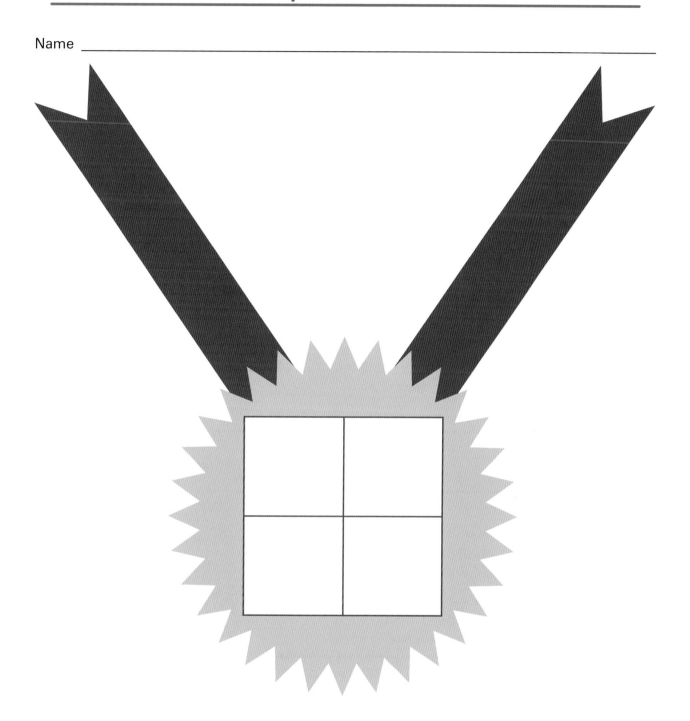

Friendship Tips Handout for Session 10

Share these **Friendship Tips** with teachers and parents who can support friendship skills at school and home. This week, Friendship Group reviewed good friendship ideas.

Remember

Good teamwork: *Join in, pay attention, support your friends.*

Take care of your friendships: *Help others, share.*

If you have a problem, think before you act:

Stop, calm down, "Take 5."

Explain the problem and how you feel. Work it out.

Try It Out

Notice how you treat others.

Make friends with good teamwork, and by helping and sharing with others.

Be ready to solve problems to help everyone have fun.

School and Home Check

- *At school:*
  Do a good deed for a friend at school.
  Help solve a problem at school.

- *At home:*
  Do a good deed for someone at home.
  Help solve a problem at home.

UNIT III

Negotiating with Friends

SESSION 11. Planning Together and Making a Deal

GOALS

1. Introduce Make a Deal (give an idea, check it out, say "yes" to good ideas).
2. Practice making a deal while working together on a collaborative project.

MATERIALS NEEDED

- Agenda Pictures: 1, 3, 5, 4, 2, and 8
- Posters: Good Teamwork, Baxter's Feeling Faces, Care for Your Friends, Traffic Light, Make a Deal
- Rock, Paper, Scissors cards (Activity Page 11.1, see p. 168; one set)
- Friendship City props (blocks, dominoes, cars, plastic animals in bags; option 1)
- Poster board with a bag of materials for sharing challenge (option 2)
- Leader Hat for Backwards Day
- Friendship Certificates and Friendship Tips Handout for Session 11 (Activity Page 11.2, see p. 169; one per child)

SESSION OUTLINE

- *Friendship Circle:* Coach's problem, Make a Deal poster, memory game (15 minutes)
- *Construction Station:* Practice Make a Deal by constructing a city OR poster (15 minutes).
- *Snack* (optional, 15 minutes)

- *Collaborative Challenges:* New games—Backwards Day; Mother, May I? (10 minutes)
- *Closing Circle:* Friendship certificates and compliment sharing (5 minutes)

ADVANCE PREPARATION

- Hang agenda pictures and posters.
- Cut out pictures of hand motions (Activity Page 11.1) and tape onto 3″ × 5″ cards.
- Complete a Friendship Certificate for each child.

DETAILED SESSION CONTENT

Friendship Circle: Coach's Problem, Make a Deal Poster, Memory Game (15 Minutes)

Greet children and invite them to share their feelings. Coaches should put up "sad" faces. Review the agenda and then explain the Coach's problem. (If there is one coach, explain the problem as a disagreement with your boss who said you could ask the group for their ideas.)

COACH 1: As you can see, Coach and I are sad today. That is because we have a problem, and we hope you can help. It is about the Friendship City we are building today. I want to use dominos and build fences, and I want to put animals in the city.

COACH 2: I don't like that idea—we already did that. I want to use colored blocks and build some houses. I want to drive the cars around the city.

COACH 1: I'm going to the red light to "Take 5" and blow off some of my stress. [Demonstrate.] Now I will explain the problem and my feelings. Coach, I want to use the dominoes and the animals. I feel frustrated that you won't agree.

COACH 2: [Demonstrate the "Take 5"/red light practice.] I know you are upset, and you are my friend, but I have feelings too, and I want to use the colored blocks and the cars. I feel frustrated that you won't agree with me.

COACH 1: We have been going back and forth about this all morning, and we just can't agree. So, you can see how we are stuck and we really need your help.

Let the children share ideas. However, don't agree too quickly with the simplest solution such as "Just do both"—use dominoes, blocks, animals, and cars—give them a little challenge. For example, in response to that solution, you might say something like "Really? Cars and animals together? The cars might run over the animals." The goal is to encourage the children to think flexibly about different ways that each coach's preferences can be met. After several ideas have been expressed, summarize the suggestions by saying something like this:

"You are encouraging us to 'Make a Deal'—and do something that will make Coach happy and something that will make me happy. That way, we have a win–win situation, and no one is a loser; both of us feel OK about the solution. I think that making a deal is a very good friendship idea. It goes with the new poster I brought today."

Review the Make a Deal poster with the children, and use choral responding to read through it with them. Note that, if you elect not to build the Friendship City but instead decide to have children decorate a cooperative poster, this "coach problem" should involve differences of opinion regarding how to construct the poster. Model your use of red light and "Take 5" as you explain the disagreement—for example, "So, I went to the red light and 'Took 5' to calm down, like this."

Next, introduce the memory version of the Rock, Paper, Scissors game. Find out if anyone knows how Rock, Paper, Scissors is played, and ask him or her to explain it to the group. If no one is familiar with this game, demonstrate the three different hand motions yourself. Review a few times so that everyone knows the hand symbol for each word. Then demonstrate how each one has power over another (i.e., paper wraps rock, rock crushes scissors, scissors cut paper). If needed, remind children to play gently so the game is fun for everyone. The memory version of the game is used here for two reasons: (1) It challenges children to use working memory, and (2) it reduces the competition associated with the game. Explain this version as follows:

> "I'm putting some cards in the middle of the circle. Each one of you will pick a card and look at it secretly. Don't let the rest of us see it. [Demonstrate.] You need to remember what is on your card, because that is the motion you will use. Once you memorize it, put the card down. When everyone is ready, we'll punch in our countdown."

To punch in the countdown, show children how to use one hand to punch into the other (like a hand in a baseball mitt), saying "one," "two," "three," "hit it." Let children practice, and "test" to see if they got it right by turning over the cards in front of each person. Then let them exchange power (e.g., paper wrapping rock). Play several rounds of the game, each time mixing up the cards in the pile, so that children select and must remember a different symbol.

Construction Station: Friendship City or Collaborative Poster (15 Minutes)

This activity provides children with an opportunity to practice negotiation in the context of planning and completing a collaborative project. Before the session, decide whether your group would be more engaged in building a Friendship City with blocks or designing a collaborative art project. If you choose the Friendship City, give each child a plastic bag with one type of material needed to build the city (e.g., one bag containing dominoes, one with colored blocks, one with plastic animals, one with poker chips and plastic trees). If you choose the collaborative poster, distribute bags to each child with different art materials (e.g., markers in one, stickers in one, stamps in one, stencils in one).

For both projects, use the following process to help the children discuss their plans and "make a deal" with each other before working on the project together. Explain that you are going to go around the circle, so that everyone can suggest ideas about how he or she wants to make the city (or poster), following the steps of the Make a Deal poster (review with the group). Then ask who would like to start. As each child takes a turn, encourage him or her to (1) give an idea about how the materials could be used in the village or poster (e.g., "We could use these dominoes to make roads and fences"); (2) check it out with friends, asking for input (e.g., "Do you like that idea?"); and (3) say "yes" to good ideas (e.g., let the children respond). After each child has shared ideas about how to use the materials and "made a deal" with friends about it, let him or her pass out the materials (e.g., distributing to each friend or placing the materials in a central location). If you opt for building the city, leave some time for the children to play with it.

Snack (Optional, 15 Minutes)

Follow the usual procedures.

Collaborative Challenges: Backwards Day and Mother, May I? (10 Minutes)

Two new active games are introduced. Each focuses on practicing positive social awareness and responding. "Backwards Day" starts out as Follow the Leader:

> "I am the leader, and you will need to follow me to play the game. Right now, my Leader Hat is on forward, so you copy just what I do. I put my arms up like this, so you put your arms up. [Put your arms up in the air, and wait for the children to put their arms up in the air.] Now I put my arms down like this, so you put your arms down." [Put your arms down next to your sides and wait for the children to copy your movement.]

Take the children through the sequence again, a little bit faster, calling out and showing them what to do, and waiting for them to copy you (e.g., arms up, arms down, arms up, arms down, arms up, arms down). Then introduce the challenge.

> "OK, here is the challenge. I am turning my hat around. Now, it is Backwards Day. This time, you do the opposite from me. When I put my hands up, you put yours down."

Go through each motion very slowly, allowing the children a chance to try it. When the coach goes up, the children go down, when the coach goes down, the children go up. As the children get more comfortable, speed up the pace a little. Once children are comfortable with Backwards Day involving two motions, add a new motion. Turn your Leader Hat around, so it is not Backwards Day anymore. Put your arms out to the side (like you are getting ready to fly) and wait for them to copy you. Then pull your arms in around yourself, and wait for them to copy you. Now take the children through the entire four-action sequence, calling out the action, showing them what to do, and waiting for them to copy you (e.g., arms up, arms down, arms out, arms in). Once they have it, turn your hat around to make it Backwards Day again. If children have any difficulty copying two motions backwards, stick with the two motions rather than going to four motions.

To play "Mother, May I?," have the children line up facing you about 10 feet away. Review the rules of the game, letting a child explain it if he or she is already familiar with the game. Then give commands one at a time—for example, "[Name], you may take one giant step forward." Wait for the child to respond, "Mother, may I?" and answer either "Yes, you may" or "No, you may not." If a child forgets to ask the question, he or she has to go back to the starting line. To make it easier, begin by giving children reminders to ask and encouraging them to support their friends by reminding each other. Use a variety of steps (e.g., baby steps, scissor steps, spinning steps) to sustain interest. Let the children take turns being Mother.

Closing Circle (5 Minutes)

During the closing circle, present each child with a Friendship Certificate (select from the Commonly Used Materials that follow Chapter 5). In your compliments, emphasize examples you saw of good teamwork, talking with a friend, giving an idea, checking it out, and saying "yes" to good ideas. Allow children to share compliments and distribute Friendship Tips Handout for Session 11.

SPECIAL ISSUES

1. The play planning discussion may be effortful for some children. Monitor the pacing of this activity. Use induction to support children who are having difficulty waiting and listening to the discussion. For example, ask them to hold materials for you or to call on others who have their hands raised. If you anticipate that this task will be especially difficult for the children in your group, consider breaking the group into dyads or triads for this activity.

2. If the children in your group find Backwards Day easy, add challenge by speeding up the game or including an additional set of motions (e.g., jumping up vs. bending down).

SESSION 12. Making a Choice for Friendship

GOALS

1. Review the concepts of fair play and negotiation.

2. Promote perspective taking and social awareness, noticing how your friend feels.

3. Practice problem solving and negotiation skills.

MATERIALS NEEDED

- Agenda Pictures: 1, 4, 7, 3, 2, and 8
- Posters: Good Teamwork, Baxter's Feeling Faces, Care for Your Friends, Traffic Light, Make a Deal
- New feelings: proud, excited, frustrated, disappointed (Activity Page 12.1, see p. 170; one per child)
- Baxter challenge cards, six cups or containers (Activity Page 12.2, see p. 171; one set)
- Physical challenge materials (tape, cotton balls, piece of paper, bowl, trash can)
- Baxter's Two Voices page and crayons/markers (Activity Page 12.3, see p. 172; one per child)
- Baxter Story 3, "Sometimes It's Hard to Share" (pp. 173–181)
- Food for a sharing trail mix snack, if desired
- Button on a long string for the button game
- Friendship Tips Handout for Session 12 (Activity Page 12.4, see p. 182; one per child)

SESSION OUTLINE

- *Friendship Circle:* Skill review, new feeling faces, Baxter's challenge course (20 minutes)
- *Construction Station:* Baxter's story, "Sometimes It's Hard to Share" (10 minutes)
- *Snack:* Cooperative trail mix (optional, 15 minutes)
- *Collaborative Challenges:* Simon Says game (8 minutes)
- *Closing Circle:* Compliments with Button, Button, Who's Got the Button? (7 minutes)

ADVANCE PREPARATION

- Prepare a set of new feelings to add to each child's feelings poster or card ring.
- Cut up the Baxter challenge cards, fold them, and place them under cups on a tray.
- Prepare the challenge course stations, numbered with an obstacle at each station.

DETAILED SESSION CONTENT

Friendship Circle: Skill Review, New Feeling Faces, Baxter Challenge Course (20 Minutes)

Greet children, invite them to share their feelings, and briefly review the agenda. Present pictures of the four new feeling cards (Activity Page 12.1), one at a time (e.g., proud, excited, disappointed, frustrated). For each face, label the feeling and ask the children to describe the feeling. See if the children can remember a time when they felt that way or if they can identify why a person might feel that way. Summarize their comments along the following lines.

> "So, when you feel disappointed, you feel a little bit sad. You might feel disappointed when you don't get to do something you want to do, or you don't get what you want. When you feel frustrated, you feel a little bit mad. Maybe you feel frustrated if someone won't let you do what you want to do, or you can't get something to work. When you feel excited, it's a really happy feeling and you might feel active and electric. You might feel excited when it is your birthday and you are getting a present. When you feel proud, you feel happy and satisfied inside—you know you have done a good job with something and put in your best effort. Right now, I am feeling excited, because it is time for us to do the Baxter Challenge Course."

Have the group find and move to Station 1 and gather in a circle or around a table. Bring out the tray that has the cups (upside down) with the Baxter Challenge Cards folded inside of them. Mix the cups around like a shell game, noting that each cup holds a picture of a friendship problem Baxter is trying to solve. The children's challenge is to explain Baxter's mistake and what he should do instead. Demonstrate the child's task as you explain it. For example:

> "When it is your turn, you'll mix the cups around like this and choose one. I'll help you read the challenge and what Baxter is thinking. This one says: 'Baxter wants to ride his bike. But his friend does not have a bike. Baxter thinks: I can ride my bike if I want to, it's my bike. My friend can find something else to do.' What do you think about Baxter's plan? [Let child respond.] What should he do to make it fair?"

Get the child's ideas. You may need to provide some additional questions or suggestions to help children understand and respond to each dilemma. A key point in each of the scenarios is that Baxter is so worried about his own feelings (he does not want to feel disappointed or frustrated) that he forgets to think about his friend's feelings. The goal of this discussion is twofold: (1) to help the children recognize how Baxter's behaviors affect his friend's feelings, and (2) to identify a fair way to behave that respects the friend's feelings. Let each child take a turn, allowing him or her to ask for help from friends if needed. As each child finishes a turn, ask the group members if they think the child's solution is fair and if it will work. Then let the child lead the group in the physical challenge at the station. After completing the physical challenge, move to the next station and repeat the process, letting each child have a turn as leader.

Set up a simple physical challenge at each station, such as (1) walking backwards on a taped line; (2) jumping in and out of a square taped on the floor three times on each foot; (3) standing behind a taped line and throwing two paper balls into a trash can; or (4) blowing a cotton ball off a table into a trash can. If space is limited, consider partner challenges, with each partner using only one hand: (1) Each child picks up a block in the free hand, and the two children clap the blocks together; (2) one partner picks up the Hula Hoop, steps through it, and passes it over to the other partner, who steps through it; or (3) one partner steps up on a chair and back down, and the other partner steps up on the chair and back down (while still holding hands). These activities break up the verbal demands of the problem discussions, and also allow children to take turns and support each other in play. Encourage them to cheer for their friends.

Construction Station: Baxter's Sharing Story and Activity Pages (10 Minutes)

Next, invite the children to sit at a table to hear another story about Baxter. Distribute copies of Activity Page 12.3, explaining that this story is about two voices that Baxter hears in his head. See if they can guess what those voices are. Note that you wonder whether they also sometimes hear different voices in their heads—or if they have different feelings about what they should do or how they should behave. As they listen to the story, they can draw a picture of Baxter's different voices and feelings, or they can draw their own. Read the story interactively, encouraging children to respond to the embedded questions. Feel free to add questions or comments to support discussion within the group.

Snack (Optional, 15 Minutes)

Consider a sharing snack for additional practice with negotiation skills. To do this, put trail mix materials into separate small baggies (e.g., raisins, Cheerios, pretzels, popcorn), and ask the group to make a plan for a fair way to distribute the snacks. Have the group "Take 5" to get calm and ready to plan, and then follow the steps on the Make a Deal poster.

Collaborative Challenges: Simon Says (8 Minutes)

Introduce the game of Simon Says. If children in the group know this game, let them explain the rules. If not, you may use the following sample dialogue to explain it.

> "In this game, the person who is Simon is the leader and wears the Leader Hat. We'll take turns being Simon. I'll go first. If I say 'Simon says . . .' before I tell you to do something, you should all do it. But if I don't say 'Simon says . . . ,' then don't do it! If you forget, and you copy me even though I did not say 'Simon says . . . ,' then the rule is that you have to sit down. The last person standing will be the new Simon. Let's try it."

Coaches should play along and, if needed, miss a cue and accompany children who are sitting down, modeling good sportsmanship. Praise joining in and playing fairly.

Closing Circle: Button, Button, Who's Got the Button? and Compliments (7 Minutes)

If time allows, introduce the game Button, Button, Who's Got the Button? with compliments. Present the long string with the button on it, and have everyone place his or her hands on the string and practice sliding the button along the string. Note that the string needs to be long enough to make it around the circle with some wiggle room, but still taunt enough that children can slide the button around. Explain that the children need to work together to pass the button from hand to hand *without showing who has it.* Say that you will turn around, count to 3, and then try to guess where the button is, as the children continue to move it (secretly) around the circle. Make a guess about who has the button. Whether or not that child actually has the button, give him or her a compliment, and let her take the next turn being "it." Proceed, stopping to give compliments as each person takes his or her turn. Then distribute Friendship Tips Handout for Session 12.

SPECIAL ISSUES

1. In a large group, children can work in pairs for the Baxter challenges and Simon Says game. In that way, everyone will get a turn before group interest diminishes.

2. If your group has trouble with transitions, consider using the Baxter Challenge Cards in the circle, giving out leader cards for each station. Then do the obstacle course afterwards.

SESSION 13. Voting to Make a Deal

GOALS

1. Work on Traffic Light, Step 2: Generating ideas and choosing solutions.

2. Introduce the idea of voting as a fair way to make decisions and choose solutions.

3. Practice coping with the everyday mild disappointment of not getting your choice.

MATERIALS NEEDED

- Agenda Pictures: 1, 3, 5, 4, and 2

- Posters: Good Teamwork, Baxter's Feeling Faces, Care for Your Friends, Traffic Light, Make a Deal

- Pretend microphone for Pass the Mike activity; flip chart or chalkboard

- Hula Hoop and Leader Hat for games

- Discussion "voting" worksheets (Activity Page 13.1, see p. 183; one per child)

- For animal games: masking tape, animal pictures (Activity Page 13.2, see p. 184; one set per group)

- Set of school supplies for negotiated prizes (optional), small plastic bags

- Friendship Tips Handout for Session 13 (Activity Page 13.3, see p. 185; one per child)

SESSION OUTLINE

- *Friendship Circle:* Introduce "Favorites Day"; play and vote on two games (15 minutes)
- *Construction Station:* Practice making a deal by voting on favorites (10 minutes)
- *Snack* (optional, 15 minutes)
- *Collaborative Challenges:* Animal Parade and Forest of Animals games (10 minutes)
- *Closing Circle:* Prize negotiation and Pass the Mike compliments (10 minutes)

ADVANCE PREPARATION

- Set up the flip chart, chalkboard, or poster paper where you will record votes.
- Cut up the animal pictures and create necklaces (with string) or badges (with tape) for the Animal Parade.
- Use masking tape to create a parade route for the Animal Parade.

DETAILED SESSION CONTENT

Friendship Circle: Favorites Day Introduction, Play and Vote on Games (15 Minutes)

Invite children to select and post a feeling face and share why they feel that way. Put up a "sad" face. Review the session agenda. Then explain the coach's problem. If there is just one coach, describe this problem as a disagreement you had with your boss.

> "As you can see, Coach and I are sad today. That is because we have a problem, and we hope you can help us with it. Today is Friendship Team Favorites Day. We want to play a favorite friendship team game, but we cannot agree on which game to play. I want to play Team Hula Hoop and Coach wants to play Backwards Day. We both 'took 5' and blew out our stress, and explained our feelings in a calm voice. But we still do not agree on which game we should play. We looked at the Traffic Light [indicate poster] and thought we should go to the yellow light. It says, give an idea, listen, and say "yes" to good ideas. But how can we do that when we want different things? We hope you have some ideas about how we can solve this problem."

Let the children share ideas. In all likelihood, they will suggest playing both games. Compliment them on their ideas for how you can Make a Deal with each other. Then explain that you would also like to find out which game is their favorite: "Let's play both games and then we will take a vote, and see which one is your favorite." Play both games (see Session 5 for Team Hula Hoop and Session 11 for Backwards Day). Then proceed with this dialogue:

> "Now, we have played both games. We are going to pass the microphone around, and let each person vote for the game that is his or her favorite. We will add up the votes and see which game is the team favorite—Hula Hoop or Backwards Day."

Proceed with the voting, announce the count and the winner, and record it on a flip chart, blackboard, or poster. Tell children you'd like to learn more about team favorites.

Construction Station: Identifying Team Favorites with Discussion and Voting (10 Minutes)

This activity is designed to help children practice problem-solving skills by giving opinions, checking out those opinions with friends, and using a voting process to select a solution. To provide a scaffold for this process, children work in pairs (or triads) to complete discussion worksheets that indicate their selections for their favorite team mascot, name, color, and lucky number. Coaches should lead children through the discussion worksheet one category at a time. Children can circle their own choice in each category first, and then ask each other what they chose, before moving on to the next category. After all the children have shared their opinions, let them give reasons to support their ideas, and also let them change their minds if they wish. Once children have made their choices and discussed them, the group should reconvene for a formal vote. Coaches should record the votes and announce the "winner" in each category, writing it down on the flip chart, blackboard, or poster paper. Some children may be disappointed if their choice did not "win," and coaches should use active listening to support their feelings of disappointment—for example: "You really liked the color blue. You're disappointed that red got the most votes. But blue is a very nice color too." However, coaches should avoid creating compromises and naming multiple choices as the winner, because we want to help children become more comfortable accepting the choice of the majority. The flexibility to accept a peer group choice (and relinquish one's personal choice) is an important skill that fosters positive peer relations. At the end of the activity, praise children for sharing their ideas, checking things out with their friends, and saying "yes" to good ideas.

Snack (Optional, 15 Minutes)

Follow the usual snack procedures.

Collaborative Challenges: Animal Parade and Forest of Animals (10 Minutes)

For the Animal Parade game, set up a "parade route" for the children to walk along. For example, make a large masking tape oval on the floor for children to march along. Hold the picture necklaces out for children to choose from, with the animal pictures face down. If children express distress about the particular animal they choose, use active listening to reflect their disappointment, but reassure them they will get a chance to try the other animals as well—for example: "You feel disappointed that you got the monkey instead of the elephant. But don't worry about it, because you will get a chance to be different animals later in the game." Explain that each person will walk along the parade route, with the special challenge of moving in the same way that their animal would move. Encourage the children to think about how their animal would move and to try out animal movements. Use praise to reinforce efforts, and invite children to ask their friends if they need suggestions about animal movements:

> "OK, everyone looks ready to try the parade. When the music starts, you parade around the route, moving like your animal. When the music stops, you freeze. Then we will trade pictures, and you will become a new animal."

The first time around, the coach should lead. As needed, support children to stay in their animal character. After they have circled around two or three times (giving them a chance to feel fully comfortable with their animal movements), stop the music, have them freeze, and have them take off their necklace and pass it around to the next person in the circle. Repeat the cycle, so that children have a chance to parade as each of the four animals.

If time allows, another game using animal movements is Forest of Animals. As with the parade, children pick necklaces (or badges) to identify their animal. First, the lights are turned off, and it is night in the jungle. Then, when the lights go on, children move around the jungle, using the movements of their animal. When night falls (lights out), the animals fall asleep again. Children rotate necklaces at night and become a new animal each "morning." As they play, praise children for their good teamwork, for joining in, and for helping their friends.

Closing Circle: Prize Negotiation (Optional) and Pass the Mike Compliments (10 Minutes)

For an optional negotiation task at the end of the session, bring a small set of school supplies (e.g., little erasers, pencils, paper clips, note cards, paper folded and stapled to create small notebooks, Post-it® notes divided into small pads). Explain that the group needs to think about a fair way to Make a Deal and decide how to divide up the supplies so that everyone gets a prize. Lead the children through the Traffic Light, going through the red light steps to calm down. Then let them know that you will to pass the microphone around the circle. Each person will have a chance to do the following (point to the poster yellow light as you say this): (1) give an idea, (2) check it out with friends, and (3) say "yes" to good ideas. As each child gives an idea, write it down on the flip chart or blackboard, and give the child a compliment about his or her negotiation skills. Once the microphone has passed all the way around the circle, you will have lots of good ideas about how to divide the supplies. Use a voting process to choose an option, and distribute the supplies in small bags, along with Friendship Tips Handout for Session 13.

SPECIAL ISSUES

1. This session sets up children for mild disappointments (e.g., they may not get their choice in the voting activities or in the Animal Parade game). It is important for children to experience these mild disappointments and to recognize that they can cope with them and still have fun with their friends. To help children who find it particularly difficult to cope with their disappointment, use induction strategies: (a) Reflect their feeling—for example, "I can see that you feel disappointed about this"; (b) express your hope and confidence in them—for example, "I know you are disappointed, but I hope you won't let that spoil your day. You can still join in and have fun with your friends. After a while, you will feel better"; (c) focus on consequences that matter for the child—for example, "You may feel disappointed for a moment, but I think you will feel happy again if you join in the play with your friends" or "I hope you can join in, because I don't want you to miss out on all of the fun with your friends"; and (d) deescalate strong feelings—for example, "I know it feels like you are mad at your friends, but I think you are just disappointed that it did not turn out the way you hoped. Your friends did not do anything mean to you, they just had a different idea. That is a small disappointment, and that feeling will pass." These emotional messages are an important aspect of the therapeutic value of these groups, so take the time to process them as mild disappointments arise in this session.

2. This session moves toward more verbal problem solving, which may be challenging for children with lower language skills. It is important to aim for the "comfort zone" of learning, in which children are challenged to work at a skill level that is near their maximal performance capacity—but not beyond. If children begin to disengage, pick up the pace and provide more direction. For groups with higher language skills, consider letting them add their own ideas to the list for team mascots, colors, and animals. This addition will extend the discussion time, but offer opportunity for problem solving.

3. Consider what level of challenge you want to set for your group in the school supply task. At the easier level of challenge, there is enough of each item to create an identical portion for each child, with minor differences (e.g., different-colored pencils). At the more challenging level, items cannot be divided to create identical portions, so the children have to determine equivalent portions.

SESSION 14. Deciding Who Goes First

GOALS

1. Consider fair ways to decide who goes first.

2. Try out fair ways to decide who goes first in the context of competitive play.

3. Practice coping with the everyday mild disappointments of competitive play.

MATERIALS NEEDED

- Agenda Pictures: 1, 3, 4, 5, 2, and 8
- Posters: Good Teamwork, Baxter's Feeling Faces, Care for Your Friends, Traffic Light, Make a Deal
- Decision wheels (Activity Pages 14.1 and 14.2, see pp. 186–187; one each per group), cardboard, spinners, brads
- Carnival games (three rings, bottles, paper balls, five pennies, plate, three little balls, mug, two cups)
- Color cards (Activity Page 14.3, see p. 188; one set) and colored tape for the Rainbow Freeze game
- Button on a string (for Button, Button, Who's Got the Button?)
- Friendship Tips Handout for Session 14 (Activity Page 14.4, see p. 189; one per child)

SESSION OUTLINE

- *Friendship Circle:* Skill review, decision wheel construction (10 minutes)
- *Construction Station:* Use the decision wheel at carnival game stations (15 minutes)
- *Snack* (optional, 15 minutes)
- *Collaborative Challenges:* Rainbow Freeze game (10 minutes)
- *Closing Circle:* Compliments with Button, Button, Who's Got the Button? (10 minutes)

ADVANCE PREPARATION

• Mount decision wheels on thin cardboard (e.g., a file folder); cut spinners from that cardboard and attached them with brads so they spin.

• Prepare carnival games; however, do not display them until time for use.

• Tape "X's" of various colors in a rainbow shape for the Rainbow Freeze game.

• Cut up the color cards and place them face down in a draw pile.

DETAILED SESSION CONTENT

Friendship Circle: Skill Review, Decision Wheel Construction (10 Minutes)

Greet children and invite them to share their feelings. Briefly review the agenda. Next, review the Traffic Light and Make a Deal posters. Remind children that they've been working on good ways to solve problems with friends, and ask who remembers what you can do to solve a problem. Let children share their thoughts, then read through the two posters together. Finally, explain the problem you want to talk about today:

> "Today, I need to talk with you about a friendship problem and get your ideas about it. The other day I was out on the playground, and I heard two kids arguing about who was going first in their game. Both kids wanted to go first. They spent so much time arguing about it, they didn't have time to play. Has that happened to you, when you and your friend both wanted to go first? How did you decide who should go first? [Let children respond.] I thought it would be a good idea if we spent some time talking about fair ways to decide who goes first, because it can be tricky. I brought a decision wheel [show the blank wheel] so that I can write down some ideas. Who has an idea about a fair way to decide who should go first in a game?"

Note that if children provided an idea in the earlier discussion, the coach can write that down on the wheel to get things started. In many groups, children may offer one or two ideas and then run out of thoughts. If so, the coach can bring out the sample decision wheel that has ideas on it, and see if the children like any of those ideas. With the group's input, the coach should fill in six different ways on the decision wheels that the subgroups can use in the following game.

> "This is great. Now we have a lot of fair ways to decide who goes first. Let's try them out. Later, I'm going to ask what way you liked best."

Construction Station: Carnival Games with Decision Wheel (15 Minutes)

Children will use the decision wheels to practice different ways of deciding who goes first as they rotate around the room in pairs or triads to play a series of carnival games. Possible carnival game stations include (1) throwing rings over bottles, (2) tossing paper balls into a garbage can, (3) throwing a penny onto a plate, (4) throwing a little ball into a mug, or (5) hiding a penny under one of two plastic cups. (In this version of the shell game, one child hides the penny and mixes the cups; the other guesses which cup the penny is under.) The goal of these brief games is to give children experience with a variety of fair ways to decide who goes first, and to gain comfort in coping with the minor disappointment of not going first.

"We are going to have our own carnival this morning, and we're going to try out four different carnival games. Each time we move to a new game, one of you will spin the wheel to see how you'll decide who goes first."

As children play, prompt and praise fair play behaviors (e.g., taking turns, following rules, refraining from teasing, cheering for friends). Make sure every child has a chance to go first at least once; if someone has not had a turn to go first by the final round, have him or her go first in that last game.

Snack (Optional, 15 Minutes)

During snack time, in addition to conversation, ask the children about the carnival games—for example: "How did the wheel work? What was your favorite way to decide who goes first?" Go around the circle to elicit two preferences from each team member. The ways they select need not be from the decision wheel, but they must be fair ways. Draw connections between group members by commenting on the similarities and differences in the preferences.

Collaborative Challenges: Rainbow Freeze Game (10 Minutes)

To play the Rainbow Freeze game, each child draws a color card, looks at it secretly, memorizes his or her special color, and then puts the color card face down. As soon as all of the children are ready, the coaches start the music. As the music plays, children move along the arc created by the colored "X's" on the floor (and across the bottom of it). When the music stops, children must remember the special color that was on their card and scramble to "freeze" on the "X" that matches their color. The coach then "checks" each person's card to see if he or she remembered his or her special color. Children take a new color card each turn. To add challenge to the game, coaches can ask children to move in a certain way to the music—such as taking baby steps, hopping on one foot, or walking backwards along the rainbow. The challenge to working memory is to remember the special color, while also concentrating on the movement task.

Closing Circle: Button, Button and Compliments (10 Minutes)

At closure, if time allows, play the game of Button, Button, Who's Got the Button? Each child takes a turn being "it," watching as the other children pass around a button on a string and trying to guess who has the button. Each time a child becomes "it," give them a compliment about his or her behavior and efforts during the session, and invite a friend to share a compliment. Make sure each child has a chance to be "it" and to receive compliments. Distribute Friendship Tips Handout for Session 14.

SPECIAL ISSUES

1. If you cannot get your decision wheel to spin, number the strategies on the wheel, have children toss a die, and try the strategy with the corresponding number.

2. If verbal discussions are a challenge for children in your group, complete the decision wheel discussion in small groups, where children have greater opportunity to be actively involved and the discussion goes more quickly. In addition, reduce the number of choices on the decision wheel if you

feel that six options are too many for your group. If needed, you can also adapt the carnival games to meet the needs of your group—reducing the number of games, changing the specific tasks involved, and/or reducing the materials involved. The critical feature of these tasks is to provide children with repeated opportunities to practice and get comfortable with the fair ways of deciding who goes first.

3. Another issue to consider prior to conducting the session is the setup for the carnival. It can be distracting for children when one coach is setting up the games while the other is trying to discuss the decision wheel. Hence, plans for quick setup and careful timing are critical.

4. If children in your group continue to experience distress when they do not get their first choice, consider introducing the "Peacemaker Award." Children earn this award by being the "peacemaker" in a conflict situation and stepping forward to agree to the other person's idea or desire. To use this award, explain that you will be looking for children who are showing excellent teamwork and resolving conflicts. Then watch for peacemaking behaviors—for example: "[Name], you let your friend go first, and that's really being a peacemaker! You may win a Peacemaker Award today." This award serves the same purpose as token rewards: It provides external motivation to encourage behavior that is difficult for some children. Do not be too specific about what is needed to win the award; if children know exactly what is needed to earn it, they may do that much and no more. However, use it generously to make sure that children who are making an effort receive recognition. As with tokens, this award should be used for a short period of time to establish the desired behavior and then faded out.

Cards for the Rock, Paper, Scissors Game

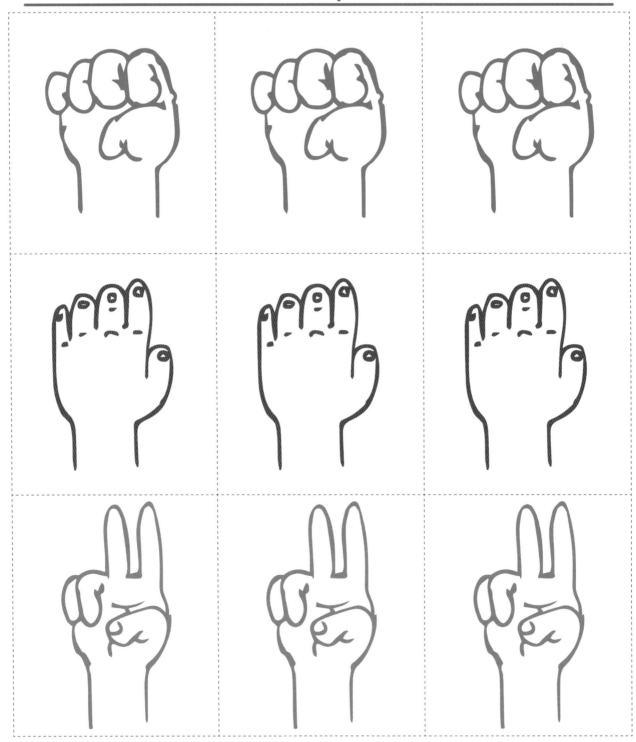

Friendship Tips Handout for Session 11

Share these **Friendship Tips** with teachers and parents who can support friendship skills at school and home. This week, Friendship Group focused on negotiating and problem solving. We talked about making plans and solving problems with others by making a deal with them.

Remember

To make a deal:

Give an idea.

Check it out.

Say "yes" to good ideas.

Try It Out

You can make plans with a friend:

Give an idea. Check it out with your friend.

You can solve a problem with a friend:

Give an idea. Check it out with your friend.

If your friend has a good idea, say "yes."

School and Home Check

- *At school:*
  Make a deal with a friend and see how it feels.

- *At home:*
  Make a deal with someone in your family and see how it feels. How did it work for you?

New Feeling Cards

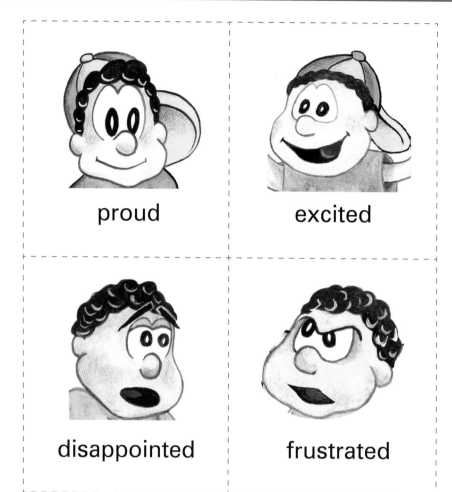

Baxter Challenge Cards

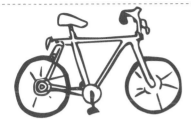

Baxter wants to ride his bike. But his friend does not have a bike. Baxter thinks: *I can ride my bike if I want to—it's my bike. My friend can find something else to do.*

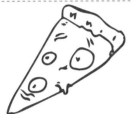

Baxter is visiting at his friend's house. He sees that there is only one piece of pizza left. Baxter thinks: *I want that pizza. I better eat it before my friend does.*

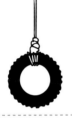

Baxter loves playing on his tire swing. But only one person can swing at a time. Baxter thinks: *If I run really fast, I can get to the tire swing first. Then I can swing as long as I want.*

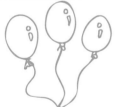

Baxter is at his friend's birthday party. They are giving out balloons. Baxter knows that blue is his friend's favorite color, but he also wants the blue one. He thinks: *I better get that blue one before my friend does, so I don't lose it.*

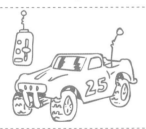

Baxter's friend has a remote control car. Baxter wants to play with it, but there is only one. Baxter thinks: *I better grab it and take the first turn. Then I can play with it as long as I want to.*

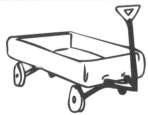

Baxter's dad gave him a wagon. He wants to ride in it. Baxter thinks: *I'll tell my friend that it's my wagon so I get to ride, and he has to pull me around.*

Finding Your Two Voices

Baxter's Two Voices

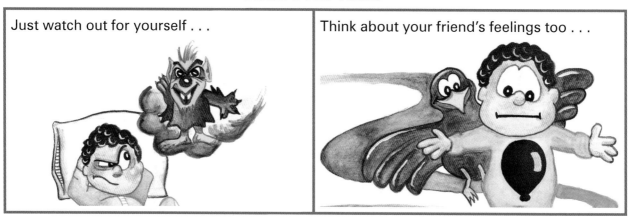

Just watch out for yourself . . .

Think about your friend's feelings too . . .

Your Two Voices

Sometimes It's Hard to Share

Text by Karen L. Bierman   Illustrations by Andy Heckathorne

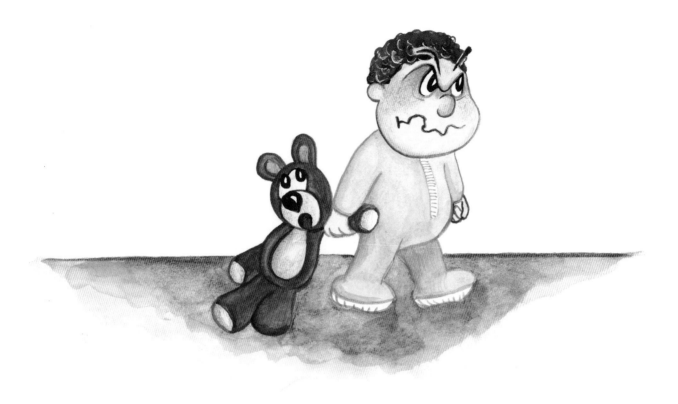

One morning Baxter woke up feeling grumpy.

Have you ever felt that way in the morning?

He tromped down the hall. When he got to the kitchen, he saw his sister using his favorite spoon.

How did he feel about that?

(page 1 of 9)

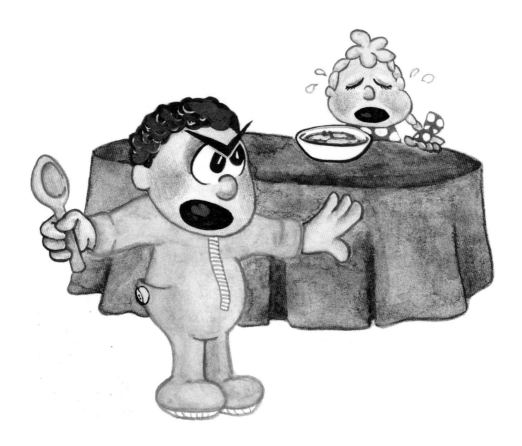

"Give it!" Baxter yelled, grabbing the spoon from her hand. "That's mine and you can't use it!" And just to make sure she heard him, Baxter pinched her. She began to cry. Baxter was sent to his room.

Why did Baxter grab the spoon and pinch his sister?

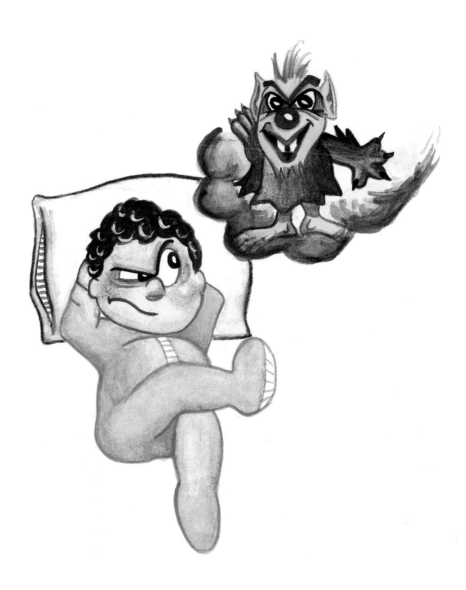

Baxter threw himself on his bed. He felt his mad power rising. "Who cares?" snarled the troll inside him, "She deserved it!" The mad power was strong and Baxter felt strong too.

What is Baxter's mad power?

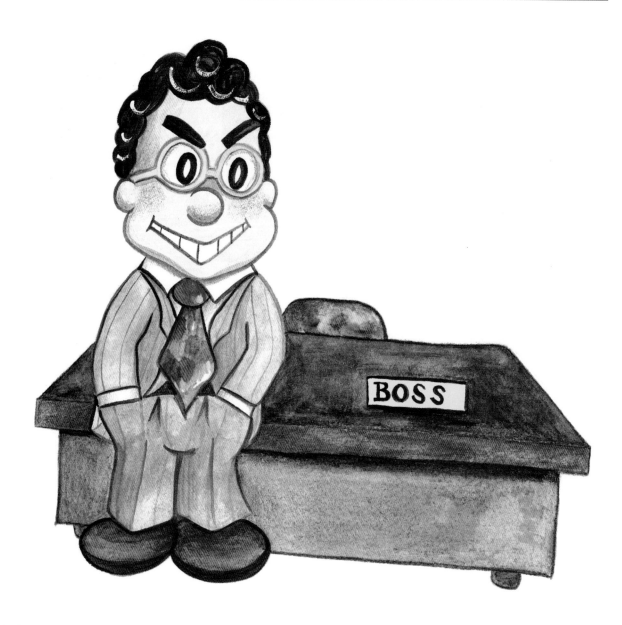

"I'm my own boss," said Baxter, "No one tells me what to do."

Have you ever felt that way when you were mad?

Downstairs, Baxter heard his sister and mom laughing. "They're having fun without me," Baxter thought, and suddenly he felt lonely and sad inside.

Why is he feeling lonely and sad?

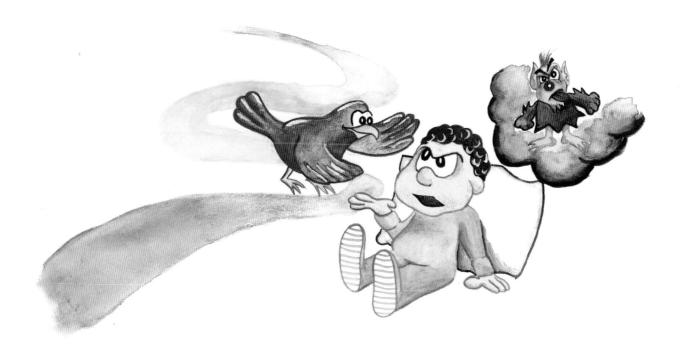

Then Baxter heard a familiar voice—his friend, the bird.

Baxter told the bird how he took the spoon and pinched his sister, and got in trouble, and got sent to his room.

The bird listened to his story and answered quietly, "You can work this out, Baxter."

What does the bird want Baxter to do?

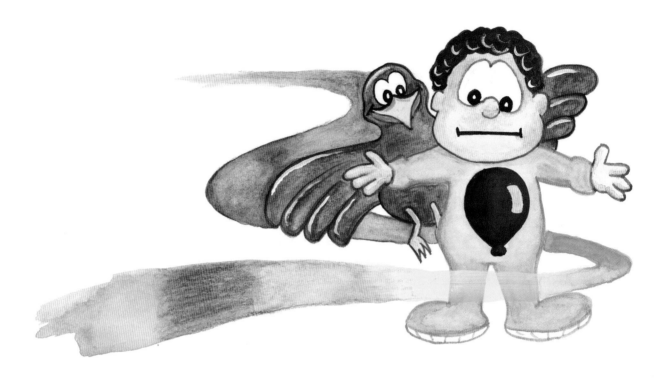

"Remember the balloon inside you," said the bird. "How does it feel now?" "Well," said Baxter, "it's very full." Baxter took a deep breath and let out the air very slowly.

How does Baxter feel now? How did the deep breath help?

"Now," said the bird, "are you ready to talk to your sister?" Baxter nodded.

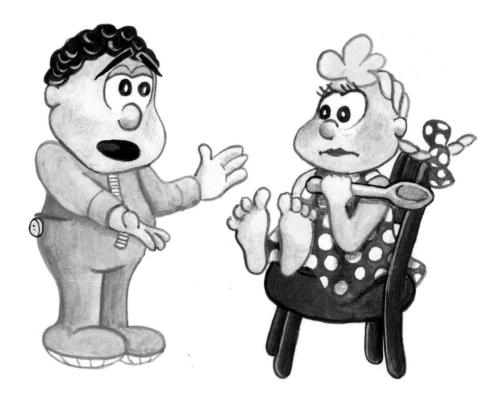

Baxter went downstairs. "The problem is," he told his sister, "I want that spoon." "Me too," said his sister, "and I got it first." Baxter heard the troll growl inside him, but he took a deep breath and tried again.

"When I can't use that spoon, I feel upset and angry." "Well," said his sister, "me too."

What should Baxter do now?

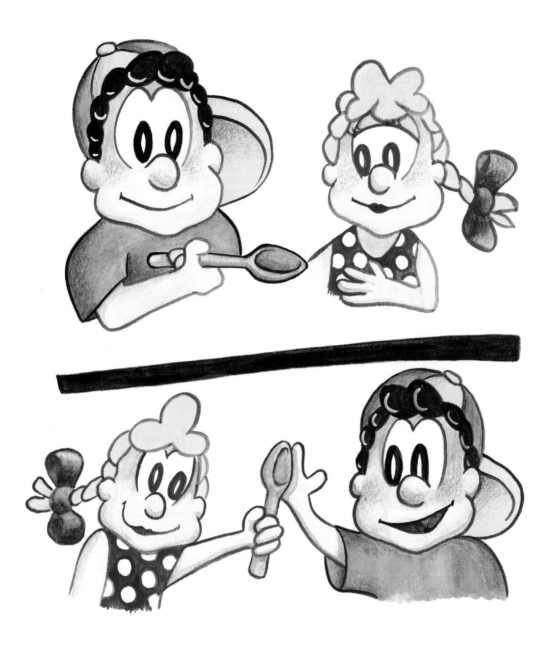

Baxter looked at his sister and then he smiled. "Let's make a deal and share the spoon," he suggested. "You use it one day, I'll use it the next, OK?"

"OK," she said, "that's fair." Baxter smiled.

What do you think of Baxter's deal?

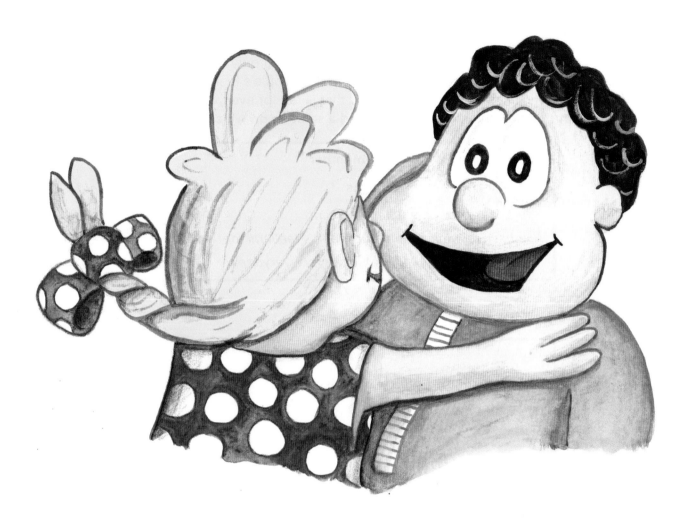

Then, to Baxter's surprise, his sister stood up and hugged him—a big, warm bear hug. "I love you, Baxter," she said. Baxter shrugged. Maybe he couldn't use the spoon every day, but it was nice to have a friend at home.

What did Baxter learn about sharing?

Friendship Tips Handout for Session 12

Share these **Friendship Tips** with teachers and parents who can support friendship skills at school and home. This week, we talked about how focusing only on getting what you want can hurt your friendships. Your behavior affects other people's feelings. It's important to think about everyone's feelings and behave in a way that is fair for everyone. Sometimes you have to talk with your friends and make a deal, to find a solution on which everyone can agrees.

Remember

Caring for your friends means:

You can't always get what you want.

You have to think about your friend's feelings too.

You have to find a plan that is fair for everyone.

Try It Out

When you make a plan with a friend:

Think about what you want to do.

Think about your friend's feelings.

Make a deal with your friend.

Check it out: Is the plan fair and fun for everyone?

School and Home Check

- *At school:*
  Make a deal to solve a problem with a friend. Tell us what you did and how you felt about it.

- *At home:*
  Make a deal to solve a problem at home. How did it go? Were you able to share ideas and make a plan together?

Friendship Team Favorites Discussion Sheet

Team Mascot:

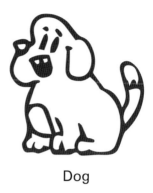

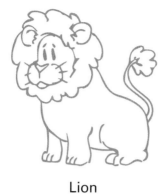

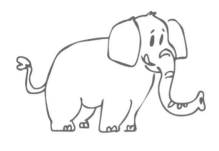

Dog   Lion   Elephant

Team Name:

Friendship Heroes

Friendship Stars

Friendship Champions

Team Color:

Red   Blue   Green

Pictures for the Animal Parade

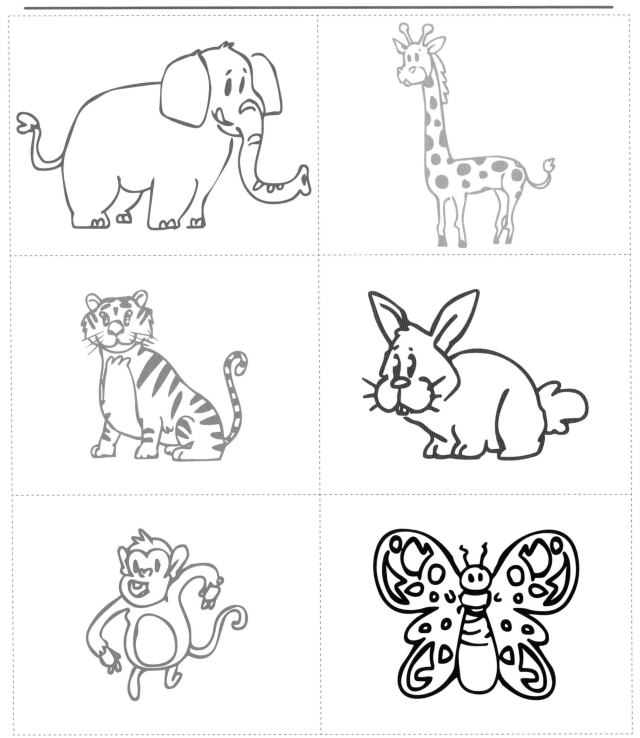

Friendship Tips Handout for Session 13

Share these **Friendship Tips** with teachers and parents who can support friendship skills at school and home. This week, we made a deal with friends by voting. Everyone gave their ideas and we took a vote to see what the group decided. We noticed that you don't always get your first choice, but taking a vote is a fair way to make a group decision.

Remember

To solve a problem or make a group decision:

Let everyone give ideas.

Listen to all the ideas.

Say "yes" to good ideas.

Try It Out

When you need to solve a problem with friends:

Give your ideas *and* ask what others think.

Take a vote to make the choice that most friends want.

It will not always be your first choice, but that is a small disappointment. Building strong friendships is the big win.

School and Home Check

- *At school:*
  Try voting to decide what game your friends want to play.

- *At home:*
  Try voting to choose a TV show or a game to play at home.

Decision Wheel

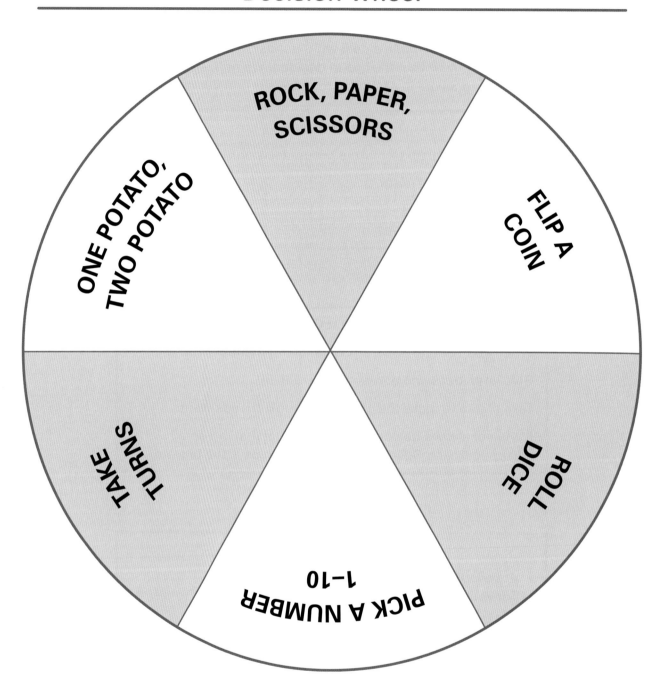

Decision Wheel

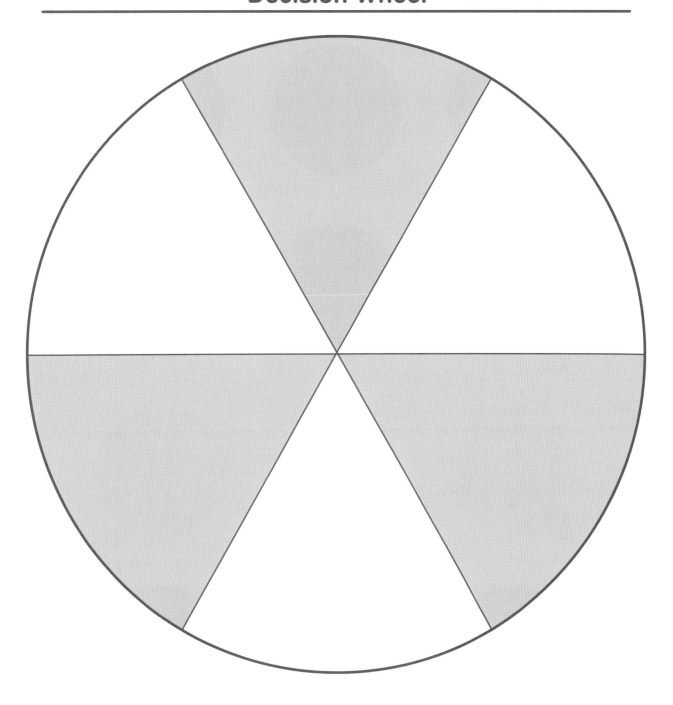

Cards for Rainbow Freeze

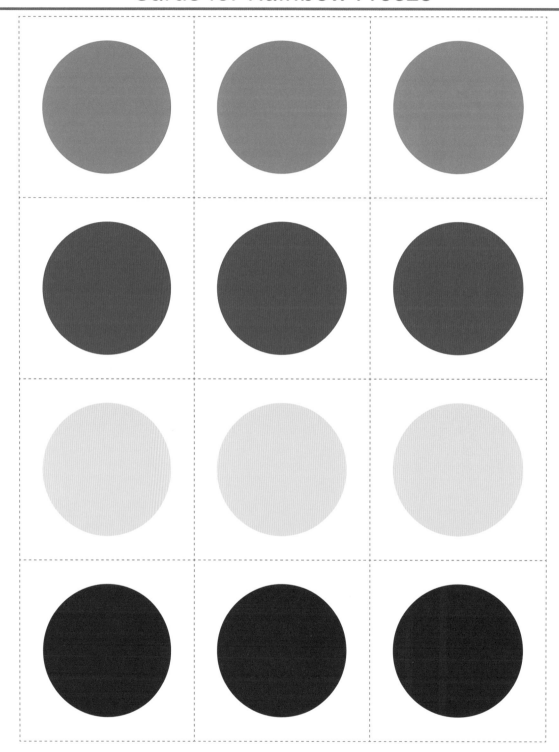

Friendship Tips Handout for Session 14

Share these **Friendship Tips** with teachers and parents who can support friendship skills at school and home. This week, we talked about fair ways to decide who goes first in a game. We came up with some good ideas. Everyone likes to go first, so it's important to find a fair way to decide, and it's also important to be a good sport when it is not your turn to go first.

Remember

There are many fair ways to decide who goes first:

Do Rock, Paper, Scissors.

Flip a coin.

Do One Potato, Two Potato.

Take turns.

Roll dice.

Pick a number.

Try It Out

When you play with a friend, use a fair way to decide who goes first.

What is your favorite way to decide who goes first?

School and Home Check

- *At school and at home:*
  Did you find a fair way to decide who goes first?
  How did you feel when someone else went first?
  Were you a good sport and fair player?

Handling Competitive Play

SESSION 15. Taking Turns and Following Rules

GOALS

1. Introduce fair play: Take turns, follow rules, treat your friends with respect.

2. Introduce the Golden Rule: Treat others as you want to be treated.

3. Practice fair play in competitive games; highlight the positive impact on friendships.

MATERIALS NEEDED

- Agenda Pictures: 1, 3, 5, 4, 2, and 8

- Posters: Good Teamwork, Baxter's Feeling Faces, Care for Friends, Traffic Light, Make a Deal, Fair Play

- Dice (one for each child), deck of cards

- Game Rules and Fair Play Score Sheets (Activity Page 15.1, see p. 208; two per child)

- Stopwatch and colored tape for the Beat the Clock group challenge

- Awards (in the Commonly Used Materials that follow Chapter 5) and Friendship Tips Handout for Session 15 (Activity Page 15.2, see p. 209; one per child)

SESSION OUTLINE

- *Friendship Circle:* Introduce fair play concepts with role plays and new poster (15 minutes)

- *Construction Station:* Practice fair play in games using a Fair Play Score Sheet (15 minutes)

- *Snack* (optional, 15 minutes)
- *Collaboration Challenges:* Beat the Clock and (if time allows) Spoons (10 minutes)
- *Closing Circle:* Compliments with awards (5 minutes)

ADVANCE PREPARATION

- Hang posters.
- Create two short stacks of cards for role play and Concentration games.
- Write children's names on the awards.

DETAILED SESSION CONTENT

Friendship Circle: Introduce Fair Play Concepts with Role Plays and New Posters (15 Minutes)

Greet children, invite them to share feelings, and briefly review the agenda. Explain that you'd like their help with some friendship problems:

> "Today, I want to show you some things that can happen during games that bother other players. Your job is to say what the problem is and how to solve it."

Give each child a die to roll to see who goes first. Have the "winner" be your role-play partner. Have children raise their hands when they recognize the friendship problem and ask your role-play partner if he or she can describe the problem and how he or she feels playing with you. Then ask the children how the problem could be solved. Repeat the dice roll and rotate your role-play partner for each problem scenario. The problems illustrate fair play concepts (e.g., take turns, follow rules, treat your friends with respect) and the Golden Rule (treat others as you want to be treated).

Problem 1

> "[Lay eight card pairs face down.] Want to play Concentration? [Let partner respond.] OK, I'll go first. [Turn over two cards that don't match.] No, wait, I messed up. That's not the one I wanted. I need to go again. [Turn over matching cards.] OK, I got a match, so I get to go again. [Turn over nonmatching cards.] Wait, no, I need to go again."

By this point, your partner may be complaining that it is his turn, and children will have raised their hands. Let your partner explain the problem and how he feels. See if any of the other children have something to add, and how the problem could be solved. Summarize by agreeing with the children—for example: "So, I wasn't playing fairly because I kept playing and playing. I needed to give my friend a turn. It's not fair unless you take turns in a game."

Problem 2

> "Let's try this Concentration game again. This time, you can go first. [Let partner take a turn.] OK, my turn. [Turn over one card, and then cover yourself with your arm while you surreptitiously peek at several cards to find the matching card.]"

Children will raise their hands. Let your partner describe her feelings and what she thinks the problem is first, and then see if others have something to add. Summarize their comments—for example: "I see, you think I was not playing fairly because I did not follow the rules. I cheated. It's not much fun to play with someone who doesn't follow the rules."

Problem 3

"OK, friend, let's try Concentration again. This time I think I've got it; I will remember to take turns and follow the rules! [This time, play by the rules, but gloat about your successes and tease your partner about his losses.] Yay, I got a match! Ha-ha! I'm ahead now. I'm better at this game than you are. Whoo-hoo, you didn't even match it—you lost again!"

As children raise their hands, ask your partner to describe his feelings and what he thinks the problem; then see if others have something to add. Ask how the problem could be solved. Summarize their statements—for example: "Yes, I think you are all correct. I was teasing my friend and making fun of him. He didn't like that. It wasn't fun for him to play with me when I did that. It's not fun to play with someone if that person doesn't treat you with respect." Point to the new Fair Play poster and read through it with the children, noting how they were just telling you the very same ideas. Then explain why it is hard for you to follow the ideas on the poster sometimes:

"The thing that's hard for me is that I really like to be the winner at games. Does anyone else feel like that? I don't really like to lose. Sometimes I want to play by my own rules, or peek at the cards, so I can win because that's fun for me. But I've learned something really important about that. Can anyone guess what it is?"

Give the children an opportunity to explain that it is not fun for the other person if he or she always loses. Let them tell you why they think it is important to play games in a way that is fair and fun for both players, rather than focusing only on winning. Then summarize—for example: "I understand what you are saying. I can't just think about myself, I have to think about my friend's feelings too. That way, we will both enjoy playing together, even if I don't win." Point to the bottom of the Fair Play poster and note that we call that the Golden Rule: "Treat others as you want to be treated." Congratulate the children for their helpful problem solving and good advice.

Construction Station: Practice Fair Play in Games Using a Fair Play Score Sheet (15 Minutes)

This session introduces competitive games with rules, which will be a challenge for some children. Have children play in pairs or triads, which is easier than playing in a larger group. To maximize the learning opportunity, coaches use a Fair Play Score Sheet to praise and comment frequently on children's fair play behaviors. This activity recognizes and reinforces fair play concepts, helping children see how it makes the activity fun for both partners (even when one doesn't win). Should any conflicts arise, the coach should encourage children to take a deep breath, calm down, say the problem, describe how they feel, and then discuss with the group what kinds of solutions would be fair, given the situation. Introduce the activity as follows:

"The first game we are playing today is Concentration, also called Memory. Who has played this game? Let's read the rules. [Read the rules.] While you play, I'll watch for fair play and give you points when I see it. Here's my score sheet. When I see you taking turns, following rules, joining in, cheering for your friend, and respecting your friend, I'll give you points. At the end of our session, you could win a Fair Play Award."

As children play, liberally label and give points for fair play. Comment on any feelings the children express and reinforce each child's efforts at fair play. For example, to a distressed child, the coach might say: "I know you're disappointed about being behind, but you're doing a great job of joining in and following rules. Maybe your luck will change." To the peers, the coach might say, "This would be a great time to cheer for Jimmy." If time allows, play dice with the Fair Play Score Sheet.

Snack (Optional, 15 Minutes)

The usual snack procedures are followed.

Collaborative Challenges: Beat the Clock and (If Time Allows) Spoons (10 Minutes)

Beat the Clock is a group challenge game. To set it up, ask the group to hold hands forming a circle. Use two different colors of tape to place "X's" at the spots where a "12" and "6" would be if the children's circle formed the face of a clock. First, give the group a practice task, which is to walk around in a circle holding hands, making a full 360-degree rotation in one direction and then a full 360-degree rotation in the opposite direction. Next, begin to give them different challenges (see below). Before and after each challenge, encourage the children to talk about their plan—for example: "What will you have to do in order to meet the challenge?" "How can you help each other keep their handgrips?" "How can you make sure that no one gets hurt, such as by being pulled down or gripped too hard?" If they have difficulty, encourage the children to discuss how they might adjust themselves to make it easier to hold hands or move together.

The challenges are twofold: (1) See how fast the group can make the full circle rotation twice around (double rotation) without anyone losing his or her handgrip with a partner. The coach should time the first, second, and third attempt to see how fast the group can go. (2) Now have the children begin in seated positions, holding hands. The challenge is to get up and make the double rotation as fast as possible and sit down again, holding hands the entire time. Again, the coach can time sequential attempts to get the group's best time.

Be sure to take time to lead the children in a preplay and postplay discussion, asking how they felt it went, what worked well, and what they might do to perform even better as a group. A key goal of this activity is to improve social awareness and communication skills, so encourage the children in the planning and reflection processes that are an important part of skill building.

If there is time for another group game, try Spoons, explaining as you set up:

"Has anyone played Spoons? Here's how it goes. We sit in a circle, and I put spoons in the middle. Everyone gets four cards. We start to pass cards around the circle, one at a time. You look at each card, and you can keep it or pass it. But you can't have more than five cards at one time. Your goal is to try to get four cards with the same number, for example, four 7's, or four 9's. When someone gets four cards with the same numbers in his or her hand, the child quietly takes a spoon. Once you see one person take a spoon, you can take a spoon. The last person goes without a spoon!

"Before we start, I'd like to tell you about something that happened the last time I played this game. One child kept cards without passing them along, so she had a lot more than five cards in her hand. She won the game, but it made others mad. Can you guess why that upset some kids? [Let children respond.] That's right, in this game you have to pass the cards along—that's fair play. It gives everyone a fair chance to win. Let's do one slow round so you see how to play. [Proceed to do a slow round, with lots of support, so that children see how the game is played. As time allows, speed up in the next round, as children begin to understand the game.]"

Closing Circle: Round Robin Compliments and Fair Player Awards (5 Minutes)

In the final friendship circle, start a round robin compliment process. Ask the child sitting next to you to identify his or her favorite game during the session. Then give that child a compliment and ask him or her to turn to the next child in the circle and do the same thing—ask about a favorite game, and then give a compliment. Give each child a coach compliment describing fair play, a Fair Player Award, Friendship Tips Handout for Session 15, and the extra copy of the Fair Play Score Sheet to use in the classroom or at home (see Friendship Tips suggestion).

SPECIAL ISSUES

1. Spoons may be too challenging for some children. Not only must they handle competition, but children must also regulate physical control in terms of moving the cards along and keeping track of both cards and spoons. If this game seems too difficult for children in your group, use an alternative game such as Go Fish.

2. In general, the goal is to provide a level of challenge that encourages children to work on new skills, at a difficulty level that allows them to attain mastery with effort. If game-playing activities are streamlined to the point that children are simply entertained, then the learning process may be minimized. On the other hand, if children are faced with too great a challenge and experience disorganization and social failure, then the learning process is also jeopardized. Hence, the success of the session rests on the coaches' ability to provide an optimal challenge in which children employ skills at the high end of their abilities without getting overwhelmed.

3. In some groups, boasting or teasing may emerge as a problem. If so, the coach has several options to deal with that behavior: (1) Ask the recipient to provide feedback to the boaster regarding how the statements affect his or her feelings. (2) Reframe and reword the boasting—for example: "You're proud that you've played so well. Let's think of a way to say that without hurting other people's feelings. You could say, 'I'm trying hard today' or 'This is my lucky day.'" (3) Redirect the behavior by encouraging the "winners" to cheer for the "losers" by saying, "I'll wait for you" or "Maybe next time you'll win."

SESSION 16. Good Things to Say When You Win or Lose

GOALS

1. Introduce the concept of good sportsmanship: good things to say when you win or lose.

2. Reflect on how the way you behave when you win or lose affects others.

3. Practice fair play and good sportsmanship in competitive games.

MATERIALS NEEDED

- Agenda Pictures: 1, 3, 4, 5, 6, 2, and 8

- Posters: Good Teamwork, Baxter's Feeling Faces, Care for Your Friends, Traffic Light, Make a Deal, Fair Play

- For discussion, a poster and strips of paper with things to say (Activity Page 16.1, see p. 210; one set)

- Cut paper strips to make paper footballs, tape

- Materials for partner challenges: paper and scissors, jar with screw top, and stickers

- Little Eddie's Dear Problem Solvers letter (Activity Page 16.2, see p. 211; one per group)

- Friendship awards (in the Commonly Used Materials that follow Chapter 5); Friendship Tips Handout for Session 16 (Activity Page 16.3, see p. 212; one per child)

SESSION OUTLINE

- *Friendship Circle:* Good things to say when you win or lose (15 minutes)
- *Construction Station:* Paper football game and partner challenges (15 minutes)
- *Snack* (optional, 15 minutes)
- *Collaboration Challenges:* Dear Problem Solvers role play (10 minutes)
- *Closing Circle:* Team wave, victory cheer, and compliments (5 minutes)

ADVANCE PREPARATION

- Hang posters.
- Cut sayings for the poster into strips and put them in a basket.
- Cut paper strips to make paper footballs.
- Put stickers in a jar for the partner challenges.
- Write children's names on the Friendship Award.

DETAILED SESSION CONTENT

Friendship Circle: Discuss Winning, Losing, and Good Sportsmanship (10 Minutes)

Greet children, invite them to share their feelings, and briefly review the agenda. It is "Sports Day" in Friendship Group, so the first task is to identify a favorite sports team. Ask the children to share their ideas and then take a vote to identify their favorite sports team. Lead a discussion about the feelings associated with winning and losing, as follows.

> "We're going to talk about winning and losing today—just like the [favorite sports team] do. Who likes to win when they play a game? How do you feel when you win? Who likes to lose? How do you feel when you lose? If everyone wants to win and no one wants to lose, how do kids have fun playing games? How come the [favorite sports team] keep on playing, even though they lose sometimes?"

The key points to draw out and reinforce in this discussion include the idea that it is fun to play the game even if you don't win every time, because the act of playing itself is fun. Some children might also recognize that if one person won all the time, other kids would stop playing with him or her. So, in order for everyone to have fun winning some of the time, everyone has to lose some of the time. Ask the following questions: "Have you ever heard someone say that it doesn't matter if you win or lose, it's how you play the game that counts? What does that mean?" Let children share their thoughts. Reinforce the idea that, when everyone plays fairly, the game is fun. Even if you lose sometimes, you can enjoy playing the game. Having fun playing with your friends is a good thing, whether or not you win. Then introduce the idea that the way you behave after you win or lose is important to friendships as well.

> "It is disappointing to lose. And when you are feeling down about losing, the way your friends treat you really matters. I am going to show you two ways that I might act when I win a game, and ask you what you think about them. Here's one way. [Pretend you are playing a card game, and you lay down your last match.] 'Yahoo! I win! I'm the WINNER! You all lose—you all are the losers!' And here is another way I might act: 'Yahoo, I won this time. But, maybe you'll win next time. Let's play again.'"

Ask the children how each way of acting would affect a friend's feelings. In which one was I being a better sport? Why? Reinforce the idea that it is OK to feel happy inside when you win, but the way that you treat your friend can be OK or not OK. You want to think about your friend's feelings before you act. Then note how the way a person behaves when he or she loses a game can also affect a friendship, and ask them to watch your demonstration again.

> "I am going to show you two ways that I might act when I lose a game, and ask you what you think about them. [Pretend you are playing cards, and your partner just won.] I might say this: 'That was a really stupid game. It wasn't really fair. It was boring, and I didn't even want to win, anyway.' OR, I might say this: 'Wow, good game. Want to play again? Maybe my luck will change!'"

Encourage a discussion about these two responses. Reinforce the idea that it is OK for you to feel disappointed and frustrated inside when you lose, but the way that you treat your friend can be OK or not OK. You can express your disappointment without hurting your friend's feelings. After getting the children's responses, explain that you are going to play a little game now to make a poster that will list good ideas about what to say when you win and when you lose. In this poster-making game, children pass a basket around the circle to music. When the music stops, they pull out a piece of paper from the basket (provide help reading the paper, if needed). The child then decides if it is a good thing to say when winning or losing, or not, and checks it out with his or her friends. If the group decides it is a good thing to say, the child tapes it onto the poster. Comment that the children will have a chance to try out the good things to say next. (Be sure to save this poster, as you will use it again in the following sessions.)

Construction Station: Paper Football Game and Partner Challenges (15 Minutes)

The first task is to create paper footballs. Each child should be given a strip of paper about 1½–2 inches wide. Ask children to watch as you demonstrate the steps in folding the football diagonally, down to the end, tucking in the final piece. Then the children should fold up their footballs. Once the footballs are done, explain how to play the game. For the game, there should be a table space to shoot the footballs across, with a tape placed about 8 inches from the end of the table. The goal of the game is to shoot the football hard enough to get it into the taped area, but not so hard that it goes off the end of the table.

Divide the children into two teams. If desired, each team can choose a name for itself or select a football team to represent. Before the game starts, demonstrate how to take a turn shooting the football across the table, and let each child take a practice shot. Encourage the children to use the "good things to say" list of ideas, as follows.

> "This game can be challenging, because you might feel frustrated or disappointed if your football goes over the table, and you don't get a point. So it is a good time to practice our fair play rules, and also a good time to remember the ideas on our list."

Read through some examples from the list of good things to say when winning or losing. Explain to the children that you will keep score in two ways. You will keep score of how many touchdown points each team gets, and you will also keep track of how many times you see the teams using fair play and encouraging their friends with the good things to say when winning or losing. The major purpose of this activity is to give the children a supportive experience with competitive play and help them practice emotional self-control and coping in the context of competition. Hence, provide reminders, support, and praise for these efforts. At any point—for example, once a team has scored three "touchdowns"—the coach can call the end of one game, announce a team winner, and let them try again. Once they have played a few times, comment on the children's scores in the area of fair play and good sportsmanship, and praise them for their efforts and good sportsmanship behaviors. Then introduce the partner challenges:

> "When you are on a team, you really have to work with your teammates. So today I brought a partner challenge that will test your good teamwork."

Demonstrate the following three steps in the partner challenge. Have the children repeat the steps and ask them what strategies they will need to use to accomplish the tasks with their partner. Be sure to ask, "What will you have to do in order to work together with your partner to complete this challenge?" To begin, each pair of children must stand arm in arm (or hand in hand), so that each child can use only one hand (the outside hand). Then the team must (1) use the scissors to cut a piece of paper in half, (2) unscrew the top of a jar, and (3) take stickers out of the jar and peel off the back to put them onto the paper. After they complete the task, ask the children: "How did you do that? What did you do to work with your partner to accomplish that challenge?" Praise the children for their communication skills and teamwork.

Snack (Optional, 15 Minutes)

Follow the usual procedures.

Collaboration Challenges: Dear Problem Solvers Role Play (10 Minutes)

Show the children the letter from Little Eddie (Activity Page 16.2, p. 211) and introduce it as follows:

> "Today I received a letter from a child who is having some friendship trouble. I'm hoping you can listen to the letter and think of some good ideas for how to solve this problem. I want to get your ideas and have you act them out and see how well they work. Then I can write back to Eddie with our suggestions. [Read the letter from Little Eddie to the group.]"

Lead a discussion. First, ask the children to talk about the problem situation and the feelings of everyone involved. Ask them how Little Eddie feels and why, how the other team members feel and why, and how Big Eddie feels and why he says Little Eddie can't play. Ask whether they think the situation is fair, and whether they have seen a problem like this at their school. A goal is to help the children think in more complex ways about difficult social problems, so encourage discussion of the problem before jumping into solutions.

Next, provide some ideas about how to solve the problem. Write down the children's ideas about the problem to get a few options. If they focus only on Little Eddie, be sure to ask what the other children on the team could do to help. Once a few ideas have been generated, ask the children which one they think is best. Ask them to think about what will happen if that solution is used. Once they have a solution, suggest that the group tries out the solution in a play.

For the first role play, the coach should play both Little Eddie and Big Eddie, and the children should play the others on the team. The following storyboard steps set up the sequence of the story, but the children need to fill in what the characters do to solve the problem.

- Scene 1: Big Eddie and the children are playing football.
- Scene 2: Little Eddie comes and watches. Then he asks if he can play.
- Scene 3: Big Eddie and the kids stop playing. They walk over to Little Eddie.
- Scene 4: Big Eddie tells Little Eddie he can't play because he is not good at the game.

The children then try out a solution that they discussed and enact the role play to see what happens. At the end, the coach should ask the children if they felt their solution worked, and whether they want to try another solution or pass that solution on to Little Eddie.

Closing Circle: The Wave, Victory Cheer, and Compliments (10 Minutes)

For this compliment circle, children need to be sitting in chairs. Explain the wave.

> "You have done such a great job of teamwork today, I want to celebrate our team support by doing the 'wave.' Who has seen fans do the 'wave'? [Let children respond and describe how the

wave is done. If none of the children knows, then the coach can explain it.] The wave is when each person standing in a line stands up and sits down right after one another, making it look like a wave of water is moving through the crowd. What do we need to do to work together to make our wave?"

Let the children offer a few suggestions and then give it a try. Praise the children for good teamwork. Once they have done one wave, try it again; then try it backwards in a sequence. If time allows, let them try the wave in playback slow motion. If you have a small group and the wave will not work well, have the children number off to identify the "odds" and the "evens." When you call them, the children are to stand up, raise their hands, cheer "YAY," and sit back down. Then call "Odds," "Evens," "Odds," "Evens," "All cheer." Try it slow once, then speed up and see how quickly the children can do this group cheer.

If time allows, you can also add the creation of a Victory Cheer to the compliment process. Ask the children if they have ever seen sports fans do a Victory Cheer when their team makes a point. As needed, explain that some fans jump up with their arms in the air, "high-fiving" whomever is nearby, and waving their hands back and forth. Have the children show some different things they have seen fans do to celebrate a touchdown. Explain that you are going to make your own Friendship Team Victory Cheer, and each person is going to add one action. Pick up a Friendship Award and read the name on it. Give that child a compliment and ask him or her to show an action that can be part of the Friendship Team Victory Cheer. Let everyone try the action. Continue in a similar manner by picking up another award, reading the name on it, giving that child a compliment, and asking him or her to show an action for the Victory Cheer. However, this time when the children copy the action, the group has to add it in sequence to the first action—again demonstrating the first action and adding this second one. Proceed in the same manner until each child has received a Friendship Award and compliments, and the whole Victory Cheer sequence is complete.

SPECIAL ISSUES

1. This session can work at two different levels. For children who are older and have a more well developed sense of social understanding, this session offers the opportunity to consider different perspectives (i.e., of winners and losers, of Big Eddie and Little Eddie). The children benefit from a discussion that considers the feelings and behaviors of the different characters in the role plays, and they may thereby fully grasp the idea that all *feelings* are OK (you can't help how you feel) but that *behaviors* can be OK or not OK (and you need to make a choice about your behavior and use self-control to avoid hurting your friendships). Younger children may not yet have the cognitive maturity needed for such a multifaceted social understanding, but the concrete guidelines for what to say when you win or lose are nonetheless beneficial.

2. There are a number of transitions in this session that may be challenging for some groups. If needed, reduce transitions by organizing the activities sequentially at a table, rather than having children move to different areas in the room. If the Problem Solvers discussion and role play seem too difficult for your group, you can replace them with alternative games or activities.

3. If desired, keep score during the football game, giving points both for winning the round and for being a good sport and a good friend in the game. This approach helps children who lose at the game feel proud of their good sportsmanship.

SESSION 17. Resisting the Temptation to Cheat

GOALS

1. Review fair play concepts and discuss following the rules (and not cheating).

2. Promote social awareness of the impact of cheating on playmate's feelings.

3. Practice fair play skills in the context of competitive games and challenges.

MATERIALS NEEDED

- Agenda Pictures: 1, 7, 3, 5, 6, 4, 2, and 8

- Posters: Good Teamwork, Baxter's Feeling Faces, Care for Your Friends, Traffic Light, Make a Deal, Fair Play

- Good things to say when you win/lose poster constructed in Session 16.

- Baxter Story 4, "Baxter's Challenge" (pp. 213–220) and storyboard pictures (Activity Page 17.1, see p. 221; one set per group)

- Partner challenge materials (book, beans, spoon, pennies, blocks), stopwatch to time races

- "Key pad" pasted on top of the materials box (Activity Page 17.2, see p. 222; one per group)

- Deck of cards, modified deck for Concentration, spoons for Spoons

- Friendship awards (in the Commonly Used Materials that follow Chapter 5); Friendship Tips Handout for Session 17 (Activity Page 17.3, see p. 223; one per child)

SESSION OUTLINE

- *Friendship Circle:* Skill review, Baxter's Challenge story, unlock the box (15 minutes)

- *Construction Station:* Competitive partner challenges (10 minutes)

- *Snack* (optional, 15 minutes)

- *Collaborative Challenges:* Baxter's Challenge play and card games of choice (15 minutes)

- *Closing Circle:* Compliments with awards (5 minutes)

ADVANCE PREPARATION

- Hang posters.

- Put materials for partner challenges in a box; cut out the Magic Code "key pad" and paste it on top of the box.

- Create a Team Challenge Rotation Chart and identify a course for the races.

- Cut apart the storyboard pictures for the Baxter's Challenge role play.

- Write children's names on awards.

DETAILED SESSION CONTENT

Friendship Circle: Skill Review, Baxter's Challenge, Unlock the Box (15 Minutes)

It's Friendship Challenge Day, with a focus on following rules and accepting a loss. Greet children and invite them to share their feelings. Ask children what they remember about the fair play ideas, and review the poster using choral responding. Ask them what they said when they won or lost a game this week, and which worked the best. Then read Baxter's Challenge story, asking the embedded questions to support discussion.

After the story, introduce the Magic Code challenge. Before starting this activity, identify a sequence of five numbers that represents the Magic Code, but keep this sequence hidden from sight. The children take turns pushing the numbers on the key pad, one by one. As long as the child is pushing the buttons in the right order (i.e., matching the Magic Code), he or she is allowed to proceed. But as soon as the child hits a number that is in the wrong order, the coach says "Beep," and it is the next person's turn. Children need to work together. They need to learn from each person's turn, and help each other remember the correct sequence as it unfolds. The team wins the challenge after each child has pressed the right sequence of numbers to open the box. Help from teammates is encouraged—working together is the goal of the exercise! After describing the game, include a pre-challenge planning discussion, as follows.

> "In this Magic Code challenge, you will need to work as a team. Each one of you will take a turn pushing the numbers on this key pad one by one. If you guess a number correctly, you will get to try the next number. If you guess wrong, I will go 'Beep,' and it will be the next person's turn. I'm going to let [Name] take one turn, so you can see how it works. [Let a child take a turn.] So, she got the first number [right/wrong], which means the first number in the code [is/is not] that number. The next person who takes a turn needs to remember that. Let's take one more example. [Name], take your turn. [Let the next child take a turn.] OK, I 'beeped' when [Name] pushed that number. What does that mean? Right, that is not the next number in the code. So, what do you know about the code so far?"

Check to see that children understand how the activity works. Then ask the preplay planning questions, as follows, letting them discuss each one: "How can you work as a team to figure out the code?"; "What can you learn by watching your friend take a turn?"; "How can you help your friends when they take a turn?" The goal is to help the children recognize that they can help each other by staying engaged and paying attention to what each child learns about the code. After the children master the code so that they can open the box, ask them how they did it—for example: "How did you work as a team to figure out the code? What did you do to help each other learn the code?" Praise their teamwork and problem-solving skills. Then open the box.

Construction Station: Competitive Partner Challenges (10 Minutes)

These partner challenges provide practice in a "team sports" context, when children need to "multitask" by supporting and working together with their teammates, and also regulating the emotions associated with winning and losing. For each challenge, pairs compete against each other to win or lose. Partner teams should be rotated each round (make a chart ahead of time). A winner should be announced after each challenge, perhaps by circling the names on the rotation schedule. The goal is to build children's capacity to cope with the feelings of winning and losing by experiencing both in this supportive group setting. As part of the learning experience, it is important to engage children in pre-activity planning and post-activity reflection, and draw their attention to strategies that help them succeed at a team challenge. Remind them to "Take 5" if they need to calm down.

> "Today you will face four challenges—three races, and a tower building contest. In the races, you will be working with a partner. You will need to follow this course. [Demonstrate the racing course. Note that it should be long enough to give the partners a chance to help each other.] Here's how it works. I'm going to go first in this relay. For this first challenge, I have to balance a book on my head and go as quickly as I can. [Name] is my partner, and if my book falls, I cannot touch it. He has to get it for me and put it back on my head. [Demonstrate.] After I finish, my partner will go and I will help."

After the demonstration, ask the children to anticipate how they will do the task before they begin—for example, ask, "What do you need to do in order to be successful at this race? How can you and your partner help each other?" Let the children do the first race and provide support as needed. Time the race, announce the winner, praise good sportsmanship (note the things that the children can say on the win and lose poster constructed in Session 16), and follow the same sequence with the next races. Possible partner challenges include (1) racing along the course, balancing some beans (or a potato) on a spoon—if it falls, the partner needs to pick it up; (2) racing along the course, balancing a penny on each index finger—if one falls, the partner needs to pick it up; and (3) working together to build the tallest block tower they can manage in 1 minute.

Following each challenge, have the children discuss what they did to make it work, or what they did that did *not* work so well. Have them share ideas about how they can improve teamwork on the next challenge. These pre-play and post-play discussions are important in building children's planning skills as well as their capacity for self-reflection.

Snack (Optional, 15 Minutes)

The usual procedures are followed.

Collaboration Challenges: Baxter's Challenge Role Play and Card Game Choice (15 Minutes)

Explain that you will be putting on a play of Baxter's Challenge story. Bring out the storyboard pictures, cut apart, and ask children if they can put them in the right order so they can enact the story. Then have children act out the characters (Baxter, John, the bird, the troll) as you read the events in the story. Encourage the children to add dialogue and show the emotions of their characters. For the role play, the narrative is as follows:

> 1. The story begins in Baxter's house. Here is Baxter. Here is his friend, the bird, who gives good advice about friendships. And here is the troll, who just cares about himself.
>
> 2. John comes over. Baxter asks if he wants to play a game. They get out a board game and begin to play. They are having fun.
>
> 3. Baxter realizes that John is ahead. Baxter does not want to lose the game. He feels upset. He hears the troll voice telling him 'Don't let John beat you.'

4. Baxter bumps the table and knocks the game. John is mad. John says Baxter did it on purpose and calls him a cheater. Baxter calls John a cheater. John leaves.

5. The troll is happy: 'Now you win!' The bird is sad: 'Who will you play with now?'

6. The bird tells Baxter that he has to make an important choice. He can cheat and win all the time—but have no friends. OR, he can play fairly and keep his friends.

7. Baxter apologizes to John: 'I didn't want to lose, but what I did was not fair to you.' John apologizes too: 'I'm sorry I called you a cheater; I still want to be your friend.'

8. Baxter and John play the game again. They play fairly and have fun."

If time allows, let children choose a favorite card game to play (e.g., Concentration, Go Fish, Spoons). Review the rules, and as children play, praise examples of fair play.

Closing Friendship Circle: Compliments with Friendship Awards (10 Minutes)

Have children Pass the Mike to music. When it stops, ask them three questions: "What was the hardest challenge for you today?"; "What did you do to beat that challenge?"; and "How did your friends help?" After answering, each child receives compliments from you and from his or her peers. At the end, distribute Team Challenge awards and Friendship Tips Handout for Session 17 to each child.

SPECIAL ISSUES

1. The group challenge of discovering the code may sound overly demanding, but most children find this novel task very interesting and engaging. They may surprise you.

2. Remember to refer to the Traffic Light and the Make a Deal posters when conflicts arise, modeling and encouraging children to "Take 5" to calm down, then explain the problem and how they feel, and finally to work out a solution.

3. If children struggle with playing fairly, consider using the Fair Play Score Sheets in this session to help children focus on their goals. As with other forms of external structure, the point is to use the score sheet for a short time to bolster children's attention to their behavior and friendship goals.

SESSION 18. Putting Your Friendship First

GOALS

1. Discuss how bossiness hurts friendships and the value of taking turns being the leader.

2. Practice fair play in competitive games with self-monitoring.

3. Promote perspective taking and social collaboration skills with group activities.

MATERIALS NEEDED

- Agenda Pictures: 1, 4, 3, 5, 6, 2, and 8
- Posters: Good Teamwork, Feelings, Care for Your Friends, Traffic Light, Make a Deal, Fair Play
- Good things to say when you win/lose poster constructed in Session 16
- Dear Problem Solvers letter (Activity Page 18.1, see p. 224; one per group)
- Tool card pictures (Activity Page 18.2, see p. 225; one set per group)
- Modified deck of cards for Concentration and Go Fish
- Game rules and Fair Play Score Sheets (Activity Page 18.3, see p. 226; two per group)
- Large jump-rope for "Big Jump"
- Cards for the "Fair or Not Fair" game (Activity Page 18.4, see p. 227; one set per group)
- Friendship Tips Handout for Session 18 (Activity Page 18.5, see p. 228; one per child)

SESSION OUTLINE

- *Friendship Circle:* Dear Problem Solvers discussion, Make a Machine (15 minutes)
- *Construction Station:* Competitive games with Fair Play Score Sheets (10 minutes)
- *Snack* (optional, 15 minutes)
- *Collaborative Challenges:* Big Jump (10 minutes)
- *Closing Circle:* Cards for Fair or Not Fair game and compliment (10 minutes)

ADVANCE PREPARATION

- Hang posters.
- Cut out tool pictures and cards for the Fair or Not Fair game.

DETAILED SESSION CONTENT

Friendship Circle: Dear Problem Solvers Discussion, Make a Machine (15 Minutes)

Greet children and invite them to share their feelings. Briefly review the session agenda. Then introduce the problem-solving challenge:

> "I need your help in answering this letter from M.J., a kid I know. Here is what he says: 'Dear Problem Solvers, I am having trouble making friends in my class. No one wants to play with me. I am really good at a lot of games. I like to choose the games, I like to go first, and I like to win. But the kids won't play with me. They say I am too bossy. I am very lonely, because I don't have any friends. What should I do?'"

Let children discuss this problem, and offer advice. Here are some discussion questions that might be helpful:

"Why don't the kids want to play with him?"

"Why do his classmates say he is too bossy to play with?"

"Why does he want to choose the games and go first all the time?"

"Why does he want to win all the time?"

"Why don't his classmates like that?"

Use active listening to summarize the children's thoughts. Draw connections between the advice they give and the Friendship Team ideas, pointing out ideas they suggest that are examples of good teamwork, caring for one's friends, and fair play. End the discussion with appreciation—for example: "Wow, you have some really good advice for M.J. I will pass that on to him." Then explain the Make a Machine challenge:

"Now I have a challenging game for you to try. This will take good teamwork! Let me show you the cards we'll use for the game. Each of these cards has a picture of a tool on it. When it is your turn, you will pick a card, tell us what you think the tool is, and show us how you think that tool moves. Ask your friends if you need ideas or help."

Children take turns drawing cards, naming the tool, and showing the motion (and if desired, also the sound) that the tool makes when it is used. Some of these are very tricky, and the coach should encourage the children to ask their friends for help or (if needed) give a suggestion about how to make the motion of that tool. Once all of the tools have been identified, continue with the directions for the game.

"Now, here is how the game works. We are going to use these tools to make a big group machine. First, [Name] is going to pick a card. She is going to start our machine by making the motion of the tool on her card. Then the next person in line will pick a card. He will make the motion of the tool on that card, and he has to connect it to [Name's] tool in order to make the machine. All of the parts of the machine have to be touching in some way. Can you guess what happens next? I will turn the machine 'on' and 'off.' Our team challenge is to stay connected and make our machine go and stop, with each person making his or her tool motion work. With everyone joined in together, we will have an awesome machine."

In addition to calling "on" and "off" to start and stop the machine, the coach can also call out other speeds for the machine, such as "low speed" (i.e., children make their motions very slowly), and "high speed" (i.e., children make their motions very quickly). At the end of this activity, praise the children for their teamwork, and note how they were able to meet the challenge of the game by paying attention, joining in, and helping their friends.

Construction Station: Practicing Fair Play with Competitive Games (15 Minutes)

Have children work in groups of twos or threes. Give them a choice of games (Concentration, Go Fish, Tic-Tac-Toe) and ask them to Make a Deal with their friends about which game to play first.

Review the rules and how each game is played. Use the Fair Play Score Sheets, but this time ask the children to score themselves. That is, after the children finish playing a game, ask them to rate themselves on the Fair Play Score Sheet before playing their next game. Should any conflicts arise, encourage children to use the Traffic Light steps (e.g., red light to "Take 5" and explain the problem and how they feel; yellow light to Make a Deal with their partner by giving an idea, checking it out, and saying "yes" to good ideas).

As in the previous session, praise instances of fair play during the game. If a child expresses distress or anger about losing the game, use your calm affect and induction strategies to support the child's self-regulation—for example: "I know you're disappointed about being behind, but you're doing a great job of joining in and following rules. Maybe your luck will change." You can also suggest that partners provide support: "This would be a great time to cheer for Jimmy." In addition, you could say "Don't worry, you might get a match next time."

Snack (Optional, 15 Minutes)

The usual procedure is followed.

Collaborative Challenge: Big Jump (10 Minutes)

Big Jump is a physically challenging activity that requires children to practice perspective taking, communication, cooperation, and helping skills. Before letting the children see the jump rope, provide an introduction like this one:

> "I have an activity for you to try today. When I show it to you, some of you will say 'Oh, great, I love this!' and some of you might say 'Oh, no, I don't like this at all.' So,you are going to have different feelings about this activity. Some of you might be really good at it, and you are going to need to help some of your friends who haven't tried it or find it more difficult. [Bring out the jump rope.] We are going to jump-rope today, but we're going to do it a little bit differently than you've done it before. The very first challenge we are going to have is to teach everyone in our group how to jump-rope."

You and your co-leader can swing the rope, or the rope can be tied at one end and swung by one coach. Or, alternatively, you can also hold the rope and spin, sending it swinging around you in a circle on the ground. By speeding up and slowing down your pace of swinging, you will be able to help children jump successfully. Generally, this challenge is done with an overhand swing, but an underhanded swing is easier, and may be the best for some children.

For the first challenge, children take turns running toward the rope, jumping over it successfully, and running out. Before beginning, let children talk about how they can help each other with this task. Some of the children can explain how to jump to less-confident others. They may be able to help by calling out a good time to start running or jumping. They might help by cheering on their friends. Once everyone has made one successful jump, the group can celebrate. Ask the children how they managed to help each other with the challenge.

The first extension activity for this task involves trying to get the whole team through the jump sequence without a miss. One person will run in, jump once, and then run out. Then the next person will run in, jump once, and run out. The children continue until all team members have gone. However, if someone misses the jump, then the whole team returns to start the sequence again. When explaining how this will work to the children, pick someone who is a good jumper: "For example, if

Susie gets too excited when she is jumping and she goes too fast and trips over the rope, then everyone has to come back to this side of the rope and try it again." Encourage the children to consider ways in which they can help their teammates—for example, "What if someone makes a mistake—how could the team help out that child?" Encourage the children to consider how they can cheer each other on and avoid put-downs.

Another extension activity is to have the whole group try to jump together. The coach can ask the group to consider how many jumps they can make together. They can talk about how they will help each other and cue each other to jump at the same time. Postplay discussions can focus on how the children solved the problem, how they worked together, and how they helped each other with the difficult challenge.

Closing Circle: Compliments and Awards (5 Minutes)

To play the Fair or Not Fair game, children pass the pretend microphone around the circle to music. When the music stops, the child holding the mike picks a card from the basket. With the help of an adult (if needed), the child reads the card and explains why he or she thinks the action described on the card is *fair* or *not fair* and why. Other children in the group give their opinions toward an effort to reach a group consensus. Sometimes you will need to ask follow-up questions, explain the scenarios, and use active listening to clarify the fair play issues. The child who answered picks a sticker, and the cycle repeats until each child has had one or two turns. Distribute Friendship Tips Handout for Session 18.

SPECIAL ISSUES

1. If personal space violations and roughhousing are problems in your group, have children make the machine motions while standing in one place, rather than connecting to each other.

2. If you have access to simple board games, these can also be used to practice fair play. Just make sure that you have a brief written description of the rules, and that the games are short enough to allow for a quick turnover in the play, so that children can practice taking turns and coping with losing.

3. If there is insufficient room for Big Jump, consider a group game like 7-Up or Spoons instead.

Game Rules and Fair Play Score Sheet

Game Rules

Concentration: The goal is to collect the most matched pairs of cards. Select the hearts and clubs, numbers 1–9, from a card deck. Shuffle the cards and lay them on the table, face down, in a pattern (e.g., 4 × 5). On each turn, a player turns over two cards (one at a time), showing all players. If the cards match, the player keeps them and takes another turn. If they don't match, the player replaces them in the same location, and it is the next player's turn. At the end of the game, the person with the most matched pairs wins.

Dice toss: The goal is to get the highest total score, after throwing five dice in three rolls. To take a turn, the player tosses five dice. For the second and third toss, the player can keep as many as he or she likes and toss the others again. The player's score is the total numbers showing on the five dice after their third roll. After everyone has had a turn, the child with highest score wins the round.

Fair Play Score Sheet

Player 1 _____

Player 2 _____

	1	2
Taking Turns		
Following Rules		
Joining In		
Cheering for a Friend		
Respecting a Friend		

Friendship Tips Handout for Session 15

Share these **Friendship Tips** with teachers and parents who can support friendship skills at school and home. This week, Friendship Group focused on the importance of fair play—taking turns, following rules, being a good sport.

Remember

Fair play:

Take turns.

Follow rules.

Respect your friends.

Treat others as you want to be treated.

Try It Out

When you play a game, take turns and follow rules.

When you play fairly, others have fun with you.

Whether you win or lose the game, you win friends when you play fairly.

School and Home Check

Use the Fair Play Score Sheet at home or in your classroom:

Did you remember to play fairly?

Was it fun for everyone?

Give yourself and your friend a compliment!

Sayings for the Win–Lose Poster

If You Win

☺ "Thanks for playing!"

☺ "Nice try!"

☺ "You can go first next time."

☺ "You were a good sport."

☺ "Maybe next time you'll win!"

If You Lose

☺ "Good game!"

☺ "Let's play again."

☺ "It's your lucky day!"

☺ "I had fun playing with you."

☺ "Thanks for playing."

Fillers

☺ "You stink at that game!"

☺ "You cheated."

☺ "That game is stupid."

☺ "I don't want to play with you."

Dear Problem Solvers Letter

Dear Problem Solvers,

I love to play football. Every day, the boys in my class have a football game during recess. But one kid, Big Eddie, says that I can't play. He says I'm not good at football and I will make the team lose. That makes me sad and lonely, and I still want to play. What should I do?

—Little Eddie

Friendship Tips Handout for Session 16

Share these **Friendship Tips** with teachers and parents who can support friendship skills at school and home. This week, Friendship Group focused on the importance of being a good sport whether you win or lose.

Remember

When you win, don't tease or boast.

When you lose, don't complain or quit.

When you are a good sport, the game is fun for everyone.

Try It Out

Choose what you'd like to say when you win:

☺ Thanks for playing!

☺ Nice try!

☺ You can go first next time.

☺ You were a good sport.

☺ Maybe next time you'll win!

Choose what you'd like to say when you lose:

☺ Good game!

☺ Let's play again.

☺ You sure were lucky!

☺ I wish I could win sometime.

☺ Thanks for playing.

School and Home Check

When you played a game at school or at home:

Did you remember to be a good sport?

Did you try out one of the good things to say?

How did it work for you?

Did your friend enjoy the game?

Baxter's Challenge
Text by Karen L. Bierman   Illustrations by Andy Heckathorne

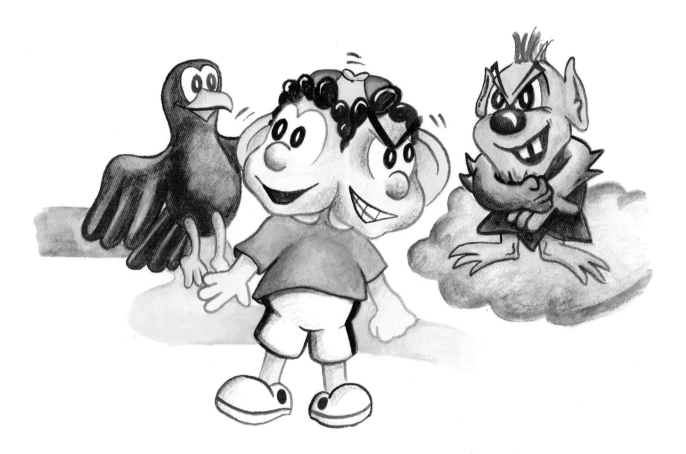

Here is Baxter.

Do you remember him?

Here is his friend, the bird, who gives good advice about friendships.

And here is the troll. The troll just cares about himself and no one else.

Do you remember the bird and the troll?

(page 1 of 8)

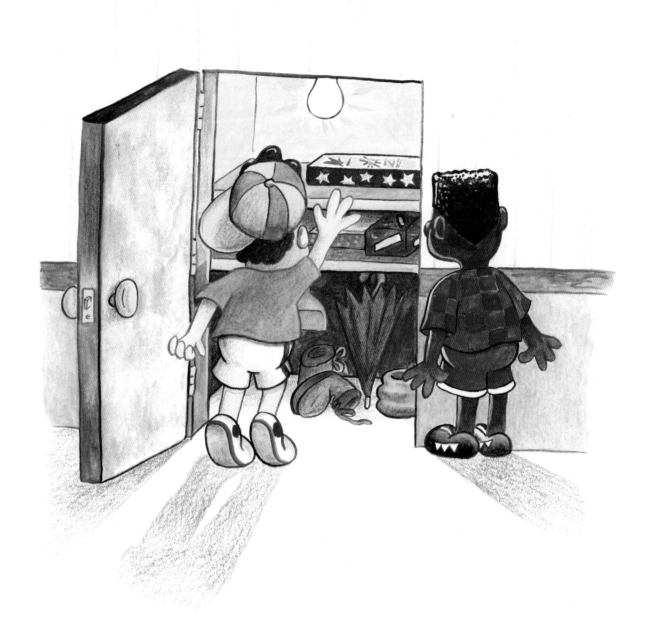

One day, Baxter asked his friend John if he wanted to play a game. They got out the game board and they were having a lot of fun taking turns in the game.

How did John and Baxter feel about playing together?

How can you tell they are friends?

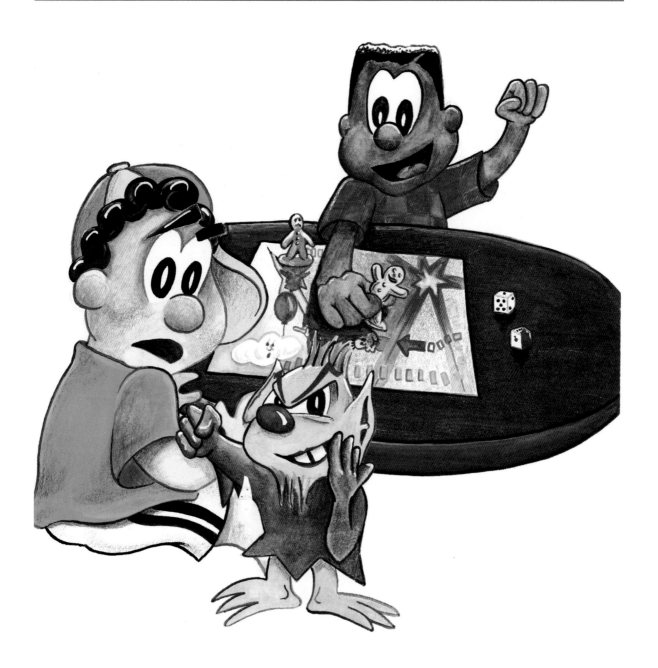

They were taking turns and everything was fine. But then Baxter realized that John was way ahead. Baxter did not want to lose the game. He felt upset. He heard the troll talking to him.

The troll wants Baxter to win, no matter what. What do you think the troll said to Baxter?

What do you think will happen next?

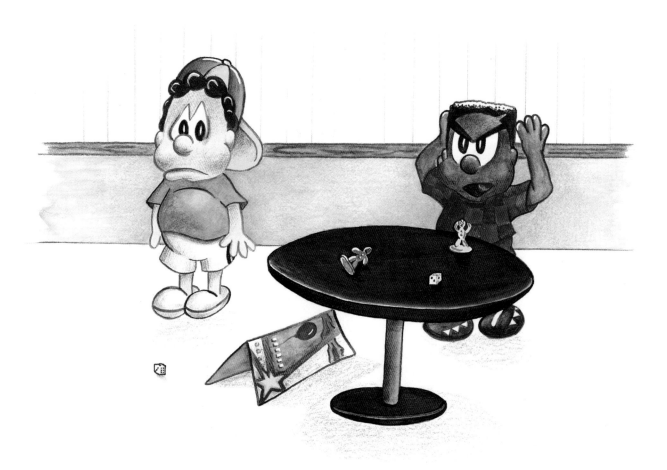

Baxter bumped the table hard and knocked the game onto the floor. John was mad. "You did that on purpose!" he said. "You are a big cheater!" "You're the cheater!" Baxter called back.

"I'm going home," said John, and he stomped out the door.

Why is John so mad? Why did he call Baxter a cheater?

How does Baxter feel?

What is going to happen to their friendship?

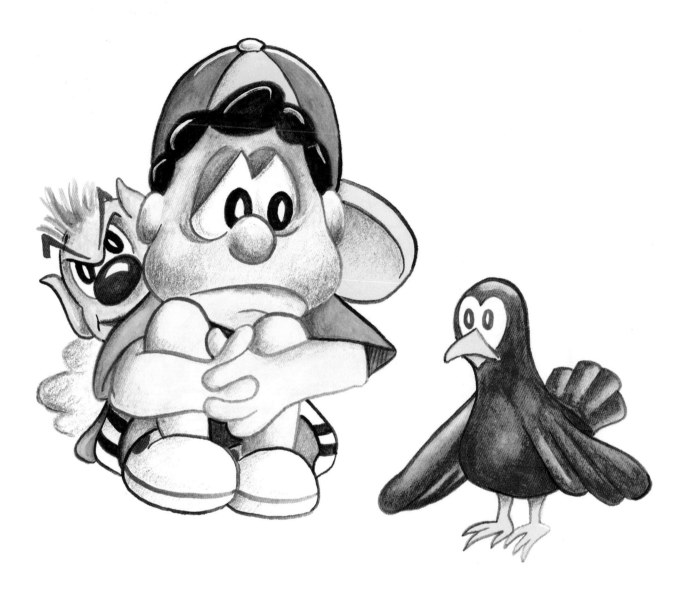

Baxter sat down by himself. The troll was happy. "Now you have the game all to yourself!" said the troll. But the bird was sad. "John was your good friend. Who will you play with now?" asked the bird.

Why was the troll happy?

Why was the bird sad?

How did Baxter feel?

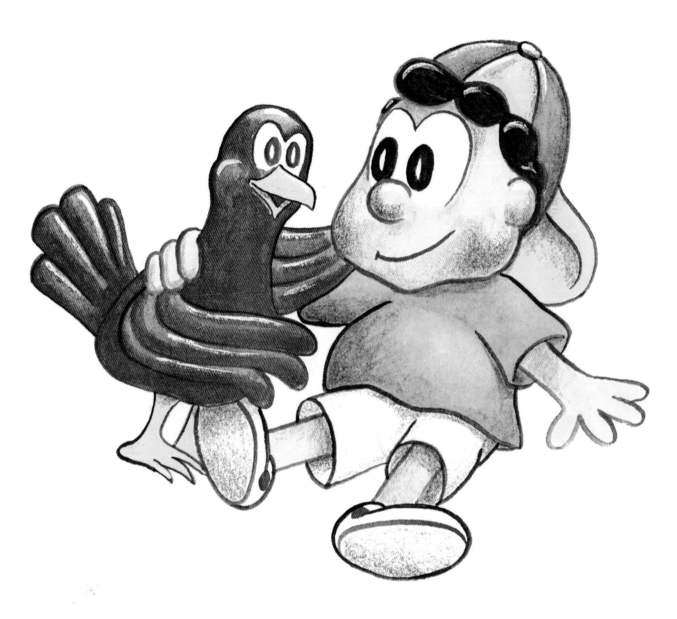

"Baxter," said the bird, "you have an important choice to make. If you want to keep your friends, you have to play fairly. Sometimes you will win, but sometimes you will lose."

Why does the bird say that Baxter has a choice? What is his choice?

What is Baxter thinking? What will he do next?

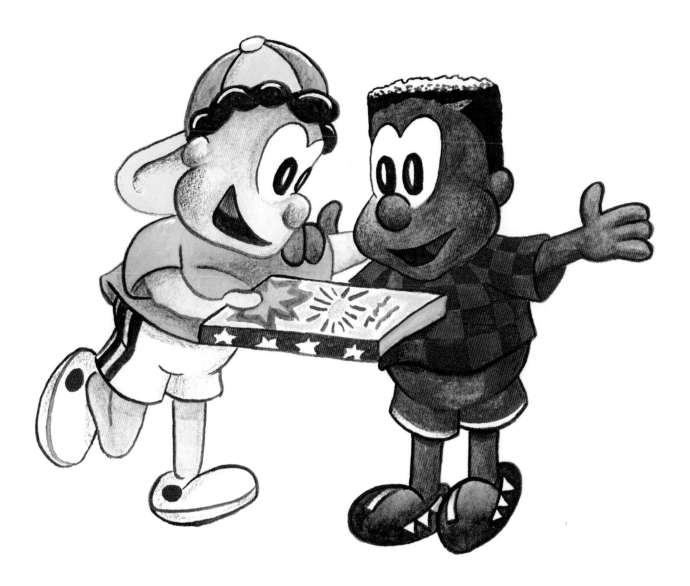

Baxter took the game to John's house. "I'm sorry I kicked the game," he said. "I didn't want to lose, but I know it was not fair to you."

"I'm sorry I called you a cheater," said John, "I still want to be your friend."

Do you think Baxter and John can still be friends? What will happen now?

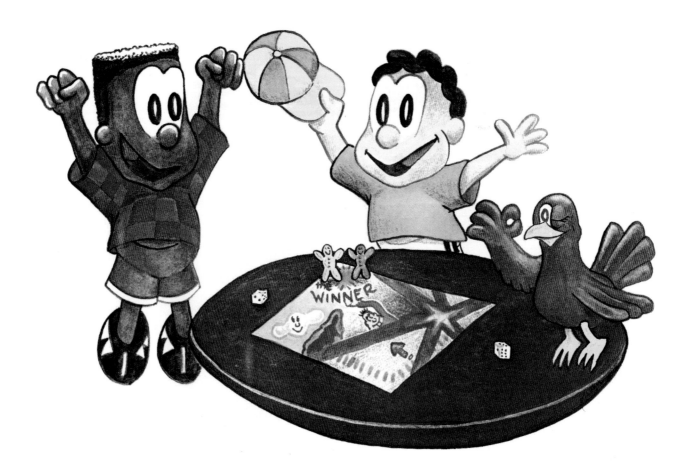

Baxter and John played the game again. They took turns. John won the first game and the second game. Baxter kept his cool, and the bird cheered him on.

Finally, in the third game, *guess what happened?* Yup, Baxter finally won.

What did Baxter learn about friendship?

Board for Baxter's Challenge Story

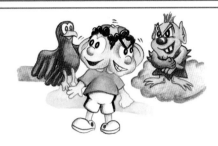

1. Here is Baxter with the bird and the troll.

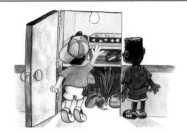

2. Baxter asked John to play a game.

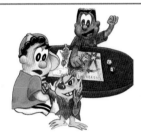

3. Baxter did not want to lose. He listened to the troll.

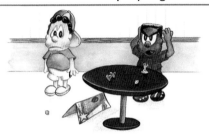

4. Baxter knocked the game down. John was mad.

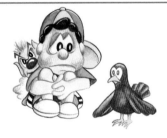

5. The troll was happy. Baxter was lonely.

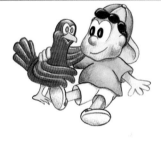

6. The bird said Baxter had a choice. Baxter chose fair play.

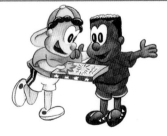

7. Baxter and John talked. They worked it out.

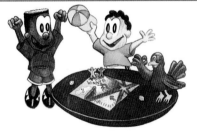

8. Baxter and John played again. Baxter played fairly and kept his cool. They had fun!

"Key Pad" for the Magic Code Game

Directions: The coach should identify a sequence of numbers that represents the Magic Code, but keep this sequence hidden from sight. The children take turns pushing the numbers on the "key pad," one by one. As long as the child is pushing the buttons in the right order (i.e., matching the Magic Code), he or she is allowed to proceed. But as soon as he or she hits a number that is in the wrong order, the coach says "beep" and it is the next person's turn. The children need to work together and watch each other. They need to learn from each person's turn, and help each other learn and remember the correct sequence. The team has won the challenge after each child has pressed the right sequence of numbers to open the box. Help from teammates is encouraged—working together is the goal of the exercise!

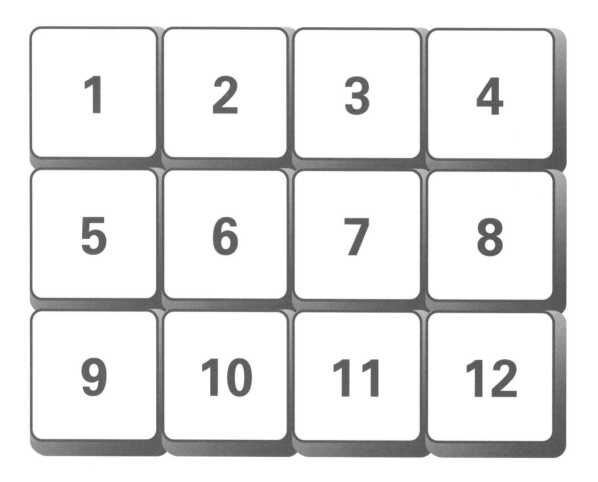

Friendship Tips Handout for Session 17

Share these **Friendship Tips** with teachers and parents who can support friendship skills at school and home. This week, Friendship Group focused on the importance of following rules in games.

Remember

If you cheat to win, it is no fun for others.

When you play by the rules, you are a fun friend.

Others enjoy playing with you.

Try It Out

When you play a game:

Try to make it fun for yourself *and* your friend.

Don't worry if you lose.

Playing fair and having fun with friends is more important than winning the game.

School and Home Check

When you played a game at school or at home:

Did you remember to follow the rules and play fairly?

Did you support your friends?

How did it work for you?

Did your friends enjoy the game?

Dear Problem Solvers Letter

Dear Problem Solvers,

I am having trouble making friends in my class. No one wants to play with me. I am really good at a lot of games. I like to choose the games, I like to go first, and I like to win. But the kids won't play with me. They say I am too bossy. I am very lonely, because I don't have any friends. What should I do?

—M.J.

Cards for the Make a Machine Game

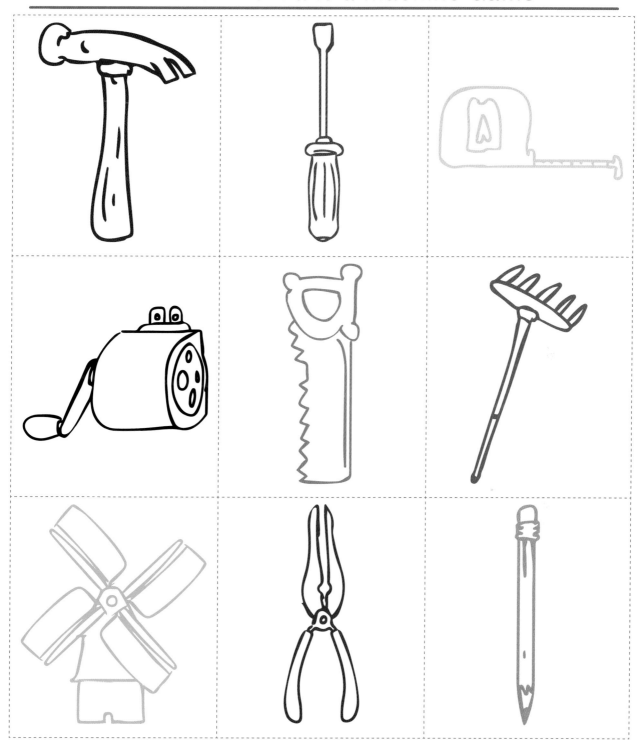

Game Rules and Fair Play Score Sheet

Game Rules

Tic-Tac-Toe

- *Preparation:* Make or use a Tic-Tac-Toe grid. Each player needs a pencil, pen, or crayon.
- *Gameplay:* The first player puts an *X* in an empty space. The second player puts a *O* in an empty space. They take turns until someone has three in a row or all nine squares are filled.
- *Winning:* Three in a row wins. If no player gets three in a row, it is a "cat game"—a tie.

Go Fish

- *Preparation:* Play with a modified deck (four suits; numbers 1–9.) Shuffle the cards, deal five to each person, and lay the rest of the pile facedown on the table.
- *Gameplay:* On each turn, a player asks another player for a specific card (e.g., "Joe, do you have any 2's?"). The partner must give the requested card(s) if he or she has it. Then the player takes another turn. If the partner does not have the card(s), the reply is "Go Fish," and the player draws a card from the pile and ends the turn. Matched pairs are placed face-up on the table.
- *Winning:* When all the cards are gone, the player with the most matched pairs wins.

Concentration

- *Preparation:* Use the modified deck. Lay the cards out in a grid.
- *Gameplay:* On each turn, a player turns over two cards. If they match, the player keeps the pair and turns over two more cards. If they do not match, the player turns the cards over again and leaves them in the grid, and it is the next player's turn.
- *Winning:* When all the cards are matched, the player with the most pairs wins.

Fair Play Score Sheet

Player 1 _____

Player 2 _____

	1	2
Taking Turns		
Following Rules		
Joining In		
Cheering for a Friend		
Respecting a Friend		

Cards for the Fair or Not Fair Game

A tall boy says: "Tallest person goes first."	At Maria's house, Maria gets to pick the games. Her friends have to do what she says.
Tom hates to lose a card game. He peeks at the cards to find the best ones.	Joe says: "Let's throw the dice. Highest number goes first."
Sasha hates to lose a game. When she loses, she says: "Rats! I hate to lose. Let's play again."	John misses the ball three times in a row. The other boy says: "Three strikes, you're out!"
Friends throw dice to see who goes first. Sam has the lowest number. "No fair," he says. "I never get to go first."	Anna is waiting in line for a turn. Another kid gets in line before her and says, "I was here first."
There are three friends, but only two cookies left. Sara says, "This one is for me."	Mark and David are playing ball. Will asks if he can play, but they say "no."

Friendship Tips Handout for Session 18

Share these **Friendship Tips** with teachers and parents who can support friendship skills at school and home. This week, Friendship Group focused on the importance of listening to everyone's ideas and points of view.

Remember

It's helpful when you share your ideas.

And it's helpful when you respect other people's ideas.

Good friends think about both points of view.

They work things out so that everyone has fun.

Try It Out

When you are making plans with others:

Give an idea and check it out with them.

Listen to their ideas.

Explain your point of view, and understand their views.

Say "yes" to good ideas.

School and Home Check

When you made plans with someone at school:

Did you share an idea and check it out with him or her?

Did you work it out and say "yes" to good ideas?

How did it work for you?

When you made plans with someone at home:

Did you share an idea and check it out with him or her?

Did you work it out and say "yes" to good ideas?

How did it work for you?

Communicating Effectively

SESSION 19. Noticing Your Friend's Feelings

GOALS

1. Introduce the idea of paying attention to your friend's feelings to prevent problems.
2. Review the importance of social awareness and communication skills.
3. Practice social awareness and communication in collaborative activities.

MATERIALS NEEDED

- Agenda Pictures: 1, 7, 3, 5, 4, 2, and 8
- Posters: Good Teamwork, Baxter's Feeling Faces, Care for Your Friends, Traffic Light, Make a Deal, Fair Play, Communication
- Baxter Story 5, "Baxter Has a Problem with His Friends" (pp. 250–256)
- Tokens or play coins (five per child)
- Pizza award and toppings (Activity Page 19.1, see p. 257; one per child), craft sticks, cotton balls, tape/glue
- Pans or pizza boxes (one per pair); red, yellow, green circles on craft sticks (one set)
- Different-colored star stickers for Hokey-Pokey Pizza (four colors, one set of four per child)
- Friendship Tips Handout for Session 19 (Activity Page 19.2, see p. 258; one copy per child)

SESSION OUTLINE

- *Friendship Circle:* Introduce communication skills with a story and poster (15 minutes)
- *Construction Station:* Partner pizza award construction communication task (10 minutes)

229

- *Snack* (optional, 15 minutes)
- *Collaboration Challenges:* Team games: Pizza Delivery Race, Hokey-Pokey Pizza (10 minutes)
- *Closing Circle:* Compliments and Friendship Tips (5 minutes)

ADVANCE PREPARATION

- Hang posters.
- Cut out the Friendship Pizza Award toppings, and make one set for each child.
- Use tape or play cones to set up a pizza delivery racecourse.
- Create "traffic signals" by taping red, yellow, and green circles on craft sticks.

DETAILED SESSION CONTENT

Friendship Circle: Introduce Communication Skills with a Story and Poster (15 Minutes)

Greet children, invite them to share their feelings, and briefly review the agenda for "Pizza Day" in Friendship Group. Introduce the idea that friendship problems can often be prevented if you pay attention to your friends' feelings and notice how your behavior is making your friend feel. Read the Baxter story, showing how it causes problems when Baxter fails to pay attention to his friends. However, when he does pay attention to his friends, he is able to change his behavior and solve the problem. The following sample dialogue introduces the idea.

> "It's great to see you all here again today. Everyone is joining in and paying attention. I can tell we're going to have a great Friendship Group today. We've been talking about how you can solve a problem with a friend. I want to talk about something a little different today, and that's how you can *prevent* problems with your friends. Does anyone know what it means to prevent something? Right, it means you notice a problem is coming and do something to keep it from happening. To prevent problems with your friends, you have to pay attention and notice how your friends are feeling. If you notice that a friend is getting upset, you can do something about it right away, and prevent a friendship problem from getting bigger."

Pull out the Communication poster and explain that communication is important to keep friendships going well and to prevent problems in friendship. Ask the children why they think the Communication poster has a picture of an ear, an eye, and a mouth. Briefly get their ideas and discuss how listening, looking, and talking help communication—how they help you know what a friend is feeling. Give an example to illustrate the concept.

> "For example, if I was playing with you, and I went like this [make a sad face], I would be communicating with you—letting you know something about my feelings. How would you know what I am feeling? [Let children respond.] Now close your eyes for a minute. See if you can tell how I am feeling by using your ears. [Call out a group member's name using a happy voice tone, then an irritable voice tone, and then a sad voice tone, each time asking children to identify your feeling.] Yes, you are guessing my feelings by using your ears and listening to the feelings in my voice."

Note that using your mouth and saying what the problem is and how you feel is also a good way to communicate with a friend. Then introduce the Baxter story and explain that they will see that Baxter gets into a problem with his friends because he forgets to communicate—he does not listen to them or look at them to see how they are feeling. Tell children that you are going to ask them for their ideas during the story, and each time you see them participating and communicating—looking, listening, and giving an idea—you will give them a token coin, which they can use later to "buy" a (pretend) set of pizza toppings for a group activity. Proceed to read the Baxter story. Try to arrange it so that each child accumulates five tokens for participation to use in the pizza-making activity, or ask the children to share so that each child has five.

Construction Station: Partner Pizza Award Construction Communication Task (10 Minutes)

This task can be done by breaking into pairs or going around the circle round robin style, as each child makes a Friendship Pizza Award for a partner. Explain that it will be like going into a pizza restaurant and "ordering" a pizza—telling the pizza maker what you want on your pizza. Ask the children, "How will you know what toppings your friend wants on his or her pizza award?" As you reflect their comments, emphasize the importance of asking questions and listening to the friend's order. Then go first to give a demonstration.

"So, watch me make a pizza award for [Name]. If you see me do something wrong, raise your hand. [Name], how many tokens do you have? OK, then you can order five toppings for your pizza. Here are the toppings you can choose. [Show the cut-out paper toppings.] Whatever you choose, I will put it on your pizza just the way you like it. What do you want first? [Let child respond.] OK, you want olives, so I am going to glue them on. Do you want them here? OK, I will put them right here. Now, I want to add some mushrooms and sausage over here, because I like them on my pizza. [Let children respond as they notice that you are not asking questions about the child's preferences but doing what you want. Let the children tell you want is wrong, but make sure that the discussion clarifies that it is the other person's pizza award, and so it needs to be made just the way the other person wants it.] Thanks for setting me straight, friends, that's how you do it!"

Proceed to let the children divide into pairs (or go round robin around the circle) and "order" their pizzas the way they want them. Provide help and guidance, as needed, to help them remember to communicate with each other during this task. Point out examples of good communication. Once the they have finished gluing the toppings onto the pizza awards to their friend's specification, give the children a chance to decorate their own certificate by adding a border of craft sticks and cotton balls. It is somewhat stressful for young children to watch someone else working with something they view as theirs (e.g., someone else making their certificate), and so giving them a chance to decorate their own certificate provides them with some closure. Encourage teamwork and the sharing of materials as the children create the certificate borders. As they are working on the borders, have each of them think of a compliment that they can give their partner, and write it on the certificate.

Snack (Optional, 15 Minutes)

The usual procedures are followed. If it is possible to provide a pizza-themed snack, it is a fun addition to this session.

Collaboration Challenges: Pizza Delivery Race and Hokey-Pokey Pizza (15 Minutes)

To play the game Pizza Delivery Race, coaches use tape (or cones) to mark a "delivery course" that the children will follow as they deliver their pizzas. As they travel each leg of their journey, the coach will hold up signs to show whether they can go fast (green), slowly with caution (yellow), or if they must stop for traffic (red). The children race in dyads: First, partner 1 races the delivery course while partner 2 watches for the speed signal, and then partner 2 races the delivery course while partner 1 watches for the speed signal. If they go too fast on a yellow light or fail to stop for the red light, they have to start the course over again. To meet the challenge, both partners must get around the course correctly, following the traffic signals. If desired, give each pair a small stack of pie pans or pieces of cardboard to carry aloft, representing the pizzas they are delivering. Explain the game, while demonstrating:

> "This is Pizza Delivery Race. You will work with a partner to deliver pizzas, and you must travel along this course to deliver them. While one partner takes this course, the other one needs to watch for the traffic signals. If the signal is green, you can move ahead at a normal speed, like this. [Demonstrate traffic light and speed.] If the signal is yellow, it is a caution, and you must move slowly, like this. If there is a red light, you have to stop until the light changes. If you don't follow the traffic signals, you have to start the course over again. Your challenge is to get both partners around the course without a traffic violation."

Have the children discuss what they will need to do in order to succeed at this challenge—for example: "What will the partner watching the traffic signals need to do? What will the partner carrying the pizzas need to do?" As you reflect on the children's answers, emphasize the importance of communication in winning this race. During the race, praise their communication efforts.

> "Wow, that was terrific. You did a great job with the Pizza Delivery Race. I really liked the way you remembered to communicate during this game. I also liked the way that all of you joined in and helped your friends—that made it fun for everyone."

If time allows, proceed to play "Hokey-Pokey Pizza." Place a sticker on the players' hands and feet to represent pizza toppings. For example, each child gets a gold star on the right hand to represent the cheese, a red star on the left hand to represent the pepperoni, a green star on the right foot to represent the green pepper, and a silver (or blue) star on the left foot to represent mushroom. (Any color–topping combination works). Directions are as follows.

> "For this game, I need everyone to stand in a circle and put their right hand in the middle. I am putting a gold star on each of your right hands, which stands for 'extra cheese.' When we play the game and I tell you to 'put your extra cheese into the middle of the circle,' you will put this hand—your right hand—with the gold star in the middle."

Continue in a similar fashion to have the children put their other hand and each of their feet into the circle to get the star sticker, and to hear what topping the sticker represents.

> "This game is a lot like the Hokey-Pokey. Who has played that before? We are going to make a Hokey-Pokey Pizza. Listen carefully, and see if you can figure out how to play."

Proceed to sing the "Hokey-Pokey" song; however, instead of the usual words involving body parts (e.g., you put your left hand in, you put your left hand out), the coach uses pizza topping labels, as follows: "You put your extra cheese in, you put your extra cheese out, you put your extra cheese in and you shake it all about. You do some pizza dancing and you turn yourself around, that's what it's all about." Most children are familiar with the Hokey-Pokey and catch on to this scheme pretty quickly. Some children will need help to remember which color star represents which pizza topping. Encourage children to help each other with this part. Then, repeat with the other verses, putting in the pepperoni, the chili pepper, and the mushroom.

If children seem ready, move on to the challenge version of this game: Hold the Toppings Hokey-Pokey Pizza. In this challenge, children must inhibit their first response and "hold" the topping called out by the leader, putting in a different topping instead. In other words, in the challenge version, they have to put in any topping *except* what the leader calls. When the leader calls "hold the extra cheese," children can put in pepperoni, mushroom, or chili peppers.

> "That was fun, and it seemed pretty easy for you. I wonder if you are ready for the Hold the Toppings Hokey-Pokey Pizza game? This is very tricky, so I am curious to see if you can do it. Here is the challenge: You have to 'hold the topping' that I call out. That means, you don't put in the topping that I call out, but you put in some other topping instead. For example, if I say 'Now hold the extra cheese,' you have to hold back on your extra cheese—don't put in your extra cheese. What could you put in?"

Walk through this example, and a few more as needed, until children have the idea. Once they can do it in a walk-through, try it with the song and faster rhythm: "Hold the extra cheese in, hold the extra cheese out, hold the extra cheese in, and shake the others all about. You do some pizza dancing and you turn yourself around, that's what it's all about." Provide help and support, as needed. You can also make this game play fun by commenting on the children's choices, such as "You remembered to hold the pepperoni! You two put on cheese, and [Name] put on mushrooms."

Closing Circle (5 Minutes)

To add novelty to the compliment routine (if desired), pass out folded pictures of the different pizza toppings. One by one, call out a topping name (or pick a topping picture out of a hat) and ask the child with the matching topping to share his or her favorite part of the session and get compliments. Give each child a turn and distribute Friendship Tips Handout for Session 19.

SPECIAL ISSUES

1. Most children prefer to make their own awards. However, making the award for someone else requires more communication. For this reason it is important to maintain the challenge as described here, emphasizing to the children that it is a Friendship Group challenge to see how well they can communicate with their friends.

2. Look for opportunities to comment aloud when you notice that children are communicating with their facial expressions or voice tone.

SESSION 20. Attending to Body Language

GOALS

1. Introduce the concept of body language as a form of communication.
2. Practice communication skills and listening skills.
3. Practice self-control in social collaboration challenges.

MATERIALS NEEDED

- Agenda Pictures: 1, 3, 5, 4, 2, and 8
- Posters: Good Teamwork, Baxter's Feeling Faces, Care for Your Friends, Traffic Light, Make a Deal, Fair Play, Communication
- Pictures in a box (Activity Page 20.1, see p. 259; one set per group)
- Puzzle Challenge answer keys, blank grids (Activity Page 20.2, see p. 260; one per child), poker chips
- Mazes (Activity Page 20.3, see pp. 261–262; one per child), blindfold
- Leader Hat, any materials needed for choice of games
- Friendship Tips Handout for Session 20 (Activity Page 20.4, see p. 263; one per child)

SESSION OUTLINE

- *Friendship Circle:* Role play, What's in the Box? communication game (15 minutes)
- *Construction Station:* Partner puzzle and blindfold maze challenges (15 minutes)
- *Snack* (optional, 15 minutes)
- *Collaboration Challenges:* Head-Shoulders-Knees-Toes Mix-Up, game choice (10 minutes)
- *Closing Circle:* Compliments and Friendship Tips (5 minutes)

ADVANCE PREPARATION

- Hang posters.
- Cut out the pictures and put them in a box for What's in the Box? charades.

DETAILED SESSION CONTENT

Friendship Circle: Role-play, What's in the Box? Charades (15 Minutes)

Following the usual routine, greet children, share feelings, and briefly review the agenda. Find out who remembers what the ear, eye, and mouth stand for in the Communication poster. Then introduce the idea that you can often tell how someone is feeling by watching how he or she looks and acts—even if no words are exchanged. Engage children in a coach's role play to illustrate the concepts. Here is a sample dialogue:

"Sometimes you can tell how your friend is feeling by watching his or her body language. What is body language? [Let children respond.] Right, it is when we use our bodies—our faces and our actions—to show our feelings, without using words. I'm going to show you some body language. Watch carefully and raise your hand when you know what I'm telling you with my body language. This is a note from someone I work with."

Open a note and start reading it silently. Look surprised. Wait for a raised hand and let children guess how you feel. Explain: "He says he is angry with me. I'm surprised to hear that." Then read some more and look guilty. Wait for a raised hand and children's input. Then explain:

"You are right, I feel bad because I said I would go to a movie with him. But I forgot and I went with someone else. I'm going to call him tonight and say that I'm sorry I forgot. I'll explain it was just a mistake and see if he will do something else with me. Meanwhile, I'm impressed that you could read my body language. How could you tell what I was feeling?"

Explain that you are going to play a game that will challenge the children to read each other's body language. To play this game of "What's in the Box?" charades, you pass around a box with cards in it to music. When the music stops, the person who has the box draws a card (without showing it to anyone else) and enacts the action in the picture (without any talking). Group members try to guess what action the child is showing (e.g., licking an ice cream cone, shooting a basket). Once someone in the group has made a correct guess, the child can show the picture to the group. Continue until each child has had one or two turns. Ask the children to reflect on what they had to do to figure out what was on the cards, and emphasize how they paid attention to their friends' body language to solve the challenge.

Construction Station: Partner Puzzle and Blindfold Maze Challenges (15 Minutes)

Partner Puzzle Challenge

In this activity, children work in dyads or triads. One child (the Helper) is given a Puzzle Challenge answer key, which shows three colored poker chips placed in different places on a 3×3 grid. The other child (the player) is given a blank grid and poker chips. Explain the nature of the challenge as follows.

"You will take turns being the player and the helper. [Name], you are the first player. You get this chart [blank grid] and these chips. Your challenge is to put each color chip in the correct square of the chart in order to solve the puzzle. [Name] is going to be your helper. He will have the answer key, so he knows where each shape goes. Here is the challenge. Your helper cannot use words to help you, and he cannot touch the puzzle pieces. He can only use body language to help you figure out where each shape goes."

Before they begin the game, encourage the children to talk with each other about how they are going to approach this challenge. Young children will often find it challenging to stay in a passive role and may want to move the pieces themselves, or show the partner the answer key. If needed, remind them that they can Take 5 and use the Make a Deal poster steps to plan the way that they will work together on this task. Only if needed, model how the Player can put a piece on the grid and ask the helper if it is correct, getting a nod or head shake in return. However, do not provide this modeling unless the children are unable to generate strategies for working together themselves. Once the player is finished, he or she can look at the answer key and check the answer. Then the children should reverse roles and try a new puzzle.

Blindfold Drawing Challenge

In this activity, children work in dyads or triads to complete simple mazes while blindfolded. Explain that the next task requires children to work together when they can't use body language—something that is quite challenging. One child is blindfolded and must rely on his or her partner's verbal directions in order to complete a maze.

> "You did a great job working together as a team on those puzzles. You really paid attention to your partner and used body language to communicate—that was nice teamwork! Now I have a different kind of challenge for you. In this challenge, you will have to communicate without any body language, because one of you will be blindfolded. The player who is blindfolded will have to ask the helper a lot of questions, and the helper will have to give directions to help the player complete the maze."

You will need to help the children plan for this task and then complete it, providing active structure to make sure the helper(s) are providing appropriate assistance. First, both children get to look at a maze sheet and run their finger through the maze. Then one child is blindfolded and must use a pencil to complete the maze. The other child, who is the helper, gives directions such as "Go straight," "Stop here," "Go up." The helper cannot touch the pencil, the paper, or the friend, only give directions verbally. The blindfolded child must work slowly and listen to the partner's directions. After completing the maze, the children switch places, and the other is blindfolded and they repeat the process. It is important to engage children in pre-activity planning and postactivity reflection in order to draw their attention to the strategies that might (or did) help them succeed at the challenge. For example, after each task, ask the children: "How did you do with that challenge?"; "What kind of help did you need from your friend?"; "What did you do to help your friend?" Praise them for listening and helping each other.

Snack (Optional, 15 Minutes)

The usual procedures are followed.

Collaborative Challenges: Head-Shoulders-Knees-Toes Mix-Up, Choice of Games (10 Minutes)

Have children stand where they can see you and where they have some room to move.

> "Today we are going to play a game called Head-Shoulders-Knees-Toes Mix-Up. I've got my Leader Hat on facing forward, so you copy just what I do. First, I touch my head. Now, I touch my toes. [Repeat these two actions a few times as the children imitate your movement.] Now

I'm turning my Leader Hat backwards. We're going to mix it up, and your challenge is to do the *opposite* of what I say. When I say 'Touch your head,' you should touch your toes. When I say 'Touch your toes,' you should touch your head. So you're doing something backwards from what I say. [Repeat these two actions a few times as the children practice doing the opposite.] OK, I'm turning my Leader Hat forward again. Now you just copy me. I'm touching my shoulders, so you touch your shoulders. Next, I'm touching my knees, so you do the same. [Repeat these two actions several times, mixing up the order, allowing the children to practice imitating you.] Now, get ready, because I'm turning my Leader Hat backwards. It is time for a backwards mix-up, so you're going to do the *opposite* of what I say. I say to touch your knees, so you touch your shoulders. [Repeat with reminders to help the children respond accurately.] Now I say touch your shoulders, so you touch your knees. Remember, you do the *opposite* of what I say."

Repeat these steps a number of times in random order, so children can practice doing the opposite of knees versus shoulders. Their goal is to ignore the impulse to copy you and instead do the opposite motion. This is challenging for young children. If the group has mastered these actions, there is an added level of difficulty you can ask them to try, as follows.

"OK, I think you are ready for the really big challenge. I still have my Leader Hat on backwards, so everything I do, you need to do backwards. There are four things I could say: If I say to touch your head, you touch your toes. If I say to touch your toes, you touch your head. If I say to touch your knees, you touch your shoulders. If I say to touch your shoulders, you touch your knees. Are you ready? Let's try it."

Give the children a series of these to try, mixing up the order of the callouts. Start slowly, so they have time to self-correct. As they get more comfortable with the game, try speeding up the cycle. If a child wants to be leader, and there is time, give him or her that chance. As you finish the game, praise the children for their great listening skills. If time allows, give them a choice of games.

Closing Circle: Compliments and Friendship Tips (5 Minutes)

In your closing comments and compliments, emphasize the communication skills your observed. Let children share compliments and then distribute Friendship Tips Handout for Session 20.

SPECIAL ISSUES

1. In the blindfold tasks, in particular, children may need explicit modeling and directions concerning the ways in which they can give their partners helpful advice and support. This task utilizes perspective-taking skills as well as practice in communication. Some children may need you to explain that pointing doesn't help because a blindfolded person can't see, but can hear.

2. Some children will not want to be blindfolded. Alternatives include pulling a knit hat down over the eyes, holding hands over the eyes, or simply closing the eyes. Cheating may become an issue, so the coach will want to be prepared to use the social problem-solving steps to negotiate the rules regarding "peeking," helping the group decide how to handle the mild violation.

SESSION 21. Asking Questions

GOALS

1. Discuss strategies for making new friends.

2. Reflect on cause–effect relationship between one's own behavior and others' feelings.

3. Practice asking questions, conversation skills, and group problem solving.

MATERIALS NEEDED

- Agenda Pictures: 1, 7, 3, 5, 4, 2, and 8

- Posters: Good Teamwork, Baxter's Feeling Faces, Care for Your Friends, Traffic Light, Make a Deal, Fair Play, Communication

- Cards for Question Ball and 20 Questions (Activity Pages 21.1 and 21.2, see pp. 273 and 274; one set per group)

- Baxter Story #6: "Baxter Makes a New Friend"

- Climb the Ladder Score Sheet and question cards (Activity Pages 21.3 and 21.4, see pp. 275 and 276; one each per child)

- Stickers, blocks, and tape measure

- Friendship Tips Handout for Session 21 (Activity Page 21.5, see p. 277; one per child)

SESSION OUTLINE

- *Friendship Circle:* Asking questions with Question Ball and 20 Questions (15 minutes)

- *Construction Station:* Social entry, Baxter Story #6 and Climb the Ladder game (15 minutes)

- *Snack* (optional, 15 minutes)

- *Collaborative Challenges:* Block Tower Challenge (10 minutes)

- *Closing Circle:* Compliments and Friendship Tips (5 minutes)

ADVANCE PREPARATION

- Hang posters.
- Cut out the cards for the Question Ball and 20 Questions games.
- Cut out the cards (if you choose to use them) for the Climb the Ladder activity.

DETAILED SESSION CONTENT

Friendship Circle: Asking Questions with Question Ball and 20 Questions (15 Minutes)

Greet the children, share feelings, and provide brief agenda review. Then introduce the session's topic of questions:

> "Last session, we talked about how important it is to pay attention to your friend's feelings. One way you can find out more about your friend's thoughts and feelings is by asking questions. Today I have a game that makes asking questions a lot of fun!"

Explain that in this game, Question Ball, children pass a ball around the circle while music plays. When the music stops, whoever is holding the ball draws a card. (As you explain what to do, demonstrate by taking the first turn.) Each card lists a category, such as "Things you do after school" and "Games." (Note that adults will need to help children read these cards.) The child who drew the card rolls the ball to someone in the circle and asks that child a question about the category noted on the card—for example: "What do you like to do after school?" or "What is your favorite game?" The child who receives the ball must answer the question to stay in the game. Then that child rolls the ball to someone else and asks a question about that same category or calls for the music. In the latter case, the music starts again, and children pass the ball around the circle until the music stops and a new category card is selected.

If the children in your group find this task easy, add a challenge. For each question category, ask them to extend the number of "turns" before choosing a new category, and see how many different questions they can ask within each category. For example, in response to the category card "Games," the first child might ask, "What is your favorite game?," the next child might ask, "What game do you like to play outside?," and the next child might ask, "What game don't you like?" The goal of this activity is to help children generate questions in common areas of conversational discourse. After a few rounds, or as child interest in this activity wanes, move on to the next game of 20 Questions.

In this version of 20 Questions, the person who is "it" draws a card with a picture on it without showing it to the other children (see Activity Page 21.2). The other children take turns (going around the circle) asking questions to try to guess the object on the card. This is a new game for most young children, and they may need some adult help. Coaches can suggest a few good questions—for example: "Is it alive?"; " Is it big or small?" Coaches may also need to help the child with the card, to make sure he or she answers the questions correctly. After a few rounds of this game, coaches can praise the children for their attention, excellent question asking, and teamwork.

If an active break is desired before continuing with the discussion of Baxter Story #6, this is a good time to replay the Head-Shoulders-Knees-Toes Mix-Up game introduced in Session 20. This game gets easier and more enjoyable for children after they practice it a few times.

Construction Station: Social Entry, Baxter Story #6, and Climb the Ladder Game (15 Minutes)

The story "Baxter Makes a New Friend" illustrates the dangers of intrusive social behavior and the value of using questions to start a conversation and gain social entry. In this story, Baxter moves to a new school. At first, his efforts to make friends are intrusive. With the help of the bird, he learns to pay attention to how other children feel and begins a conversation to make a new friend. If desired, you can give children the score sheet for the Climb the Ladder game to color while you read and discuss the story. Some children are better able to listen when they have something to do with their hands. A sample wording for how to introduce the story follows.

> "Today I have a new story about our friend Baxter. Do you remember him? This story is about a time Baxter moved to a new school and wanted to make a new friend. I want you to see if you can tell how he felt when he arrived at the new school. He made a few mistakes when he first tried to make friends, and I'd like to see if you can spot what went wrong for him. In the end, he finally figured out a way to make a new friend. I'll be interested to see if you can tell how he did it. After the story, we are going to play a game called Climb the Ladder. If you want, you can color your ladder while you listen."

Read through the story with the children, using the embedded questions to engage them in the storytelling and discuss their ideas about making new friends. Help children understand the story by asking them about Baxter's feelings at various points in time, what he tried to do, how the other children felt, what happened then, and so on. The goal is to foster the children's perspective-taking skills (i.e., the ability to recognize and understand the thoughts and feelings of others); their understanding of cause–effect relationships in interpersonal interactions (i.e., in Baxter's case, understanding how certain things he did led to poor outcomes, whereas other things he did led to good outcomes); and their recognition of the importance of asking questions, sharing information, and listening to others when making friends.

Following the story, you can ask children to generate ideas about things they could tell or ask others in order to make new friends, and then introduce the Climb the Ladder to Friendship activity. This game can be played in two ways to serve different purposes. (1) It can provide a scaffold to help children role-play the process of making friends themselves. To use it in this way, review the steps for friendship making written on each step in the ladder. Then, give each child a turn to role-play the process, pretending that he or she is meeting a new friend. You can give them a star sticker to put on each step in the ladder that they remembered to include in their role play. Alternatively, (2) the ladder activity can be played using the cards. This version of the activity adds an element of additional skill difficulty, as the cards present a range of more challenging friendship situations that require perspective taking and sensitivity. To use the cards, have children take turns drawing cards and giving answers. Each time a child can answer the question on his or her own card, or offer an additional response to the card someone else drew, he or she earn a star sticker to add to the steps of their ladder.

Snack (Optional, 15 Minutes)

The usual procedures are followed.

To provide them with an opportunity to practice conversation skills, encourage the children to share information, ask others questions, and listen to what their friends have to say. To support this natural conversation, suggest topics that they might talk about—for example: interesting experiences they had in the past week; plans they have for the coming week; something they are looking forward to; something coming up that they are worried about; things they did with a friend during the past week or things they are hoping to do with a friend in the coming week; and so on.

Collaborative Challenges: Block Tower Challenge (10 Minutes)

This challenge involves cooperative block building and provides practice in problem-solving skills and planning. Children work in dyads or triads.

> "I brought a special challenge for the group today, and I wonder if you are ready for it. The challenge is to see if you can make a plan and work together to build a very tall tower with these blocks. To meet the challenge, we need to build one that is _____ tall."

Choose a height that seems reasonable, given the size of blocks available to the children. The goal height should be a challenge, but not an unattainable one. Indicate with a tape measure just how high you'd like the group to aim. Depending upon children's responses, you can raise or lower the standard until they feel comfortably challenged by the task.

> "Now, this is not going to be easy, and you probably won't be able to get it this high the very first time you try. But you'll get a second try after that. So here's what I'd like you to try. While you are building the tower the first time, take the time to notice what your friends do. You might really like some of the things they do because they are very helpful for building a tall tower. You might see a friend do something else that you think is not helpful. If you don't meet the challenge the first time, you'll be able to talk about what you and your friends can change the second time to make it a little taller."

Ask the children to make a plan for how they want to approach the task before you give them the blocks. Once they have a plan, let them start building. If they are successful at meeting the standard, ask them to comment on what they did that worked so well. If they are not successful, ask them to share their feelings about things that could be done differently and help them come up with an improved building plan. Then let them try again.

Closing Circle: Compliments and Friendship Tips (5 Minutes)

Following the usual procedures, finish with a compliment circle and distribution of the Friendship Tips handout for this session.

SPECIAL ISSUES

1. It may be useful to use a less-than-bouncy ball for the Question Ball activity.

2. The 20 Questions game may be difficult for some children. Be prepared to give concrete prompts, such as "You need to find out if it is an animal or a thing." Ask, "Is it an animal?"

3. Cooperative block building can be a challenge because some children prefer to make their own structures and resist involvement, whereas others dominate the task without involving others. If needed, consider (a) providing a recognition award or prize for pairs who achieve a certain height, or (b) allowing children to build something on their own after they achieve their group goal. In addition, prompt group communication and problem-solving efforts among the group members.

SESSION 22. Listening

GOALS

1. Introduce and discuss good listening skills.

2. Reflect on the role of listening skills in friendship and problem solving.

3. Practice listening skills in collaborative activities.

MATERIALS NEEDED

- Agenda Pictures: 1, 3, 5, 4, 2, and 8

- Posters: Good Teamwork, Baxter's Feeling Faces, Care for Your Friends, Traffic Light, Make a Deal, Fair Play, Communication

- Follow the Leader Friendship Awards (Activity Page 22.1, see p. 278; one per child), star stickers, markers, clipboards (one per child)

- Hat with poker chips (two colors, one per child)

- Land Your Plane Safely (Activity Page 22.2, see p. 279; one blank and one map per child)

- Marshmallows and uncooked spaghetti for cooperative bridge construction

- Friendship Tips Handout for Session 22 (Activity Page 22.3, see p. 280; one per child)

SESSION OUTLINE

- *Friendship Circle:* Listening skills demonstration, Time Beaters Challenge (10 minutes)

- *Construction Station:* Follow the Leader and Land Your Plane Safely games (15 minutes)

- *Snack* (optional, 15 minutes)

- *Collaborative Challenges:* Team construction, marshmallow and spaghetti bridge (15 minutes)

- *Closing Circle:* Round robin compliments and Friendship Tips (5 minutes)

ADVANCE PREPARATION

- Hang posters.

- Put two colors of poker chips in a hat, with one chip for each child.

- Copy Land Your Plane Safely pages and create varied maps for the control tower.

DETAILED SESSION CONTENT

Friendship Circle: Listening Skills Demonstration, Double Time Beaters Challenge (10 Minutes)

Greet children, share feelings, and briefly review the agenda. Tell them that you are going to ask someone a question, and you want him or her to watch you as you listen to the answer. Ask the children, "Who can think of a special day when they did something really fun?" Let children respond. "OK, [Name], please tell me all about what you did on this special day." As the child tells you about the day, listen for a minute, and then start to rustle around in your seat, as if trying to get more comfortable; look distracted and avoid eye contact with the speaker. When the child stops talking, ask the group, "How did I do as a listener?" Let the children tell you what you did wrong as a listener, and what you should have done. In the course of the discussion, summarize the advice the children give to highlight good listening skills: (1) Look at the person, (2) be quiet when he or she is talking, and (3) pay attention to what he or she says. If desired, write these three guidelines on a flip chart. Then, tell them you are going to try out these ideas, and ask another child to tell you about their special day. Listen carefully, and when the child is done, ask the group how you did. Ask them to consider the listening skills (did you look at the person, were you quiet when they were talking, did you pay attention to what they said.) Then, proceed to introduce a listening problem you had with a co-worker. (If you have a co-leader, do this as a role play; if you are a single leader, explain what happened when you were planning with a coworker and describe both points of view.)

> "[Co-leader's Name] and I had a problem the other day that I'd like to tell you about. Maybe you can give us advice. [Co-leader's Name] came to my house to plan our session and choose games for today. I told her that we were going to play a Follow the Leader game, and I would show her how to do it. But, she wanted to do something else. I explained that, since we were at my house, we were going to do things my way."

Next, the co-leader should explain his or her point of view, as follows.

> "We were at [Coach's Name's] house, but I didn't think that I should have to do everything his way. I wanted to give my ideas too. But, he did not listen to me. I did not have much fun, and I don't think it was fair. We want to know what you think."

Facilitate a discussion among the children about what is unfair in this situation, and what fair alternatives are possible. Often, children will immediately respond by saying that the coach should let the co-leader choose as well. Encourage children to think through the problem by challenging this response—for example: "Well, I had really thought about it a lot, and I felt that the Follow the Leader game was the right game for us to play. So I did not want to spend our time doing other things. And it seems like I should decide what we do when we are in my house." The goal is to encourage the children to think through the challenge of dealing with strong personal preferences, in order to listen and accommodate the preferences of another. The goal is to help the children put their ideas into words and draw connections with their own lives. To extend the conversation, ask if they have faced a similar situation when they had a friend play at their house (or when they played at a friend's house), how it felt, and how it was resolved. As you summarize, emphasize the points the children made regarding the importance of listening to a friend and taking the friend's perspective into account.

At the end of this discussion, introduce a brief group challenge activity called Double-Time Beaters, which requires controlling and shifting the pace of a beat, thereby exercising inhibitory control and attention set-shifting skills. In this activity, children pick one of two different-colored poker chips from a hat (e.g., red and white). Children who choose white chips are going to be the Beaters, and they will make a beat (clap hands) to a slow, steady rhythm (e.g., equivalent to quarter-note beats). Children who choose red chips are going to be the Double-Time Beaters, and they will make a beat (clap hands) to a double-time rhythm (e.g., equivalent to eighth-note beats—such that they clap twice for every one time the other group beats). To teach children this game, lead each group separately at first.

> "Everyone with red chips is going to be a 'Beater' and clap a beat like this. [Illustrate a slow, steady beat, let the children on the white team join in, and then stop.] Everyone with white chips is going to be a 'Double-Time Beaters' and clap a beat like this. [Illustrate a beat that is twice as fast as the first group, let the children on the red team join in, and then stop.] OK, now here is our challenge. We have to put those beats together. [Start out with the Beaters doing a slow, steady beat, and then have the Double-Time Beaters join in. If you have two coaches, each one should lead a group. Then let children switch team and try playing the other role.]"

Construction Station: Follow the Leader and Land Your Plane Safely Games (15 Minutes)

Follow the Leader Certificate Decoration

For the next task, each child should have a Friendship Award, which presents an array of shapes on it, a page of star stickers (four different colors), and four different-colored crayons. Each child will have a chance to be the leader. The leader should be seated back-to-back from the other three children, with his or her own table or clipboard. The leader gets to put one sticker on his or her Friendship Award and color one shape (e.g., putting a red sticker on the triangle at the top of the page and coloring the heart red). The other children should be at another table or with their own clipboards, seated so that they cannot see what the leader is doing. As the leader does something, he or she describes it to the other three children, and their challenge is to listen carefully and do the exact same things on their awards. That is, they have to copy the leader—but without looking. The children can ask questions, and the leader should try to answer the questions as well as he or she can. The goal is to practice listening and effective communication skills. When everyone is done, the children can turn around and compare what they did with the leader's work. Each child takes a turn as leader, adding cumulatively to the Friendship Award. At the end of the session, children take the final awards home.

To introduce this game, take the role of leader and demonstrate how to explain where you are placing your sticker and what you are coloring. This task is quite difficult for younger children, so it is helpful for them to see a demonstration as well as hear your directions. After you have demonstrated, you can ask the following questions to help them plan how they will approach the task: "What does the leader need to do to make sure everyone can copy him or her? What do the followers need to do to make sure they follow the leader correctly? How can you help each other?" Following each leadership turn, have the children discuss what they did to help them make a good copy of the leader's award, and what happened that led them to make a mistake. If they had difficulties, have them think of ideas that might help them succeed on the next turn. When children have finished the challenge, let them add a few final decorations of their own choice to their awards.

Listen and Land Your Plane Safely Game

To prepare for this task, create a "map" for each child to guide the "control tower" by drawing a line that goes from the plane in the upper corner through different pathways around the birds, tress, and buildings to arrive at the landing strip in the lower corner of the page. To play, children divide into pairs or triads. One child (the pilot) is given a map showing an airplane and several obstacles. The other child (the "control tower") has a map showing the safe route for the plane to land. The children must be separated so they can hear each other, but the "pilot" cannot see the map in the hands of the control tower. The control tower gives directions (e.g., "First, go straight ahead and over the top of the fireworks. Then go down between the fireworks and the bird"). The pilot uses a pencil to follow the directions. To draw the correct, safe route for the plane, the pilot must listen carefully to the directions given by the control tower, and then check it out with the control tower (e.g., "OK, I go straight ahead over the clouds, right?"). When the plane is safely "down," the pilot can check the plane's "route" with the map of the control tower to see if he or she made it down correctly. Let children reverse roles and try it again.

Snack (Optional, 10 Minutes)

The usual procedures are followed. Encourage children to share information about themselves, ask others questions, and listen to what they had to say. To support natural conversation among group, introduce topics such as plans they have for the coming week, something they are looking forward to, something coming up that they are worried about, things they did with a friend during the past week, or things they are hoping to do with a friend in the coming week. The goal is to use snack time to practice the conversation skills targeted in the program in the context of naturalistic interaction.

Collaborative Challenges: Team Construction, Marshmallow and Spaghetti Bridge (15 Minutes)

In this task, children construct bridges together using marshmallows and uncooked spaghetti. Split the children into groups of two or three before starting this activity. Each team is given 10 minutes to build the highest structure in the room or the widest bridge or tallest arch. Teams build by sticking the raw, uncooked spaghetti sticks into marshmallows. In order to foster productive communication, make it clear that the members of each team must work together to build one structure, and include a planning discussion before the building starts. Without these supports, children will often start building by themselves. Encourage them to talk with each other and make plans about how they will approach the task and help each other before they start building. As they build, praise good teamwork and communication. If they start to have difficulties, ask them to talk about what they are doing that is working (and not working) for them. If they get frustrated, remind them to use the Traffic Light steps to calm down and think about how to solve the problem. At the end, ask them what they did to communicate effectively and work together successfully.

Closing Circle: Round Robin Compliments (5 Minutes)

For the round robin compliment process, ask the child sitting next to you to identify his or her favorite game during the session. Then give that child a compliment and ask him or her to turn to the next child in the circle and repeat the process (e.g., ask about a favorite game and give a compliment). Once the circle is completed, distribute Friendship Tips.

SPECIAL ISSUES

1. The Follow the Leader certificate decoration can be difficult because it requires children to inhibit their desire to decorate their award in their own way. Instead, they have to listen carefully, communicate clearly, and follow the leader. If they complain about this task, explain that this is the way the team challenge works. It is a challenge because you have to listen to the leader. You can also let them know that, at the end of the team challenge, they will have an opportunity to add a decoration or two of their own choosing.

2. The marshmallow bridge-building task requires verbal skills for planning and problem-solving skills. If you feel that this task will be too difficult for children in your group, choose a game or activity used earlier in the program and repeat it for skill practice.

SESSION 23. Working Collaboratively

GOALS

1. Review the communications skills that were a focus of this unit.
2. Provide practice in the communication skills in a variety of activities.

MATERIALS NEEDED

- Agenda Pictures: 1, 3, 5, 4, 2, and 8
- Posters: Good Teamwork, Baxter's Feeling Faces, Care for Your Friends, Traffic Light, Make a Deal, Fair Play, Communication
- Friendship Bingo cards for interview game (Activity Page 23.1, see pp. 281–282; one card per child)
- Bandanas or strips of cloth for pirate headwear, clues for treasure hunt
- Maze forms, several blank and several with answer keys (Activity Page 23.2, see p. 283)
- Newspaper and tape for cooperative tower construction
- Sharing snacks in plastic bags (e.g., crackers and peanut butter, raisins, peanuts, Cheerios, chocolate chips)—optional
- Pieces of paper in a hat (or cup); one with *captain* written on it
- Friendship Tips Handout for Session 23 (Activity Page 23.3, see p. 284; one per child)

SESSION OUTLINE

- *Friendship Circle:* Friendship Bingo, pirate treasure hunt (15 minutes)
- *Construction Station:* Collaborative mazes (10 minutes)
- *Snack:* Negotiation snack (optional, 15 minutes)
- *Collaborative Challenges:* Team construction, pirate lookout tower (15 minutes)
- *Closing Circle:* Pirate captain, compliments, and Friendship Tips (5 minutes)

ADVANCE PREPARATION

- Hide a pirate headband (bandana, strip of cloth) for each child around the room.
- Write a clue for each headband (e.g., "Look below a window and behind a can").
- Create an answer key on a maze form, showing the secret pathway through the maze.

DETAILED SESSION CONTENT

Friendship Circle: Friendship Bingo, Pirate Treasure Hunt (15 Minutes)

Greet children, invite them to share feelings, and briefly review the agenda. Explain that today is Pirate Day in Friendship Group, and the children are going on a treasure hunt to find their pirate headbands. However, first they have to earn their treasure hunt clues.

Show them the Friendship Bingo game cards. Depending upon the verbal skills of the children in your group, you might want to let each child complete his or her own card (for children with more well-developed verbal skills), or have the children work in pairs to complete their cards (for children with less well-developed verbal skills). To play this game, children take turns asking each other about categories on their Bingo card (e.g., "Who likes to play soccer?") and writing down the initials of children who agree. Note that some children will need an adult to help them with the reading. The goal is to get a Bingo "blackout"—finding one or more children in the group who fit in each square of their cards. Once the children have completed their cards, they each receive a clue that will lead him or her to the pirate bandanna. Along with the clue, you can support children's search for the treasure by noting when they are getting "warmer" or "colder." Once they have found the headbands, you can tie them on, pirate-style.

Construction Station: Collaborative Mazes (10 Minutes)

Before the session, create a secret pathway through the maze form with a marker. This pathway should start at the bottom, move through the squares in the middle, and end at the top. If you want to play the game multiple times, draw several different pathways on several different maze forms to serve as the answer keys. These are for you to refer to as you play the game; do not show them to the children. Explain to the children that the pirates have set up booby traps on their island to keep strangers away. The team's challenge is to figure out the right way through a maze on the island that avoids the booby traps. As a group, the children are presented with one blank copy of the maze form (without the secret pathway showing). Each child is given a "token" to move through the maze (e.g., a game piece or penny). To find the right way through the maze, the children take turns. One at a time, they move a token onto one block in the maze. If their choice is correct, they get to move a second time. If their choice is incorrect, you give them a signal (a beep) to indicate a false move. After a false move, the next child in the circle takes a turn. If the children work together and pay attention to each other, they can learn from each other's trial-and-error mistakes to master the maze. This game challenges children to focus on the group, regulate their behavior, attend to every player's actions, and support each other. If your space allows, consider making the maze with carpet squares or colored paper taped to the floor and letting children find the way through by taking turns walking through the maze.

As the children contemplate the task, encourage them to talk about ways that they can help each other with the challenge. Use specific praise and reflective comments to support good team-work and effective collaboration during this task. When the children are successful, ask them what they are doing to help themselves solve the maze. If desired, let the children try a second maze. Encourage them to discuss what they learned from their first experience, and to make plans for working together as a group the second time.

Snack: Negotiation Snack (Optional, 15 Minutes)

Explain that the pirates gathered different supplies on their travels across the sea. Pull out snack materials that are in separate clear plastic bags (e.g., raisins, peanuts, Cheerios, chocolate chips). Explain that each pirate is going to get some crackers and peanut butter, and each is going to get one "treasure bag" of toppings to share with the group. They are going to need to bargain with the other pirates to agree on a method to share the toppings and make sure every pirate gets his or her fair share. If needed, review the steps of the Traffic Light and Make a Deal posters to remind them of the steps they can use to make a plan together. During this process, support the children in the problem-solving and negotiation process.

Collaborative Challenges: Team Construction, Pirate Lookout Tower (15 Minutes)

This task requires group planning, communication, and problem-solving skills, as well as frustration tolerance. If this kind of task has been challenging for your group in prior sessions, consider having them work in pairs. If you think they are ready for the challenge, ask them to work as a single team in this session. Explain that the pirates want to protect the treasure they have placed on this island. They need to build a tall watchtower, so that they can see anybody who tries to sail to their island. The team has 10 minutes to build the highest tower they can out of newspapers and tape. Before the children begin to build, encourage them to share ideas about how they can build a tall tower and work together. This preplay discussion is particularly important, because once children have materials in their hands, they will often start building by themselves rather than working as a team. Encourage them to talk about how they want to approach the task, and how they will help each other before they start building. As they build, praise good teamwork and communication. If they start to have difficulties, ask them to review what they are doing that is working for them, and what they are doing that is not working very well. If they become frustrated, encourage them to follow the Traffic Light steps, "Take 5" to calm down, and Make a Deal about how to solve the problem. As they finish the task, ask them to talk about what they did to communicate effectively and work together success-fully. Let them know that they have successfully protected the treasure!

Closing Circle: Find the Pirate Captain and Closing Compliments (10 Minutes)

If time allows, Find the Pirate Captain is a group game that fits thematically with this session and offers a novel structure for compliments. To play this game, one child is declared the "finder." The others draw a folded piece of paper from a hat; one paper has the word *captain* written on it. While the finder closes his or her eyes, the others show their papers, so everyone else knows who is cap-tain. The group then begins to copy the captain, who does repetitive clapping and body motions that change occasionally (e.g., clapping hands, patting knees) The finder tries to guess which child is the captain that everyone else is copying. Once the child guesses correctly, he or she receives compliments from the coaches and peers. The game continues until everyone has been the finder. Distribute Friendship Tips Handout for Session 23.

SPECIAL ISSUES

1. This session builds upon the previous sessions that target communication and collaboration skills. If your group has struggled with the collaboration activities in the prior sessions, you can reduce the level of demand by providing more direction or having children work in pairs. In general, planning and collaborating with a partner is easier than with a group, so working in pairs simplifies the task. However, children who have progressed well through these activities are ready for the challenge of problem solving in a larger group. Positive support, emotion coaching, and reminders to follow the Traffic Light steps for problem solving will help children master these skills. The goal is to set the demands at a level that challenges children's skill development, but still keeps them engaged and motivated.

2. The purpose of the pirate theme is to add fun. If children do not want to be pirates, do not force the issue. If children escalate into play pirate fighting, remind them that these pirates are in hiding, so they must stay calm and quiet in order to build their tower together and keep safe.

Baxter Has a Problem with His Friends

Text by Karen L. Bierman   Illustrations by Andrew Heckathorne

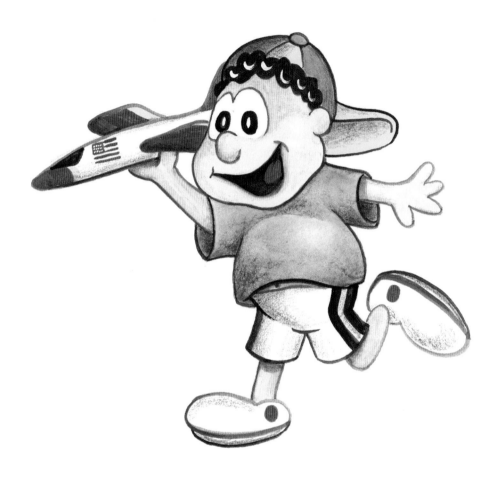

One morning, Baxter was walking to his classroom. He was thinking about the kids in his room and hoping they would notice him. He had an idea! "Wait till the kids see what I have here," he thought. "This will really surprise them." As quietly as he could, Baxter slipped into the classroom and began to sneak up behind a group of kids.

What is Baxter going to do?

(page 1 of 7)

From *Social and Emotional Skills Training for Children* by Karen L. Bierman, Mark T. Greenberg, John D. Coie, Kenneth A. Dodge, John E. Lochman, and Robert J. McMahon. Copyright © 2017 The Guilford Press. Permission to photocopy this material is granted to purchasers of this book for personal use or use with students (see copyright page for details). Purchasers can download additional copies of this material (see the box at the end of the table of contents).

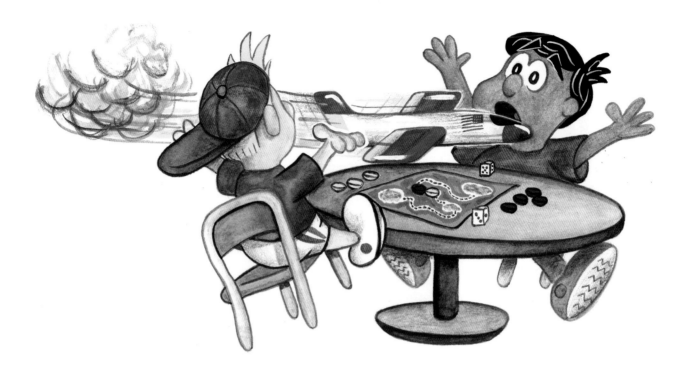

"HEY, EVERYONE!" Baxter shouted suddenly, holding his airplane up high in the air. "AIRPLANE COMING!" No one looked at Baxter's plane. No one said "Hi" to Baxter. They just played their game. "Here it comes," shouted Baxter, "It's going to crash!" and Baxter slid the airplane onto the table, scattering the pieces of the game everywhere.

How do the kids feel about that? What's going to happen next?

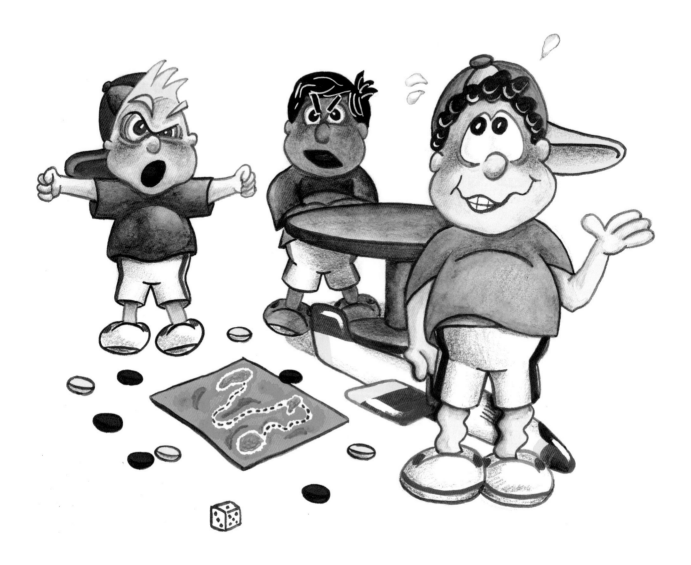

Now the kids looked at Baxter, and they were mad. "BAXTER!" Billy and David yelled together. "You ruined our game," said Billy. "I'm sorry," said Baxter, "I didn't mean to spill it. I just wanted to show you my airplane."

"We don't care about your plane," said David, "Just leave us alone." Then the kids turned their backs and started to pick up their game. Baxter ran to his desk and put down his head. No one cared about him or his plane.

How does Baxter feel? What went wrong?

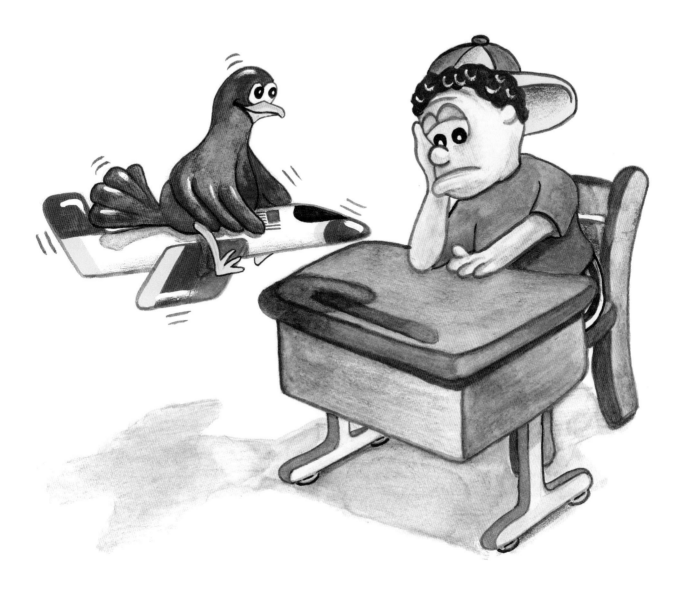

Baxter sat at his desk trying not to cry. He heard a gentle voice inside his head.

"What happened?" asked the bird. "I tried to make friends today, bird, but no one liked my plane," Baxter answered. "They told me to leave them alone. They don't like me, Bird, and I don't like them." "I see," said the bird. "That is a problem. What about your balloon?" the bird asked.

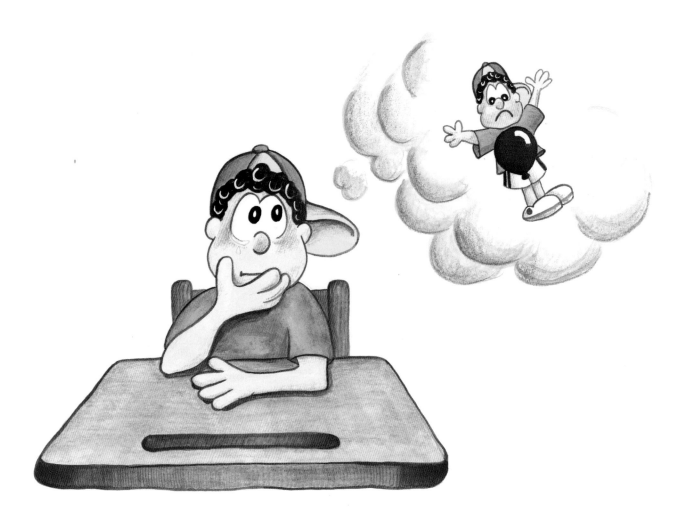

"It's full," gulped Baxter, "very full and about to burst." "What should you do, Baxter?" asked the bird. Baxter took a long deep breath. He felt a little calmer. He took another breath. "I'll talk to them," said Baxter.

What should Baxter say to the other children?

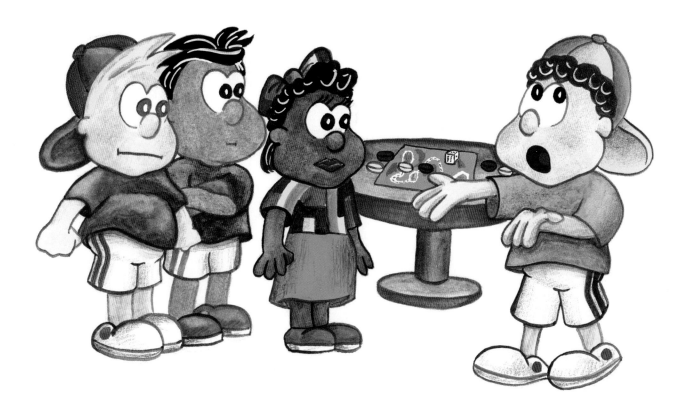

Baxter walked to the back of the room. The kids were getting ready to play the game again. "I'm sorry about the game. I didn't mean to bump it—honest," said Baxter. "You barged in," said David, "You weren't careful." "I just wanted to show you my airplane," explained Baxter. "Next time, you have to wait," said Tasha. "OK," said Baxter, "Can I play the winner when you're done?"

What will the kids say?

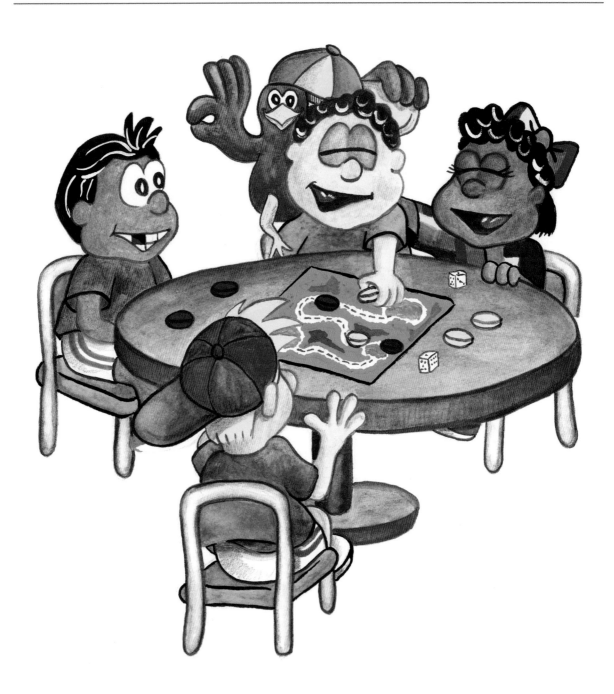

Baxter waited, and when it was his turn, he joined the game. He heard the bird whisper gently in his mind. "You did that well, Baxter. You calmed down, you told your classmates your feelings, and you paid attention to your friends. You had a problem, but you worked it out."

What did Baxter learn?

Pizza Toppings and Friendship Pizza Award

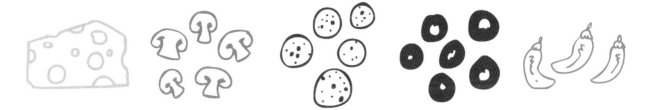

Friendship Pizza Award

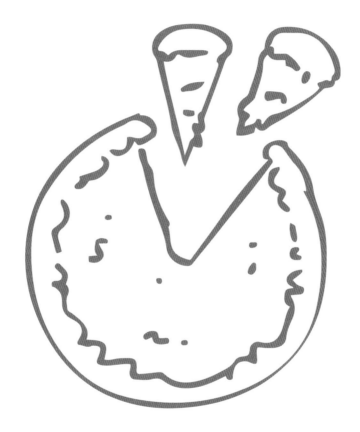

To: _____   From: _____

You are a good friend.

Friendship Tips Handout for Session 19

Share these **Friendship Tips** with teachers and parents who can support friendship skills at school and home. This week, Friendship Group focused on preventing friendship problems by paying attention to your friend's feelings.

Remember

It is important to look and see how your friends are feeling, and listen to hear what your friends have to say.

If there is a problem, use your words to say the problem and how you feel.

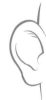 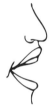

Try It Out

See if you can tell how people feel by:

    The look on their face

    The sound of their voice

    The things that they say

School and Home Check

Think about a time when your behavior affected someone's feelings:

    How did you notice the person's feelings?

    How did your behavior make him or her feel?

    Did you take action to prevent a problem?

    Did you do something to strengthen your friendship?

What's in the Box? Charades

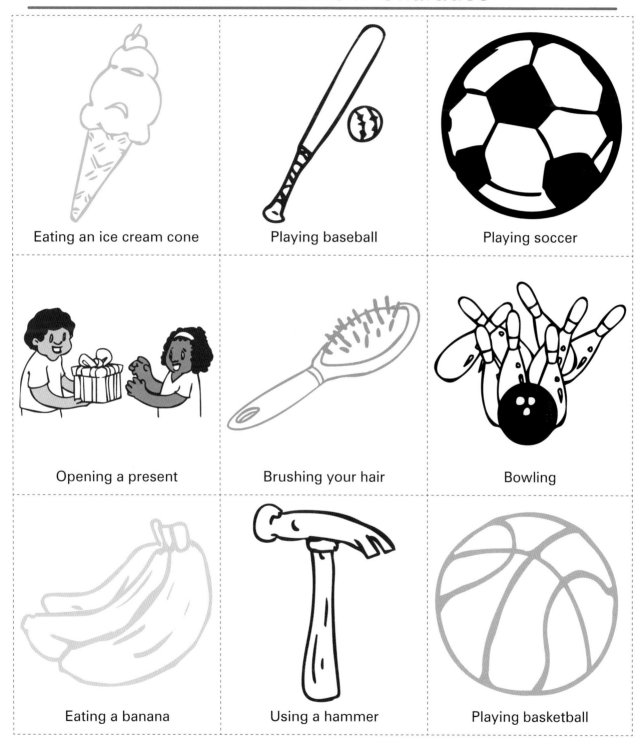

Eating an ice cream cone	Playing baseball	Playing soccer
Opening a present	Brushing your hair	Bowling
Eating a banana	Using a hammer	Playing basketball

Puzzle Challenge Answer Keys and Blank Play Sheet

Puzzle Challenge Answer Key 1

●	●	○
○	●	●

Puzzle Challenge Answer Key 2

●		●
	○	
●		●

Puzzle Challenge Blank Play Sheet

Maze 1

Maze 2

Friendship Tips Handout for Session 20

Share these **Friendship Tips** with teachers and parents who can support friendship skills at school and home. This week, Friendship Group focused on reading body language and nonverbal communication skills.

Remember

People communicate by the way their face looks, and by the way their body moves.

You are a good communicator when you look and listen, and also when you use your words.

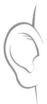 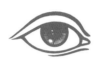 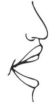

Try It Out

Take time to notice how your friend feels by:

  The look on his or her face

  The sound of his or her voice

  The things that he or she says to you

School and Home Check

See if you can say or do something that makes someone else feel better. What can you do to:

  Make someone smile?

  Show someone you are his or her friend?

  Make someone feel happy?

Baxter Makes a New Friend

Text by Karen L. Bierman   Illustrations by Andy Heckathorne

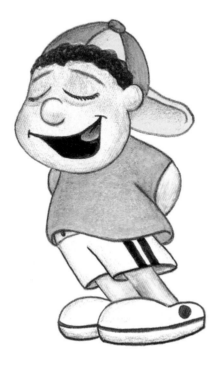

Over the summer, Baxter's family moved. Now he's going to a new school. He doesn't know what it will be like. He hopes he'll find a friend, but he's worried—what if the kids are mean? How will he make friends?

Have you ever felt like that?

(page 1 of 9)

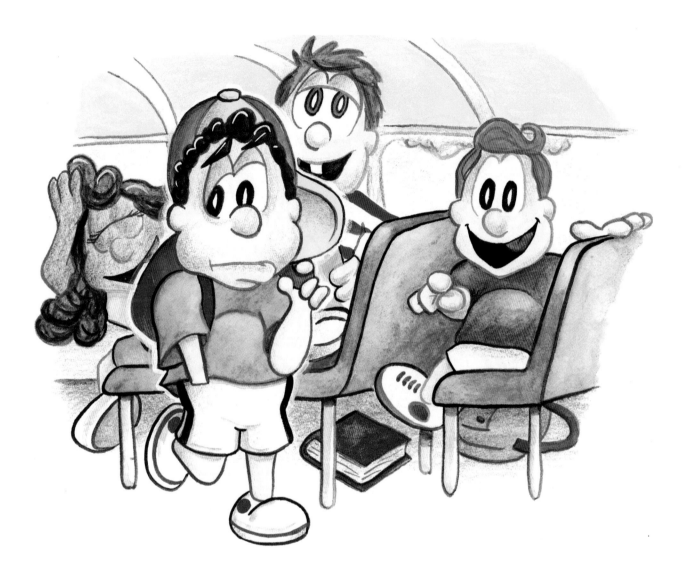

On the first day of school, Baxter saw the bus coming. It was full of kids laughing and talking, but Baxter didn't see anyone he knew. He forgot to look where he was going and he tripped over a backpack. Someone giggled. Baxter found an empty seat and hid his head.

How does Baxter feel? Why did someone giggle? Why did Baxter hide his head?

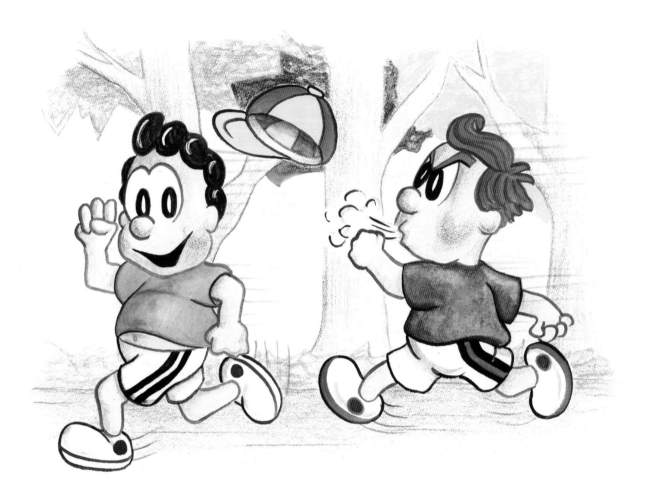

Baxter hid all the way to school. Then he thought, "I should show these kids what I can do." He tagged the boy next to him. "Wanna race?" he asked, "I can beat you." And fast as he could, Baxter ran toward the school. "Hey, slowpoke, I beat you!" Baxter called. "So what!" said the kid as he turned his back and walked away.

Why did Baxter race the other kid? How does the other kid feel? What went wrong for Baxter?

266

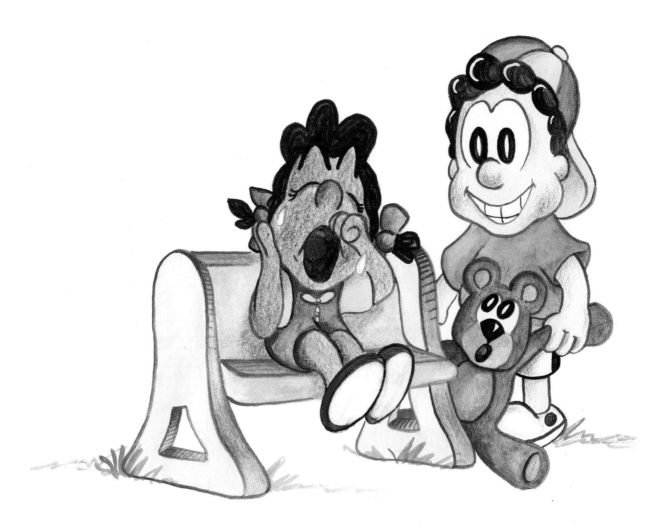

Baxter looked around the playground for a friend and saw a girl sitting on a bench. Baxter ran up to her and grabbed the bear. "I've got your bear," he called, "try to get it."

Why did Baxter grab the girl's bear? How does she feel?

The girl began to cry. Baxter threw her bear back. "It was just a joke," he thought, "doesn't anybody at this school know how to joke?"

Why didn't the girl like Baxter's joke? What will happen to Baxter now?

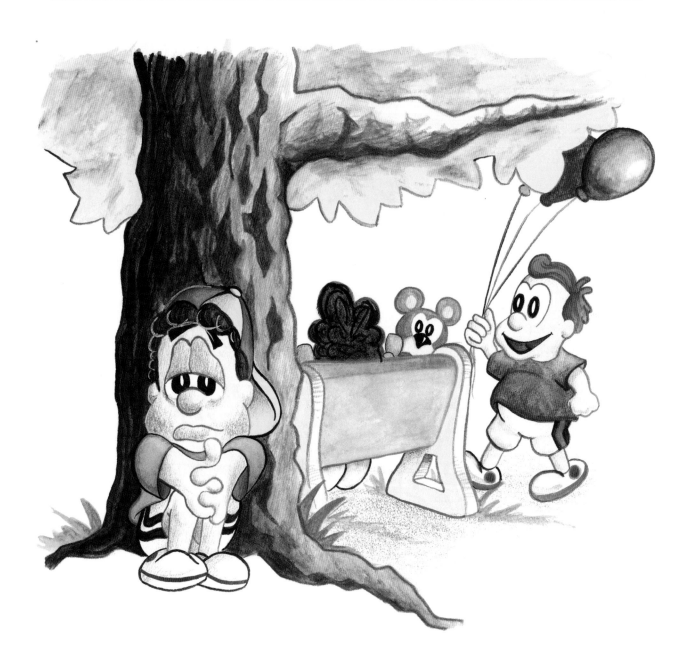

Baxter sat down and watched the kids playing around him. "I'll never fit in here," he thought, "They'll never like me."

How does Baxter feel? What is his problem?

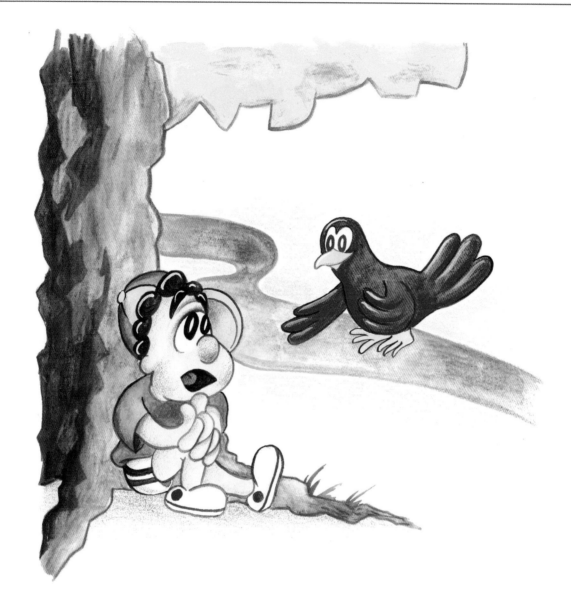

Baxter heard a familiar voice in his mind.

Who was it? What will the bird do?

"Oh, Bird," sighed Baxter. "I tried to make a new friend, but no one here likes me.

"Well," said the bird, "perhaps you're not trying the right way."

What does the bird mean? What is Baxter doing wrong?

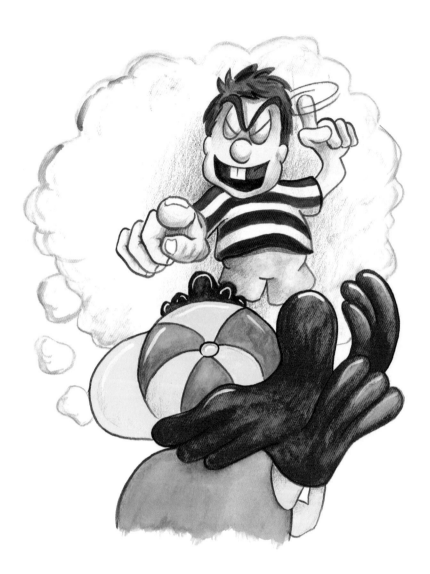

"What if a new kid called you a 'slowpoke' or took something from you—how would you feel?" asked the bird. "Well," said Baxter thoughtfully. "I'd think they were a big show-off." "Try this," suggested the bird. "Think about how you wish someone would treat you."

How does Baxter want to be treated? What should he do?

"I wish someone would come up to me and say 'Hi' and ask my name," said Baxter. "Try doing that yourself," suggested the bird.

Will it work? What will happen?

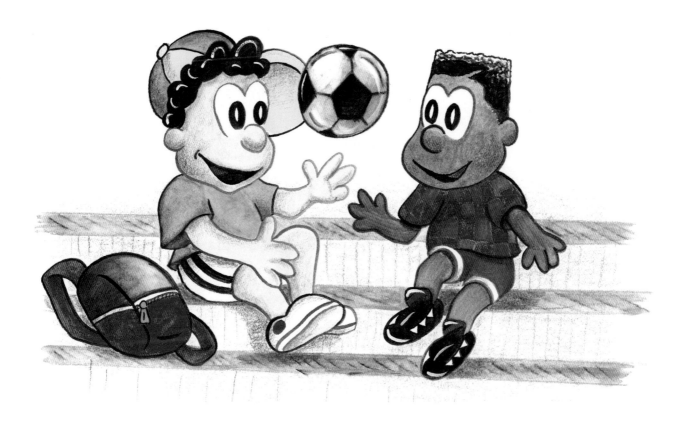

Baxter saw a boy and walked over to him. "Hi, my name's Baxter. What's your name?" "John," said the boy. "Who's your teacher?" asked Baxter. "Mrs. Smith." "Me too," said Baxter. "We're in the same class!" Baxter and John talked for a while. They sat together at lunch. At recess, they played ball.

How did Baxter make friends with John? What did he do to make John like him?

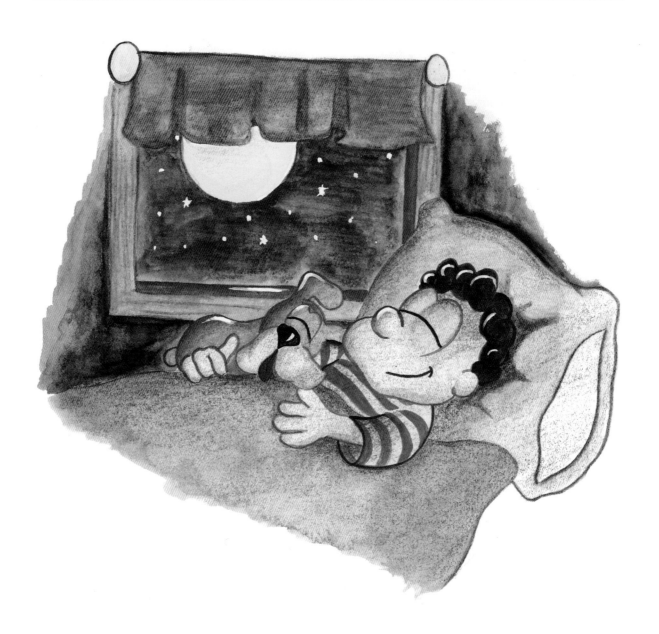

At the end of the day, Baxter lay in his bed thinking about his new friend John. "I guess making friends is not too hard," he thought, "as long as I remember to treat others the way I want them to treat me." Baxter fell asleep and had good dreams all night long.

What did Baxter learn?

Cards for the Question Ball Game

Things you do after school	Games
Things that scare you	Things you are excited about
Things on TV	Music
The weather	Sports
Pets	Food
Party	School

Cards for the 20 Questions Game

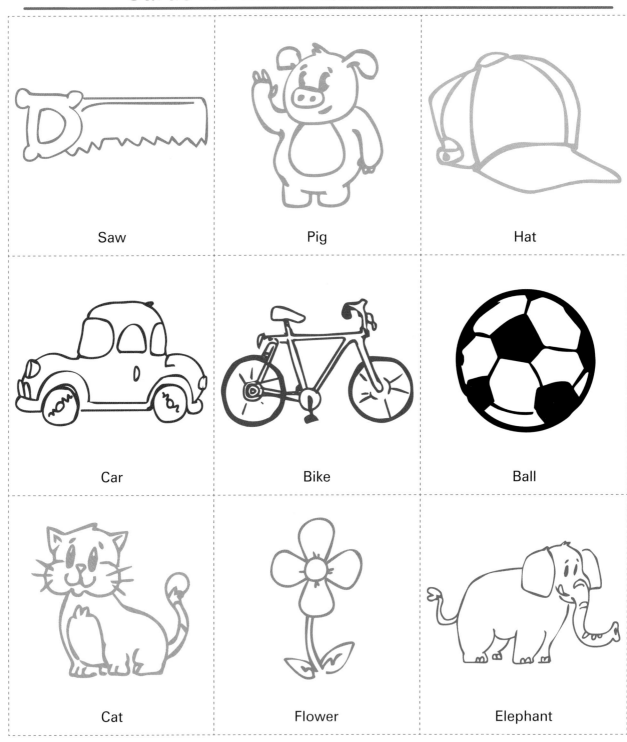

Saw	Pig	Hat
Car	Bike	Ball
Cat	Flower	Elephant

Score Sheet for the
Climb the Ladder to Friendship Game

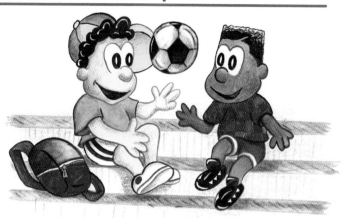

Step 6: Keep the conversation going.

Step 5: Invite the other person to play.

Step 4: Ask about the other person.

Step 3: Tell about you.

Step 2: Ask his or her name.

Step 1: Introduce yourself to someone.

Cards for the Climb the Ladder Game

It is your first day in a new school. Show us how you would introduce yourself to another student in your classroom.	Choose a partner. Tell this partner your favorite game and find out what game he or she likes best.
You see a new kid on your bus. Show us how you would find out his or her name.	Find out if anyone in the group has a dog and a cat.
Tell us three things you could tell someone about yourself, to help that person get to know you.	You want to introduce your friend to your cousin. Tell us what you would say.
A group of children is playing ball, and you want to join. What would you say to those kids?	A friend gets a new hat and asks if you like it. You don't like it, but you don't want to hurt your friend's feelings. What could you say?
You meet a new boy on the playground. You introduce yourself and he tells you his name. What can you say next?	You tell a new friend that you like to play soccer. She says that she likes to play soccer too. What could you say next?
By accident, you run into a girl on the playground and knock her over. What should you say?	Two children are playing with the ball. You ask if you can play too, but they say "no." What do you say?
You are waiting at your bus stop in the morning. Your friend comes to wait for the bus too. Tell us what you say to your friend.	Your friend asks you to play at her house. But you are going to play with a different friend. What do you say?

Friendship Tips Handout for Session 21

Share these **Friendship Tips** with teachers and parents who can support friendship skills at school and home. This week, Friendship Group focused on asking questions and making new friends.

Remember

The ladder to friendship:

1. *Introduce yourself to someone.*
2. *Ask his or her name.*
3. *Tell about you.*
4. *Ask about the other person.*
5. *Invite the other person to do something.*
6. *Keep the conversation going.*

Try It Out

Try starting a conversation with someone.

Keep the conversation going.

Tell about you, and ask about the other person.

School and Home Check

Find a time that you can make a new friend, or get to know someone better.

Start a conversation.

Invite him or her to do something with you.

Tell us how it worked out.

Friendship Award

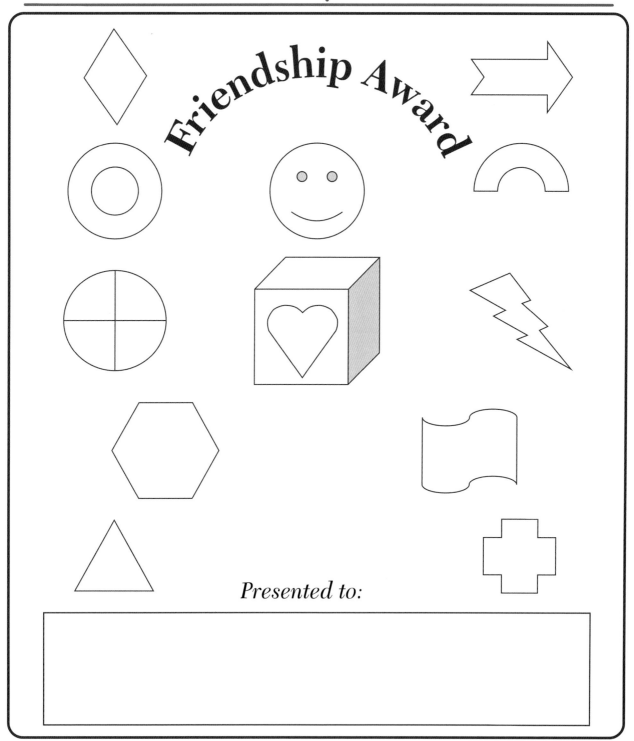

Friendship Award

Presented to:

Listen and Land Your Plane Safely

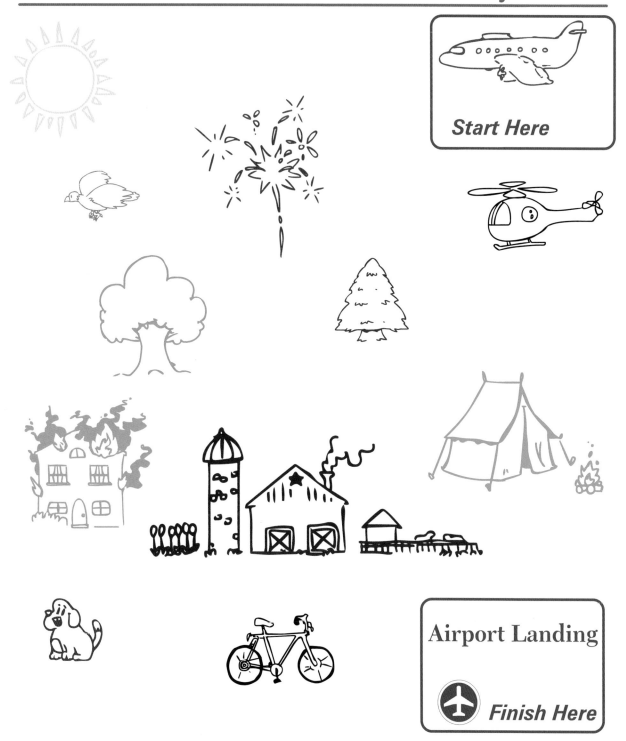

Start Here

Airport Landing

Finish Here

Friendship Tips Handout for Session 22

Share these **Friendship Tips** with teachers and parents who can support friendship skills at school and home. This week, Friendship Group focused on reading body language and nonverbal communication skills.

Remember

To be a good listener:

1. *Look at the person who is talking.*
2. *Be quiet when he or she is talking.*
3. *Pay attention to what he or she says.*

Try It Out

Try using your good listening skills.

How does it feel?

How do others look and feel when you listen to them?

School and Home Check

See how many times you can use good listening skills this week. Try listening carefully:

To your friend.

To your teacher.

To your parent.

How did it work?

Cards for Friendship Bingo

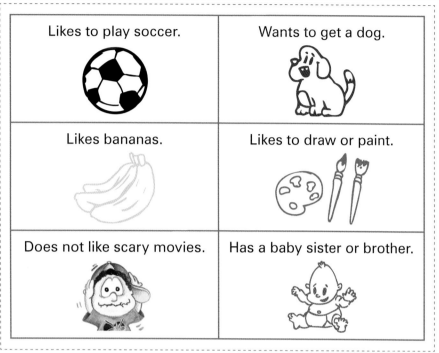

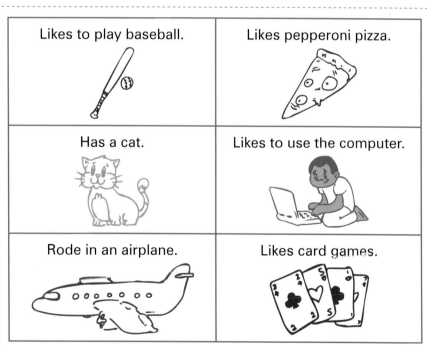

(page 1 of 2)

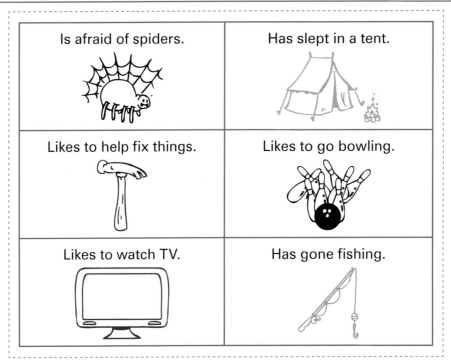

Is afraid of spiders.	Has slept in a tent.
Likes to help fix things.	Likes to go bowling.
Likes to watch TV.	Has gone fishing.

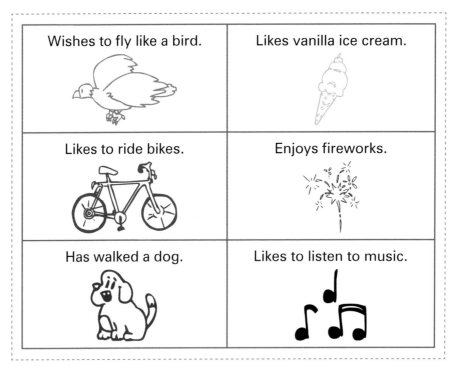

Wishes to fly like a bird.	Likes vanilla ice cream.
Likes to ride bikes.	Enjoys fireworks.
Has walked a dog.	Likes to listen to music.

Maze Form

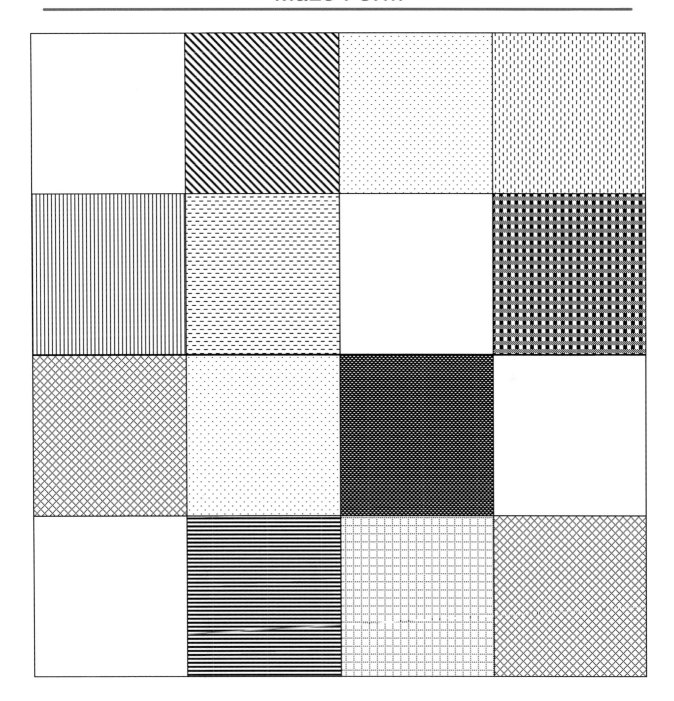

Friendship Tips Handout for Session 23

Share these **Friendship Tips** with teachers and parents who can support friendship skills at school and home. This week, Friendship Group focused on reading body language and non-verbal communication skills.

Remember

A good communicator:

Joins in and tells about him- or herself.

Ask questions and learns about others.

Shares feelings.

Gives ideas for how to solve problems.

Says "yes" to good ideas.

Try It Out

Try out your communication skills.

You will make friends.

You will have fun.

You will learn new things.

You will help solve problems.

School and Home Check

See if you can start a conversation with someone and keep it going.

　　What did you learn?

　　How did it feel?

See if you can help solve a problem and make a plan.

　　What did you do?

　　How did it feel?

Coping with Tough Stuff

SESSION 24. Coping with Provocation or Bullying

GOALS

1. Discuss the problem of bullying and different ways to respond.
2. Identify effective strategies to cope with different kinds of bullying.
3. Practice communication and negotiation skills in collaborative challenges.

MATERIALS NEEDED

- Agenda Pictures: 1, 7, 3, 5, 4, 2, and 8
- Posters: Good Teamwork, Baxter's Feeling Faces, Care for Your Friends, Traffic Light, Make a Deal, Fair Play, Communication
- Baxter Story 7, "Baxter Faces a Bully" (pp. 298–305)
- Array of small objects on a tray, along with a towel, for Bug in a Rug game
- Keep Your Cool game board and question cards (Activity Pages 24.1 and 24.2, see pp. 306 and 307; one per dyad/triad)
- Negotiation snack items (optional)
- Carpet squares or colored paper for All Aboard
- Button on a string, Friendship Tips Handout for Session 24 (Activity Page 24.3, see p. 308; one per child)

SESSION OUTLINE

- *Friendship Circle:* "Baxter Faces a Bully" story, Bug in a Rug team game (15 minutes)
- *Construction Station:* Keep Your Cool game and discussion (10 minutes)
- *Snack:* Negotiation snack (optional, 15 minutes)

- *Collaborative Challenges:* Friendship Charades, All Aboard Challenge (15 minutes)
- *Closing Circle:* Button, Button, Who's Got the Button?, compliments, and tips (5 minutes)

ADVANCE PREPARATION

- Hang posters.
- Set up items on the tray for the Bug in the Rug game.
- Cut out the cards for the Keep Your Cool game.

DETAILED SESSION CONTENT

Friendship Circle: "Baxter Faces a Bully" Story, Bug in a Rug Team Game (15 Minutes)

Greet children, invite them to share feelings, and briefly review the session agenda. Next, present the Baxter story, as follows:

> "You remember Baxter, right? Today I brought a story about a very difficult problem that Baxter had. Someone at school was being mean to him and he had to figure out what to do about it. Some of his ideas didn't work very well. While you're listening, see if you can figure out how Baxter tried to solve his problem and what solution finally worked."

During and after the story, encourage discussion that focuses children on the salient events, helps them think about Baxter's feelings and motivations, and helps them follow the cause–effect sequences in the story—for example: "How is Baxter feeling now?"; "Why did he take the little boy's cookies?"; "What will happen next?" In addition, explore the children's personal impressions, experiences, and opinions—for example: "Has something like this happened to you?"; "What would you do?"; "What should Baxter do now?" Some children may disagree with Baxter's solution, or say that they would use aggression to protect themselves. If so, respond with care. Bullying can be very difficult to handle effectively, and so it is important to empower children to use problem solving and to think about their various options, rather than relying on one solution. The goal is not to tell them what to do in a situation like this, but rather to help them *think through* their options. You should avoid taking the stance that fighting is never an appropriate response to provocation (there may be times when children have to defend themselves). On the other hand, you want to empower children to think first (rather than retaliate first), encouraging them to consider other alternative responses to provocation that may be more effective and more self-protective than fighting. In these discussions, the coach can refer back to Baxter—for example: "When Baxter tried to fight someone, he ended up in trouble with the bus driver. Fighting at school can get you into trouble"; or "Baxter thought about punching Bugsy, just like you're suggesting, but Bugsy was bigger than him. He thought he'd get hurt. So he tried to outsmart Bugsy, didn't he? He figured out a way to use his head to fight back instead of using his fists."

Next, play the Bug in a Rug game, which provides an activity break. Children sit in a circle and a tray of objects is placed in the middle of the circle. One child is designated as the "hider" and another as the "seeker." All children have a chance to study the objects on the tray. Then the tray is covered and removed from the circle. Out of eyesight from the others, the hider removes an object from under the covered tray and wraps it in a hand towel. Then the tray is placed back in the middle, and everyone chants: "Bug in the rug, bug in the rug, what is that bug in the rug?" This is the signal to remove the cover, so that the seeker can study the objects on the tray and guess which object has been removed and hidden in the towel (e.g., the rug). After a guess is offered, the object is revealed. The cycle is repeated, with new children assigned to the roles of hiders and seekers, until all children have had a turn. The difficulty level can be adjusted by adding (or subtracting) items and shifting their locations over time.

Construction Station: Keep Your Cool Game and Discussion (10 Minutes)

The Keep Your Cool game provides children with opportunities to practice good teamwork and talk with each other about staying calm and coping effectively with provocation. It works best to have children divide into dyads or triads, each getting a game board, pair of dice, and two pennies for markers. One coach should help each small group. Coaches will need to read the cards if the children do not yet read. The directions are as follows:

> "Here is how you play this game. First, you each shake the dice, and the child with the highest score goes first. When it is your turn, you shake the dice and move forward that many spaces. When you land on a smiling space, you pick a card. If you answer the question on the card, you stay on the space. If you have trouble thinking of an answer, ask your friend."

As you will see, about two-thirds of the challenge cards ask questions about keeping calm and responding thoughtfully to provocation. The other cards involve funny physical challenges, designed to foster engagement in the game. You can play with the children, providing a model, and also praising good teamwork and positive behaviors. If a child has difficulty thinking of an answer to a card, encourage him or her to ask a friend for help.

Snack: Negotiation Snack (Optional, 15 Minutes)

To provide practice in negotiation, this snack needs to include several different options that are not easily divided. For example, snack options could include two packages of cheese crackers, two packages of pretzels, and two packages of fruit snacks. Using the Make a Deal steps as a guide, encourage children to (1) stay calm and describe their own preferences for snack, (2) suggest ideas about fair ways to decide who gets what or ideas about how to divide up the snack materials evenly, and (3) check out the plan by questioning their friends and saying "yes" to good ideas. If groups stonewall in this process because of a lack of willingness of group members to negotiate, the leaders should comment on the group process and clarify the options—for example: "You all did a good job sharing your feelings and giving ideas, but you are having trouble saying 'yes' to good ideas. I can tell that John and Sue are feeling frustrated and hungry. You've got two good ideas to choose from—doing One Potato, Two Potato to see who gets the fruit snacks or opening both packages and dividing up the fruit snacks. What is a fair way to decide which idea to use?" If children remain stonewalled, offer your solution (e.g., "Let's vote and the majority rules"), but do not do so before giving them a chance to resolve things themselves.

Collaborative Challenges: Friendship Charades, All Aboard Challenge (15 Minutes)

In larger groups, divide children into two teams of two or three children each for Friendship Charades; in smaller groups, let the children work together while you guess what they are modeling.

The teams need to think about something they have learned about friendship during Friendship Group, and come up with a short skit that allows them to enact and demonstrate the friendship idea or behavior. If children have difficulty with this task, suggest that they look at the skill posters to generate ideas (e.g., friends share, help each other, take turns, cheer for each other, show good sportsmanship). When each team has selected a friendship idea to demonstrate, the Charades begin. Each team puts on their short skit for the other pair (or for the coach). The observers try to guess what friendship idea or behavior is being demonstrated.

If time allows, introduce the All Aboard challenge. Explain that this challenge is for the whole group and will require good teamwork and problem-solving skills. Begin by spreading out carpet squares or pieces of paper. Start with two squares per child, and have each child put one foot on one square. All the squares should be lined up next to each other to create a "boat." (If the floor is slippery, you may want to tape them down.) Each child needs to stand on the boat. At each "turn," you will remove one square from the boat. The children need to reorganize themselves to stay together on the ship and keep all feet on some part of the carpet squares or paper. As more and more pieces are moved, children need to discuss how to adjust themselves and physically support each other to remain on the boat. The challenge is to see how long they can stay on the boat as pieces are removed (e.g., how small of a boat they can fit themselves onto). As the game moves forward, support children in the problem-solving process as they discuss how to fit onto a smaller space, and praise them for staying calm, giving ideas, listening to friends, and saying "yes" to good ideas.

Closing Circle: Button, Button, Who's Got the Button?, Compliments, and Tips (5 Minutes)

Review the game Button, Button, Who's Got the Button? (introduced in Session 12). See if any child remembers how to play and let him or her explain it to the group. Children work together to pass the button around the string without showing who has it. The person who is "it" must turn around and count to 3, and then turn around again to look at the circle and guess who has the button. Whether or not the guess is correct, give the person who was chosen a compliment and tell him or her to choose who is "it" next. Stop to give compliments and ask for a compliment from a peer as each person takes their turn. At closure, distribute Friendship Tips Handout for Session 24.

SPECIAL ISSUES

The Baxter story can elicit discussions of problems that are hard to solve, especially when children are living in dangerous neighborhoods. Offer support as children discuss the problems. Do not attempt to offer any "quick fix." It is always unwise to offer a potential solution without having a clear-enough grasp of the situation to know whether the solution is viable. For example, "just walk away" may work in some situations but not in others. In some cases, it will be helpful to have the group brainstorm about possible ways to deal with a bullying situation away from school, such as planning ahead, walking another way, walking with someone else, staying away from the area, or staying in at night. In other cases, if adult intervention appears needed, it is important to follow up with parents or teachers.

SESSION 25. Managing Disappointments

GOALS

1. Discuss friendship disappointments that may emerge and cannot be changed.

2. Promote adaptive appraisals in such situations (avoiding blame).

3. Discuss strategies for coping with these disappointments.

4. Practice teamwork and self-control in competitive games.

MATERIALS NEEDED

- Agenda Pictures: 1, 3, 5, 4, 2, and 8
- Posters: Good Teamwork, Baxter's Feeling Faces, Care for Your Friends, Traffic Light, Make a Deal, Fair Play, Communication
- Letters for Dear Problem Solvers (Activity Page 25.1, see p. 309; one per group)
- An array of stickers to share
- Craft sticks, tape, note cards for house building
- Friendship Tips Handout for Session 25 (Activity Page 25.2, see p. 310; one per child)

SESSION OUTLINE

- *Friendship Circle:* Dear Problem Solver letters, Beat Around the Circle game (15 minutes)
- *Construction Station:* The Big Wind Blows friendship skill review (10 minutes)
- *Snack* (optional, 15 minutes)
- *Collaborative Challenge:* Building a house with craft sticks and tape (15 minutes)
- *Closing Circle:* Plan a fair way to divide stickers, compliments, and Friendship Tips (5 minutes)

ADVANCE PREPARATION

- Hang posters.
- Cut out Dear Problem Solver letters.

DETAILED SESSION CONTENT

Friendship Circle: Dear Problem Solver Letters, Beat Around the Circle Game (15 Minutes)

Greet children, invite them to share feelings, and briefly review the session agenda. The session begins with a discussion about coping with disappointments when the situation itself cannot be changed, so put up your "sad" face. Start by sharing a memory of this kind of problem (see the following example) and then introduce two Dear Problem Solvers letters. In both of the situations described in these letters, the problem cannot be prevented or resolved by talking things out with the friend. Children are asked to identify the feelings of the children who experienced the events, analyze why the events occurred, and think about how the children might cope with their feelings of distress, when they can't change the situation itself. In comparison to other problem-solving discussions in the program that have focused on solving the interpersonal problem in order to feel better, this one focuses on managing the internal feeling itself. Key ideas are that (1) you can reduce your stress and distress (e.g., by taking a deep breath and telling yourself to calm down; by distracting yourself); and (2) you can adjust your interpretation about the cause of the distress by recognizing that no personal ill will was intended, and by telling yourself that it is OK and you can move on from the situation. This session introduces the idea that you can choose to ignore a feeling or manage a feeling by choosing a coping action (e.g., choosing to be a peacemaker, choosing to put friendship first).

A related theme is to avoid hostile interpretations when disappointments arise. Here is a sample introduction:

> "Did you notice that I put up my sad face today? I was remembering something that happened between me and my friend when we were your age. My friend was very good at spelling, but I wasn't. She got her spelling homework done quickly and always got 100% on the spelling tests. After a while, I stopped being friends with her, because I didn't like it when she was better than me. Now, when I think back about it, I don't think that was a good reason for me to give up on a friendship. It makes me feel sad. What do you think?"

Encourage children to respond to the scenario. Ask follow-up questions to focus the discussion on the key issues:

> "I felt sad that I wasn't as good a speller as my friend. Was that my friend's fault? Was it a good idea to leave the friendship so that I felt better? Why or why not? Why do I feel sad about it now? What else could I have done? Has this happened to you?"

As children respond, use active listening to emphasize the key points: Sometimes you feel sad about something that happens in a friendship, but it is not your friend's fault. Then you want to find a way to cope with your feelings and to keep your friendship going.

> "Sometimes things don't work out the way we want them to, and there is nothing we can do to change it. When that happens with a friend, it is easy to give up on the friendship. Sometimes breaking off contact with the friend can help you feel better at first. That's what happened to me. But, later, I was sorry that I gave up on my friend. I could have kept that friendship if I had handled my feelings differently. I could have said to myself 'Take 5,' blown a little bit of my sadness and disappointment out like this [model taking a long, deep breath], told myself 'I'm disappointed, but I can handle this. It's not anyone's fault, it just worked out this way.' Maybe I could have saved that friendship. [Pause and ask the children if they would like to take a deep breath and blow a little sadness out with you.] I want to read you a letter from Mary, who needs help from Dear Problem Solvers. I hope that you have some ideas for her. Here is her problem:

Dear Problem Solvers,

I have two best friends, Natasha and Keisha. Keisha's family is going to the beach. She can take one friend. She picked Natasha. I am left out. I feel very upset. I don't know how to stay friends with them when I feel like this."

—Mary

Explore the story with the children before you ask them to give advice. Ask them:

1. *How is Mary feeling? Why?* She says she is "upset," but ask the children to identify more specific feelings. Mary might be disappointed to miss going to the beach, and feel lonely and left out, and she might feel jealous that Keisha picked Natasha.

2. *Is this a problem that Mary could have prevented or that she can solve?* The children might say that Mary could try to talk Keisha into picking her, but if they do, point out that then Natasha would have the problem—it would not really solve the problem, just move it around.

3. *Since Mary cannot change the situation, what can she do to feel better and save her friendship?* Children may suggest coping strategies that involve distractions that would help Mary feel better, such as doing something else or finding a new friend. Use active listening to accept any ideas. If they do not mention it, ask them how she can cope with her feelings of anger toward Keisha, so that those feelings don't hurt her friendship. Your goal is to help children recognize that sometimes disappointments occur as a function of a situation, and not because of ill will on the part of a friend. In a case like that, it is important to find a way to cope with the feelings of disappointment and jealousy, so they do not end a good friendship. Key coping strategies include trying to reduce feeling intensity (e.g., "Take 5"), remember that no ill will was intended, and choose coping behaviors (e.g., tell Keisha it is OK and you understand, invite her to do something special with your family). If Mary can put her friendship first (even though she is disappointed), she will not lose her important friendship. If time allows, continue to the next Dear Problem Solvers.

"I have one more letter to share with you. This one is from John; he also needs help from Dear Problem Solvers. I hope that you have some ideas for him. Here is his problem.

Dear Problem Solvers,

My school had an awards ceremony. All my friends won races and got awards. I did not win anything. My teacher put the awards up on the wall in our classroom. I feel upset when I see them. I think my friends might laugh at me. I don't even want to go to school anymore."

—John

Explore the story with the children before you ask them to give advice. Ask them:

1. *How is John feeling? Why?* He says he is "upset," but ask the children to identify more specific feelings. John might be disappointed or embarrassed that he did not win any awards, and he might feel incompetent or jealous of his friends. He might be worried that other kids will tease him because he did not win anything and they did.

2. *Is this a problem that John can solve?* The children might say that John could try to win an award next year. If they do, note that he could work harder next year, but there is nothing he can do about the awards this year.

3. *Since John cannot change the situation, what can he do to feel better and save his friend-ships?* Use active listening to accept any ideas about how John could cope with his feelings and feel better. Key ideas to emphasize include: (1) ideas about how John can calm down, (2) what he can say to himself about the event (e.g., his friends did not do this to make him feel bad, no one wants him to feel bad), and (3) how he can save his friendships (e.g., tell his friends he is proud of them; remind himself that his friendships are more important than getting an award and that he is a good friend). The important point is for John to find a way to set aside his feelings of disappointment, worry, and jealousy, so they do not keep him from enjoying the time he has with his friends at school, and the important support that his friends provide.

The Beat Around the Circle game provides a brief, active break after the discussion. Sitting in the circle, children cross arms and lay their hands flat on the table or floor. It is important that they cross arms so that each child's hands are in front of a neighbor (one on each side), and each of the two neighbor's hands are in front of the child. Someone is picked to start the pat, and each hand pats the table in its turn. If someone pats his or her hand twice, then the direction changes and the patting goes the other way. Because the children's arms are crossed, they have to watch carefully to determine when it is their turn to pat. If someone lifts her hand to pat when it is not her turn, or if someone does not pat when it is his turn, that hand is out. Play continues until there is only one hand that has not made a mistake left in the circle. Although the game can be played cooperatively (e.g., simply drop the rule that a hand is out when a pat is missed), the use of a competitive game in this session allows for more practice with the skill of coping with disappointment. To help children cope with a loss, remind them to "Take 5" and use one of the "Good things to say when you lose" statements from Session 16 to express their disappointment.

Construction Station: The Big Wind Blows Friendship Skill Review (10 Minutes)

A group game, the Big Wind Blows, is used to help children review Friendship Group skills and to identify friendship ideas, plans, and intentions regarding the use of friendship skills in the future. To play this game, players sit in chairs forming a circle (one chair fewer than the number of play-ers), with one person in the center as the "Big Wind." You ask the child in the center a question (see examples in the next list) and he or she answers—for example: The coach asks, 'When you feel angry, what do you do?,' and the child answers, "Take a deep breath and calm down." Then the child in the center raises his or her arms and twirls around while the coach says "The Big Wind blows everyone who . . . ," filling in the statement with the child's intention—for example: "The Big Wind blows everyone who is going to take a deep breath and calm down when they feel angry. Go." Once the coach has finished the statement and says "Go," the child in the center stops twirling and all of the children who agree with that statement stand up and look for a different seat. Whoever fails to find a new seat and is left in the middle of the circle gets the next question. Here is an example of how this game can be presented to the children:

> "I hope that all of you will remember our Friendship Group ideas for a long time. Friendship Group is coming to an end, but the ideas you learned about friendship in here will help you make friends and keep friends forever. We're going to play a new game today called the Big Wind Blows. As part of the game, I am going to ask you questions about how you will use the friendship ideas in your life."

As you describe the game, demonstrate in a slow walk-through of the steps of the game, to show children how they should stand in the middle, answer a question, and then spin around. Possible questions for the Big Wind Blows game include:

"What will you do to show Good Teamwork?"

"What will you do to make a new friend?"

"What will you do if you see a friend crying?"

"How will you cooperate with others?"

"What will you do if you feel angry?"

"How will you make a new friend?"

"How will you decide who goes first at a game?"

"How will you solve a problem with a friend?"

"How will you make a deal with a friend?"

"How will you show your friends that you care about them?"

"What will you do when you feel lonely?"

Snack (Optional, 15 Minutes)

The usual procedures are followed.

Collaborative Challenge: Build a House with Craft Sticks and Tape (15 Minutes)

This activity provides children with an opportunity to practice cooperation, problem-solving skills, and collaborative planning. If you have a large group, split the children into dyads or triads. Show them the materials—craft sticks, tape, and a note card for each group. Note that you can make this challenge more difficult, if desired, by (1) providing toothpicks, rather than craft sticks, to build with; or (2) asking children to make a two-story house.

> "I brought a special challenge for the group today, and I wonder if you are ready for it. The challenge is to see if you can make a plan and work together to build a house with these craft sticks and tape. To meet the challenge, you need to build a house that has four walls and can support this note card roof."

Have the children talk with their partners about how they want to approach the task before you give them their pack of craft sticks and tape. The goal is to have them discuss a plan with each other before they start to build. Once they have a plan, give them their materials and let them get started. Once the houses are done, give them the note card to see if their house can support a roof. Then ask a few questions designed to encourage their self-reflection regarding their performance as a team—for example: "How did they do working as a team?"; "What did they do to help each other in this task?"; "What was most challenging about the task?": "How did they overcome the difficulty to succeed?" Use specific praise to support positive teamwork, problem-solving efforts, and self-regulatory behaviors observed during the task. Encourage the children to clap for themselves in recognition of their good teamwork and finished products.

Closing Circle: Plan a Fair Way to Divide Stickers, Compliments, and Friendship Tips (5 Minutes)

If time allows, use a sticker sharing activity to provide practice in problem solving. Display a set of varied stickers and ask the children to generate ideas for fair ways to divide the stickers and Make a Deal with each other, so that each person has some nice stickers to take home him or her. After the children generate ideas about good ways to share the stickers, summarize the suggestions and integrate them into a plan of action. "Check it out" with the group. Then let the children proceed with their plan and divide the stickers. Share compliments and distribute Friendship Tips Handout for Session 25.

SPECIAL ISSUES

1. The specific problems that serve as discussion examples can be modified to make them relevant for your particular group of children. Children who are older (ages 7 and 8) are more likely to be distressed by friendship issues that involve performance comparisons (e.g., a friend being a better speller or a better runner), whereas younger children (ages 5 and 6) are more likely to be distressed by an unequal distribution of resources (e.g., a friend getting a new game or toy that the child does not have). You can modify the specific examples used in this discussion to fit your group.

2. In the scenarios described in this session (as in many situations in life), it's not possible to change the situation. So, the child must make an "internal" adjustment in the way he or she is thinking and feeling. You want to focus children's attention on how to do that: how to adjust their goals, attributions, and stress level to better cope with the disappointment. Sometimes it helps to focus on an alternative goal, such as choosing to be a peacemaker. Children can say "I'm choosing to be a peacemaker" and move toward that, while letting go of the goal that led them to feel disappointed and upset.

SESSION 26. Closing Friendship Group

GOALS

1. Review the skills covered and the goals of Friendship Group.

2. Share favorite memories as a review and a closure activity.

3. Promote feelings of self-efficacy for future friendship experiences.

MATERIALS NEEDED

- Agenda Pictures: 1, 3, 5, 4, 2, and 8

- Posters: Good Teamwork, Baxter's Feeling Faces, Care for Your Friends, Traffic Light, Make a Deal, Fair Play, Communication

- Microphone, What I Learned in Friendship Group cards (Activity Page 26.1, see p. 311; one set)

- Poster board or flip chart to create list of favorites
- Friendship Group Memory Book forms (Activity Page 26.2, see p. 312; one per child)
- Printed compliments (optional; Activity Page 26.3, see p. 313; one per child), star stickers, markers
- Materials for favorite games
- Friends Forever awards (Activity Page 26.4, see p. 314; one per child)
- Friendship Tips Handout for Session 26 (Activity Page 26.5, see p. 315; one per child)

SESSION OUTLINE

- *Friendship Circle:* Pass the Mike memories, favorite game selection (15 minutes)
- *Construction Station:* Memory Book construction (15 minutes)
- *Snack:* Usual procedures (optional, 15 minutes)
- *Collaborative Challenges:* Favorite games (10 minutes)
- *Closing Circle:* Friends Forever awards, compliments, and tips (5 minutes)

ADVANCE PREPARATION

- Hang posters.
- Cut out cards for the What I Learned in Friendship Group game.
- Cut out compliments for the Friendship Group Memory Books.
- Fold books into quarters, with *Friends Forever* printed on front, bottom edges cut, edges stapled.

DETAILED SESSION CONTENT

Friendship Circle: Pass the Mike Memories, Favorite Game Selection (15 Minutes)

As the children arrive, greet them and invite them to share their feelings. Put up two faces, sad and happy, to introduce the mixed feelings associated with the group closure.

> "I put up two different feelings today— sad and happy. I'm sad because today is our final Friendship Group. I know I'm going to miss seeing you. But I also put up 'happy' because I feel very happy that I got to know each of you as friends this year, and had such fun times with you. Does anyone else feel that way? [Let children respond and provide active listening to support their expressions of feeling.] Today I want to share Friendship Group memories. I hope you will all help me remember the things we did together and the fun times we had."

Explain how the game is played. Like other Pass the Mike games, the children pass the mike while the music plays. When the music stops, the child holding the mike picks a card from a hat with a question (e.g., the What I Learned in Friendship Group cards). The child answers the question by stating what he feels, and then picks a friend and asks her the same question. After that child answers, the mike is passed around again. Once each child has had a chance to answer one or two questions from the hat, move on to discuss favorite activities.

Explain that you want to make a special poster to help remember fun times the group has had together. The first step is to brainstorm as a group, and write down a list of activities in Friendship Group that this group really enjoyed doing together. Proceed to write down on poster board, with a heading at the top, "Our Friends Like to. . . ." If needed, you or the co-leader can suggest some activities to write on the list to get the discussion started, such as "Play games together" or "Pretend together, and put on shows." Ask the children for their ideas about things they enjoyed doing together in Friendship Group, and write down their answers. If children focus narrowly on one dimension of group activities, such as listing favorite games, encourage a broader view by suggesting some alternatives, such as helping each other, talking with each other, sharing feelings, and so on. Any ideas children offer are acceptable, as long as they are not inappropriate; do not write down inappropriate or unfriendly suggestions. Once there are six suggestions, or so, on the list, continue with the selection of favorites:

> "Wow, those are great ideas. Here is what we have on our list of things that we have enjoyed in Friendship Group. [Read through the list.] I am going to pass our microphone around one more time, and ask each one of you to tell us a game or activity that you like best on this list. I'll give you this marker, and you can put a star by your favorite thing and then sign our poster. Later today, we'll play a favorite game one more time."

As each child identifies his or her favorite activity, let the child make a star on the poster by that activity and sign his or her name on the poster. Praise the children for their teamwork.

Construction Station: Memory Book Construction (15 Minutes)

Children construct Friendship Group Memory Books for each other. Each child has a Memory Book, and these are passed around the table. Markers and small heart or star stickers should be provided. A child's name is written on the front of each "book," and the books are passed around so that each partner can write a compliment or other friendly statement on a page of the book. Coaches should lead a brief discussion to help children think about messages they could write for each other, and some children may need adult assistance to write their message. It might be helpful to create an example by filling out one "book" so that the children can see how compliments from friends are written into the book. If needed (for younger or less verbal children), you can provide printed examples of affirmations. Children can select one of these printed affirmations for a particular friend, cut it out, and paste it into the friend's book. Each child is left with a Memory Book to take home that includes affirmations from each of his or her friends. There is also a page in their own books for children to write or draw a picture of something they learned in Friendship Group that helped them with their friendships and that they plan to remember and use in the future. Here is a sample of an instruction for this activity:

> "We're going to do something today that will help us remember the friendly times we had in our Friendship Group. We're going to make Friendship Group Memory Books for each other. Each one of you will get a book with your name on the front, like this. We will pass your book around the table. Each of your friends will have a chance to write a friendly comment inside, and add a sticker to decorate his or her message. At the end, when your book comes back to you, you will be able to read the messages from your friends and draw a picture to show a favorite memory

you have of Friendship Group. Before we start, let's talk about what you might write in your friend's Memory Book. Try to think about what makes that person a good friend—something you saw him or her do that was friendly, nice, or helpful."

Encourage the children to think about positive messages that they can write in the books, such as "You shared with me," "You are helpful," or "You are a good friend." Some children will need adult help throughout the process, in order to think of varied compliments for the partners and to write them down.

Snack (Optional, 15 Minutes)

The usual procedures are followed. This can be a good time to talk with children about what they learned in Friendship Group that was most helpful to them. You can ask them how they used the friendship ideas in their friendships at school or home. You can also ask if they have suggestions for you—things to do more (or less) of in future Friendship Groups to make them helpful for children. If desired, a special snack can be served in celebration of the group's accomplishments.

Collaborative Challenges: Favorite Games (10 Minutes)

Play one or two of the favorite games chosen by children in the initial discussion. Be prepared to review the game procedures and rules with the children if it has been a while since they played the games.

Closing Circle: Friends Forever Awards, Compliments, and Tips (5 Minutes)

In the final compliment circle, the coaches should give each child a Friends Forever Certificate of Participation, with a personalized commendation recognizing a particular strength and area of growth the child showed during his Friendship Group participation. As each child's commendation is read, ask for group applause. End with a positive sentiment:

> "It is always sad to say goodbye to a friend, but the feelings of friendship can go on and on, even when we are not together. We can remember the fun times we had together."

SPECIAL ISSUES

Groups will vary in terms of the amount of time they spend discussing group memories. For groups that have been together for a longer period of time, and for children with more advanced verbal skills, the discussion and peer affirmation activities (e.g., Memory Book construction, snack discussion) can fill the session time productively. For other groups, discussions will be shorter, and there will be more time for the activities and opportunities to practice skills.

Baxter Faces a Bully

Text by Karen Bierman   Illustrations by Andrew Heckathorne

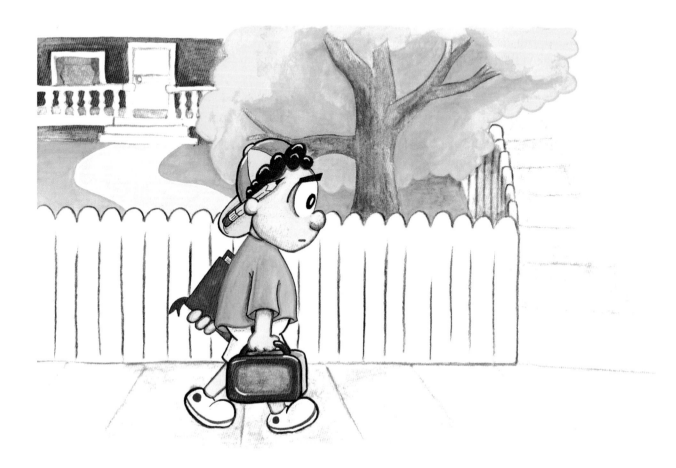

"I don't want to go to school today," said Baxter to his mom. "I'm sick." "You look find to me," said his mom. "But I can't go, Mom. Something bad might happen." "Oh, don't be silly, Baxter, you'll be fine."

A few minutes later, walking to the bus stop, Baxter didn't feel fine. His hands were sweating, and his heart was pounding.

Why are Baxter's hands sweating and his heart pounding? How does he feel?

(page 1 of 8)

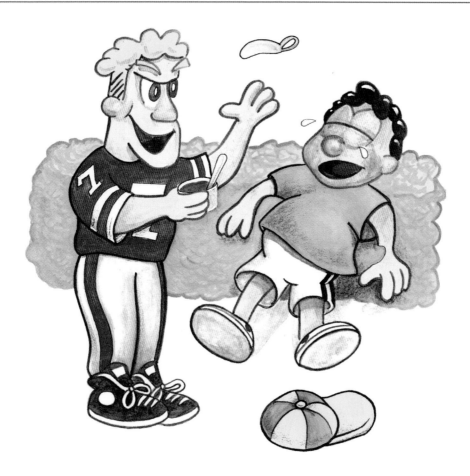

He turned the corner and there it was—the bus stop, the kids, and Bugsy.

"Here comes Baxter," yelled Bugsy, and Baxter's heart dropped. Bugsy grabbed Baxter's lunchbox.

"Whatcha' got for me today?" he said, taking Baxter's pudding. "Gonna cry?" Bugsy laughed and ate the pudding. Baxter shut his eyes as tight as he could, but some tears spilled out.

What is happening to Baxter? Why is he shutting his eyes? Why are tears spilling out?

"Crybabies wait in the bushes," said Bugsy, pushing Baxter down. The kids laughed.

Why are the kids laughing? How does Baxter feel? Do you know anyone who acts like Bugsy?

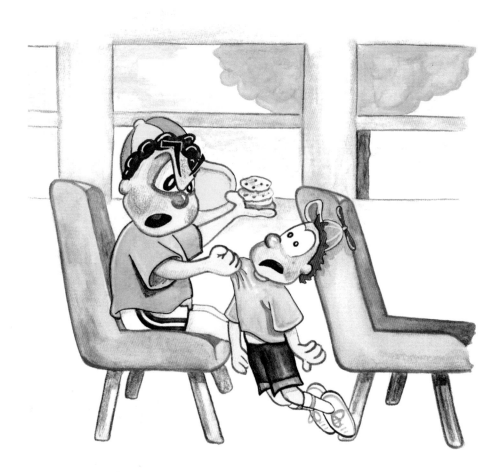

The bus came and Baxter got on. His face felt red and hot and his legs were still shaking. A little kid sat down next to him. "How come you're crying?" he asked. "I'm not crying, stupid" growled Baxter, "let me see your lunch."

Why does Baxter look so angry? Who is he mad at?

"I've got cookies," said the kid. "Not anymore—they're mine," said Baxter, grabbing the cookies, "and if you tell, I'll beat you up."

Why did Baxter take the little boy's cookies? What do you think of Baxter's behavior? What will happen next?

At first the kid just looked surprised. But then his face turned red, his fists came out, he screwed up his mouth, and he screamed at the top of his lungs "GIVE THEM BACK!"

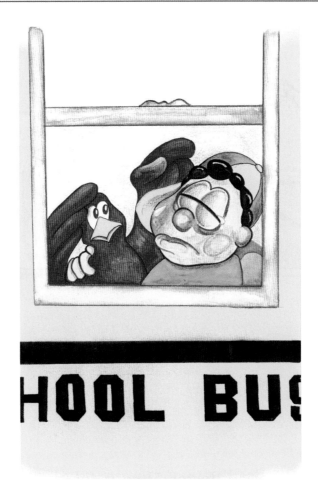

The brakes on the bus screeched, and the bus driver turned around. "Get up here," he snarled, pointing to the front seat. "You're in big trouble now."

Why did the bus driver make Baxter go to the front seat? Why is he in trouble?

Baxter sat behind the driver. He pressed his hot face against the cool window. "Please let this be a dream," he thought, "don't let me be in trouble again."

How does Baxter feel now? Why is he upset?

Then, in his mind, Baxter heard a familiar voice. "Baxter, can I help?" "Oh, Bird, I'm so glad you're here. I'm in terrible trouble," Baxter whispered. "I can see," said the bird, "you lost your cool."

What does it mean to "lose your cool"? What advice will the bird give Baxter?

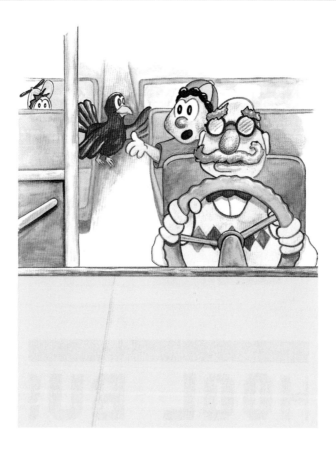

"It wasn't my fault, Bird!" cried Baxter, "Bugsy did it!" "Well, Bugsy scared you, that's true," said the bird. "He's a scary guy. But that's not why you're in trouble."

"You mean the cookies?" said Baxter, sheepishly. "I don't know why I took them. Bird, I don't even like oatmeal-raisin."

Why did Baxter take the cookies from the little boy? Do you think it is Baxter's fault that he is in trouble or Bugsy's fault? Why?

"And how do you feel now?" asked the bird, "any better?" "No, not really," said Baxter, doubtfully. "I think I feel worse."

Why does Baxter feel worse now?

All the way to school, Baxter and Bird talked about the bully problem. By the time the bus arrived, Baxter felt better.

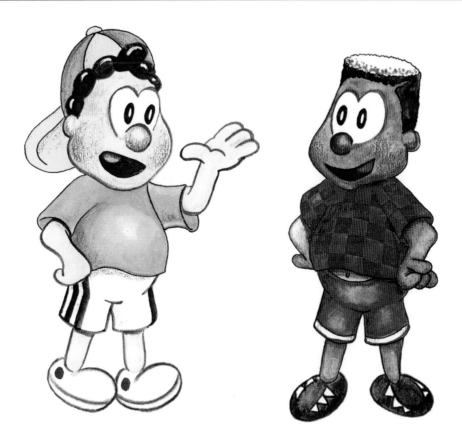

Later that day, Baxter talked to his friend John to get ideas about how he could handle Bugsy. "I think staying calm is important," said Baxter. "If I don't get upset, maybe teasing me won't be fun." "Maybe," agreed John, "but you need a friend too. He won't tease you if we stick together. And maybe you should tell a teacher," suggested John.

"Maybe I need to," said Baxter, "but I think I'll try this plan first."

What is Baxter's plan? What do you think Baxter should do?

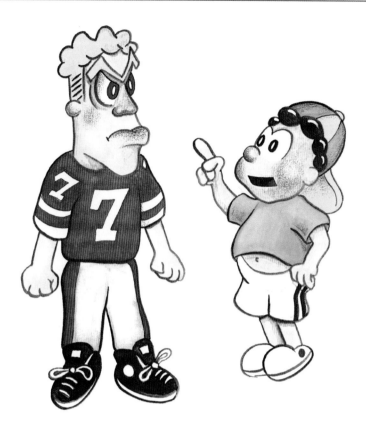

After school, Baxter walked to the bus stop with John. He saw Bugsy waiting. Baxter took a deep breath and let it out slowly. "That's right, Baxter" he heard the bird say in his mind, "Stay calm."

"Hey, Baxter" called Bugsy with a sneer. "Did you get the letter I sent you?" "No," said Baxter. "That's 'cause I forgot to stamp it" laughed Bugsy and he stamped his foot down onto Baxter's toes. It hurt—a lot! Baxter bit his lip to keep it from trembling.

"That's an old joke," he said in a quiet voice "and it's not very funny." Then Baxter turned toward the bus with his friend John.

"Wait till tomorrow, Baxter" Bugsy called after him "I'll get your pudding again." Baxter didn't even turn around. "I think I'll buy lunch tomorrow," he said in a low voice and the kids in the bus line giggled.

What did Baxter do to make Bugsy stop teasing him? Is it working? What would you do?

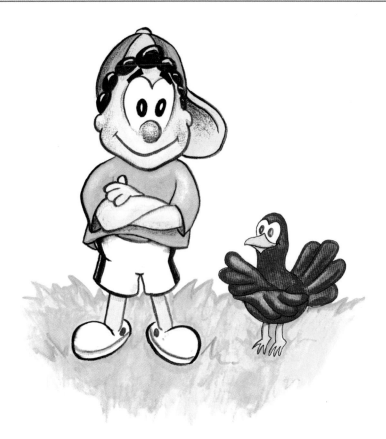

"WOW, you really kept your cool," said John. "I did," Baxter nodded, feeling very proud of himself.

Why does Baxter feel proud of himself? What do you think about what Baxter did?

But then he thought with dismay, Bugsy will be back again tomorrow. "Just remember your plan" he heard the bird inside. "Stay calm, stick with your friends, and tell an adult if you need to."

Baxter smiled to himself. Bugsy was a big guy with a loud voice, but when you got right down to it, Bugsy wasn't very smart. If he just kept his cool, Baxter thought, he could outsmart Bugsy 9 times out of 10.

ACTIVITY PAGE 24.1 (One per Group or per Pair)

Game Board for the Keep Your Cool Game

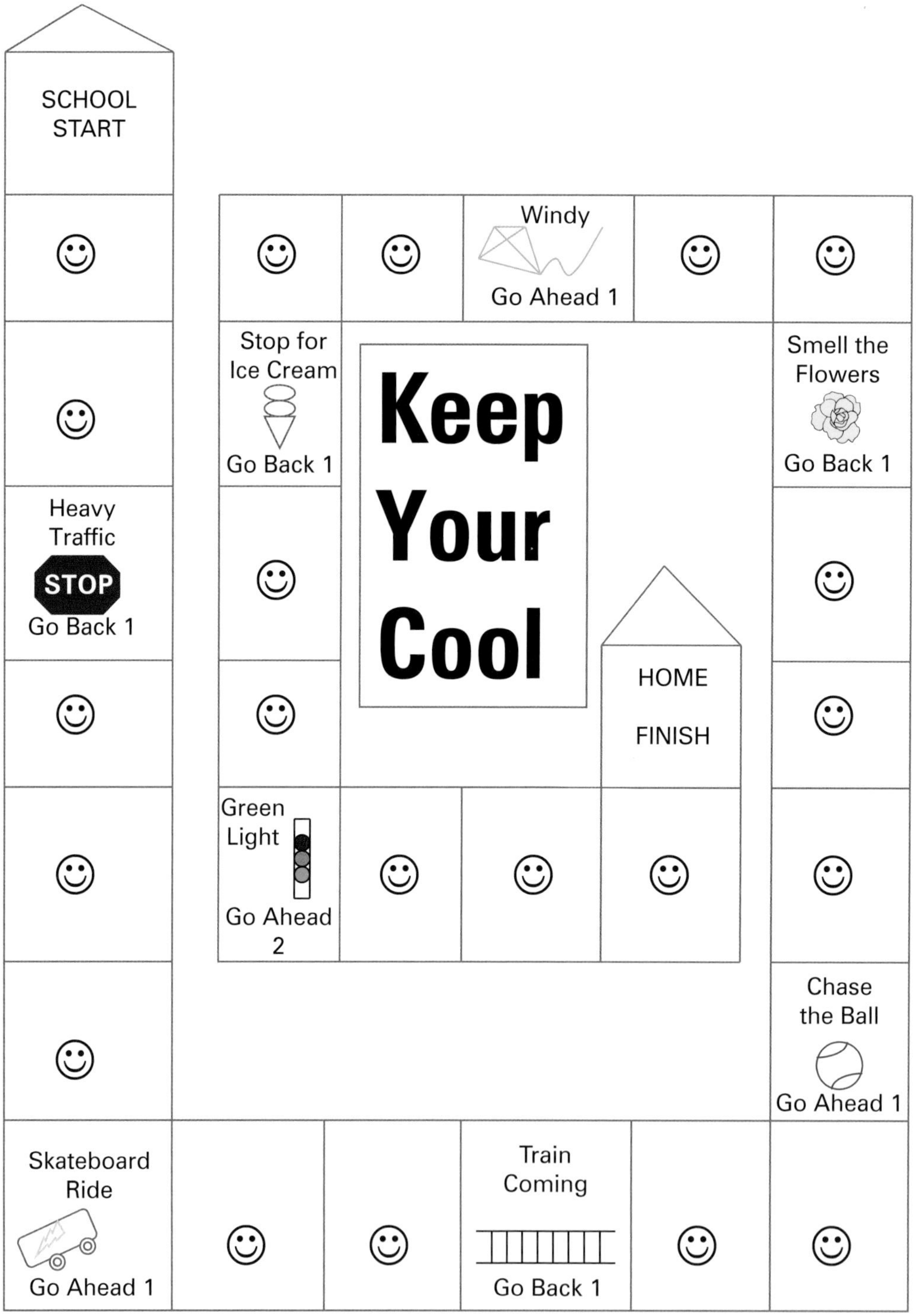

SCHOOL
START
Windy
Go Ahead 1
Stop for
Ice Cream
Go Back 1
Keep
Your
Cool
Smell the
Flowers
Go Back 1
Heavy
Traffic
STOP
Go Back 1
HOME
FINISH
Green
Light
Go Ahead
2
Chase
the Ball
Go Ahead 1
Skateboard
Ride
Go Ahead 1
Train
Coming
Go Back 1

Game Cards for the Keep Your Cool Game

Tell about something you do to calm down when you are upset.	If someone calls you a name, how do you keep your cool?	Put your hands on your shoulders. Try to touch your elbows together.
If you could turn into an animal, which animal would you choose? Why?	Tell about a time someone was mean to you. What did you do?	Tell about a time someone teased you. What did you do?
If you are upset, how can a friend help you feel better?	Show a mad face and tell what you are thinking of.	Try to twiddle your thumbs forward and backwards.
If someone starts a fight with you, how do you keep your cool?	See if you can stand on one foot and touch your other foot.	If someone is mean to you, what can you do about it?
What does it mean to hurt someone "by accident" or "on purpose"?	What's your favorite dessert to eat?	Give two reasons why it is not a good idea to fight at school.
If someone makes you mad by cheating in a game, what can you do about it?	If someone bumps you and says it was an accident, what would you do?	Try to pat your head and rub your tummy at the same time.
Make a silly face.	What is something you worry about at school? How do you cope with your worry?	Show a scared face and tell what you are thinking of.
When you feel frustrated or upset at a friend, how do you calm yourself down?	Tell about something that made you feel proud.	If you got into a fight with a friend, how could you make up?

Friendship Tips Handout for Session 24

Share these **Friendship Tips** with teachers and parents who can support friendship skills at school and home. This week, Friendship Group focused on keeping your cool when someone teases or bullies you, and on making a plan for how to manage the situation.

Remember

If someone teases you or bullies you:

1. *Stay calm and keep your cool.*
2. *Talk with someone you trust about the problem.*
3. *Think about different ways to solve the problem.*
4. *Make a plan and try it out.*
5. *Get help from an adult if you need it.*

Try It Out

If someone teases you or bullies you, follow the Traffic Light.

Stop, calm down, "Take 5."

Tell what the problem is and how you feel.

Thinks of ideas for how to solve the problem.

Listen to others' ideas.

Make a plan and try it out.

If you still need help, talk to an adult.

School and Home Check

Did someone tease you or bully you this week?

Did you stay calm and keep your cool?

Did you talk with someone and make a plan?

How did your plan work?

Was a friend teased or bullied this week?

Did you help the friend stay calm, talk about the problem, and make a plan?

Dear Problem Solvers Story Letters

Dear Problem Solvers,

  I have two best friends, Natasha and Keisha. Keisha's family is going to the beach. She can take one friend. She picked Natasha. I am left out. I feel very upset. I don't know how to stay friends with them when I feel like this.

—Mary

Dear Problem Solvers,

  My school had an awards ceremony. All of my friends won races and got awards. I did not win anything. My teacher put the awards up on the wall in our classroom. I feel upset when I see them. I think my friends might laugh at me. I don't even want to go to school anymore.

—John

Friendship Tips Handout for Session 25

Share these **Friendship Tips** with teachers and parents who can support friendship skills at school and home. This week, Friendship Group focused on coping with a friendship disappointment.

Remember

Sometimes . . .

things don't go the way you want in a friendship.

you feel disappointed or jealous.

you have to accept the situation and move on.

Try It Out

When you feel disappointed or jealous in a friendship, try to:

"Take 5": Relax, take a deep breath, and tell yourself to calm down.

Tell yourself it is OK, and you can still be friends.

Do something else.

Choose to be a peacemaker

Give it time; you will feel better after a while.

School and Home Check

How did you handle your feelings this week?

Did you remember to "Take 5"?

Did you tell yourself, "I can handle this"?

Were you able to move on and keep your friendship?

Cards for
What I Learned in Friendship Group Game

What is your favorite Friendship Group game?	What did you like most about Friendship Group this year?	Tell about a problem you had with a friend. How did you solve it?
Show how your face looks when you lose a game. What do you say when that happens?	Show how your face looks when you win a game. What do you say when that happens?	How can you make a friend feel special?
How do you show your friends that you like them?	Tell about a time when you got mad at a friend. How did you solve the problem?	What do you like to do with your friends?
What is the best thing about having friends?	What is one important thing you learned about friendship this year?	Give your friends some "high fives."
If you feel sad, how can a friend help?	Why is it important to share?	How can you be a peacemaker?

Memory Book Form

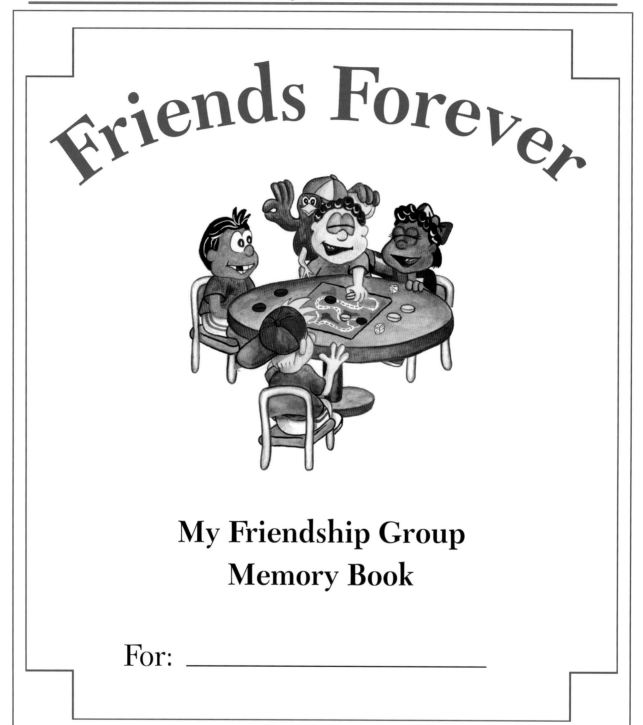

Friends Forever

My Friendship Group Memory Book

For: _____

Printed Compliments for Memory Books

You are a really good friend!	I like the way you share and help.
I like to play with you.	You are a good problem solver.
You keep your cool. You are a peacemaker.	You are a good sport and a fair player.
You are kind. You care about your friends.	I will miss you. You have been a good friend!
You are fun to play with. You are nice to others.	You have great ideas! I'm glad I met you.

Friends Forever Award

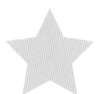 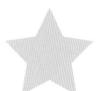 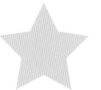 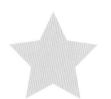

Friends Forever
Certificate of Participation

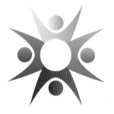

Name: _____

Dates of Participation: _____

Coaching Staff: _____

Commendation

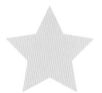   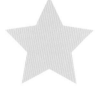

Friendship Tips Handout for Session 26

Share these **Friendship Tips** with teachers and parents who can support friendship skills at school and home. This was the last week of Friendship Group and we focused on celebrating our time together and what we learned.

Remember

Friendships are special.

Take care of your friendships.

Then your friends will take care of you.

Try It Out

You know how to make a friend:

Talk with someone. Ask questions. Listen.

Play fairly.

Cooperate, help, and share.

Keep your cool, "Take 5," and solve problems.

You will make new friends and keep your old friends!

School and Home Check

You are ready to make friends at school and at home.

You are ready to be a peacemaker and a problem solver.

Let your Friendship Star shine.

Friendship Group Manual
ADVANCED ELEMENTARY SESSIONS

Cooperation and Conversation Skills

SESSION 1. Meeting and Greeting: Friendly Face, Tell about You

GOALS

1. Introduce Friendship Group, explain the purpose, identify participants.
2. Introduce and practice two conversation skills: friendly orientation and self-disclosure.
3. Practice cooperation skills in collaborative group activities.

MATERIALS NEEDED

- Poster: Friendship Group Guidelines
- Category cards (Activity Page 1.1, see p. 339; one set), poker chips, and basket for Discovery Circle
- Poster board prepared with categories or one copy of Activity Page 1.2, see p. 340
- Markers (for Friendship Discovery poster), masking tape (for Line-Up), soft tossing objects (for Group Juggle)
- Friendship Tips Handout for Session 1 (Activity Page 1.3, see p. 341; one per child)

SESSION OUTLINE

- *Friendship Circle:* Introduce group purpose and guidelines, Discovery Circle (15 minutes)
- *Construction Station:* Friendship Discovery poster construction (10 minutes)
- *Snack* (optional, 15 minutes)

- *Collaborative Challenges:* Line-Up and Group Juggle (12 minutes)
- *Closing Circle:* Compliments, Friendship Tips, and assignment (8 minutes)

ADVANCE PREPARATION

- Hang Friendship Group Guidelines poster.
- Cut out category cards, fold, and put in basket for Discovery Circle.
- Write categories on poster board or copy Activity Page 1.2.

DETAILED SESSION CONTENT

Friendship Circle: Introduce Group Purpose and Guidelines, Discovery Circle (15 Minutes)

Invite the children to sit together in a group, forming a "friendship circle." Introduce yourself and provide a brief description of the group schedule and purpose.

> "Hello, everyone, my name is _____, and I'm going to be the coach of this Friendship Group. I'm glad to see you all here today. We are going to meet in our Friendship Group every week. We'll get to know each other and have fun together."

Explain that the purpose of the group is to talk about how to build good friendships and to try out new activities and games. Note that many children their age have some worries about friendships, getting along with others, and fitting in, and that the group will give them a chance to talk about how to deal with some of those social challenges and worries. Also, a big goal is to make sure everyone has fun! Ask the children to introduce themselves. Then discuss the Friendship Group Guidelines and invite children to comment or add to the list.

> "Before we get started with today's activities, let's talk about a few important guidelines for our group meetings. [Point to the Friendship Group Guidelines poster.] In Friendship Group, we listen to each other, support each other, and respect each other. What do those words mean to you? How will those guidelines help us in friendship group?"

Encourage children to discuss and give examples of each guideline. Be prepared to offer a few ideas to help the children get started, if needed. For example, if the children do not mention it, suggest that supporting each other includes helping and sharing. Respecting each other means no put-downs, and no gossip outside of the group. That means that what is said in the group stays in the group. Respecting the coaches means following the rules of Friendship Group. Let the children add to the guidelines if they have other suggestions that they want to write down on the list. During this discussion, look for opportunities to recognize children's positive participation and contributions—for example: "Thank you for sharing your thoughts, [Name]"; "I appreciate your participation, [Name]; you are supporting the group with your attention and good listening." Then, introduce the idea that *telling about yourself* is a good way to make new friends; it is a good way to start a conversation, and it helps others learn more about you.

"Telling about yourself is a good way to help others learn more about you, it makes conversations go well, and it can help you become better friends with others. You can tell all kinds of different things about yourself, such as your name, grade, where you go to school, and your hobbies. What other kinds of information could you share that others would be interested in? What do you like to learn about children you meet?"

Let the children add their suggestions for information that can be shared with others. Explain that, in addition to what you say, it is important to think about the way you look when you are talking with someone and trying to make a friend. We constantly communicate through body language without even thinking about it. Ask the children what message you are sending, and illustrate an introduction with poor body language (e.g., telling someone your name and where you are from, with eyes downcast, a somber expression, and body turned away). Then ask the children what message you are sending when you make the same introduction with eye contact and a smile. Ask the children to define what was different about your body language in the two examples. Summarize the point by noting that a friendly face is an important way to show that you are interested in becoming friends, and that you would be a nice person with whom to talk. Introduce the Discovery Circle activity as a fun way to practice telling about yourself and showing a friendly face.

In the Discovery Circle activity, children sit in a circle and take turns picking up a card that lists a category of information (e.g., brothers and sisters, favorite food; Activity Page 1.1). Each child is given a pile of poker chips (or other tokens) and there is a bucket in the middle of the circle. Once a child has selected a piece of paper, he or she reads the category and shares personal information that fits in that category (e.g., tells how many brothers and/or sisters he or she has, describes a favorite food). The other children in the circle throw their poker chips into the bucket in the middle of the group to indicate that they share the quality or characteristic or agree with the speaker's opinion. In addition to praising children for their participation, friendly faces, and listening skills, emphasize how much the children have in common by calling attention to the growing number of poker chips in the bucket at the end of the activity. Continue until children have each had a couple of turns, or until interest is diminishing. Use specific praise to underscore the value of the target skills, pointing out how children's friendly faces, positive body language, and sharing information about themselves is helping the group members make new friends and learn about each other.

"In this next activity, I'm giving you the challenge of finding out more about each other. I'm going to sit back and see how well you can tell about yourselves and learn about each other on this friendship challenge."

Construction Station: Discovery Poster Construction (10 Minutes)

This activity can be done in dyads or triads or altogether as a larger group (the task is easier for children when it is done in smaller groupings, but allows practice of more advanced conversation skills when done in the larger group). Each group is given a poster and told that partners must talk with each other and share their ideas, working together to fill in the poster. The poster should be divided into boxes, with a category title at the top of each box (see Activity Page 1.2). Category examples include total number of pets among group members, band or singer everyone likes, food no one likes, place everyone wants to visit, good things about school (list five good things), games everyone likes (list three), total number of brothers and sisters among group members, place no one has ever been, favorite summer activities (list three), and favorite after-school activities (list three).

Let children take leadership roles and work on this task together, without your intervention, to the extent that they are able. Provide support, encouragement, and organizational suggestions only as needed.

Snack (Optional, 15 Minutes)

If desired, used the Snack Jobs chart from the Early Elementary Session 1, and let children discuss which roles they want to take in this session (e.g., distributing plates, napkins, drinks, food, or helping with cleanup). Snack time provides an informal opportunity for conversation among the children and with the coaches. In addition, snack time can be used to discuss how children enjoyed the Friendship Discovery poster activity and what they learned about each other that they did not know. Coaches can comment on positive features of their teamwork and conversation skills they noticed as the children worked on the poster together. At the end of snack time, the upcoming challenge activity can be described, and the children's ideas for how to help each other meet the challenge can be reviewed. (Note that, if your group does not include a snack break, you can discuss the Friendship Discovery poster and praise the children's teamwork at the end of that activity, before moving on to the collaborative challenges.)

Collaboration Challenges: Line-Up and Group Juggle (12 Minutes)

Two collaborative challenge games are described. Depending on the time available, choose one or do both. Save 7–8 minutes for the closing compliment circle and skill review.

Line-Up

Collaborative challenge games such as Line-Up provide naturalistic opportunities for children to practice social problem solving and cooperative skills. In this game, the coach uses masking tape to mark a line on the floor and gives the team the challenge of getting everyone lined up along the line in alphabetical order by using the first letter of each team member's *middle* name. Before they start the challenge, ask the children how they plan to organize themselves to master the challenge—for example: "Who has an idea about how you can do this?"; "What do others think of that idea?" "Does anyone have another idea of how to go about this challenge?" The goal of this planning discussion is twofold: (1) It gives children an opportunity to practice their conversation and cooperation skills, and (2) it encourages them to plan an approach before starting the challenge. After children complete the group challenge, check their work by going down the line and asking the middle name of each child. Congratulate the group members on their good teamwork and ask them to reflect on their success—for example: "How tough was the challenge?"; "How did you solve the problem?"; "What did you have to do to master the challenge?" Extending this activity, children can be asked to line up in the order of other characteristics, such as the number of brothers and sisters they have, or the months of their birthdates. An additional challenge is to ask the children to line up according to their shoe size or hand size, but with the caveat that they cannot use talking to communicate with each other. In a small group, extend the challenge by using the "no talking" options or seeing how fast they can do a sequence of line-ups as you call out the categories (e.g., middle name, number of siblings, birthdate months). Ask a few questions before the group starts each challenge to encourage anticipatory planning and ask a few questions after they finish to encourage self-reflection and to reinforce effective teamwork. Additional postchallenge questions include "How did you communicate with each other?"; "How did you feel when you first started [e.g., frustrated]?"; "How did you feel when you got it?"; "How could you tell that others in the group were feeling frustrated [or excited]?"; "What made this challenge easy [or difficult] for you?" It is important to include the discussion questions before and after the children finish a challenge, even though many children find it less interesting to talk about it (they would rather just do it). The discussion amplifies the learning potential of the activity. However, use your judgment and pace the discussion so that children's interest and engagement are sustained.

Group Juggle

Children sit in a circle with their hands in front of them. A bag within reaching distance should contain several soft, non-bouncing objects (e.g., beanbags, squoosh balls, small stuffed animal). To start the juggle, toss one object gently to the child sitting across from you, calling his or her name ("Hi, [Name], here you go"). The child should respond "Thank you, Coach," and then toss the object to another child in the circle, calling his or her name. That person says "Thank you, [Name]," and then calls out the name of another child who has not yet had a turn. Children should leave their hands out until they have had a turn, so it is easy to spot the children who have not yet had a turn. This process continues until each person has had a turn.

Tell the group that they have just made a juggling pattern. The first challenge for them is to see if they can remember their juggling pattern, and throw the beanbag around the circle in the same order that they just used. After a successful go-round, you can compliment the children and ask them a few questions to help them reflect on the teamwork that allowed them to succeed—for example: "How did you remember who to catch from and throw to?"; "What did your friends do to help you out?" If time allows and the children are still engaged, you can introduce a second challenge: either (1) seeing how quickly the group can remember and complete the naming and tossing sequence, or (2) adding a second object around the circle in the same sequence midway through the first sequence, so that two objects are circling around the circle, one after the other. If you choose the latter option, start the juggle the same way you did the first time. However, when the first beanbag is approximately midway through the sequence of people, pull out a second object and start it in the same sequence. Possible postplay discussion questions include "How did you feel when you suddenly saw the second thing coming?"; "How did you keep your focus—what did you do to remember who to catch from and throw to?"; "What happened when someone made a mistake—how did you get back on track?"; "How did your teammates help each other out?"

Closing Circle: Compliments, Friendship Tips, and Assignment (8 Minutes)

Join in a friendship circle and distribute copies of the Friendship Tips Handout for Session 1.

> "Have you guys had a good time in our Friendship Group today? I really enjoyed spending time with you today and getting to know you. I can tell you are going to be a very special team! We end each Friendship Group by talking about some friendship tips and ideas about how you can work on your friendships at home and school."

Review the handout with the children, highlighting the skills they worked on during the group. Read through the suggested practice activities for children to try at home, and let them know that you will be interested in hearing about their experiences with these skills when you all get back together next week. Then proceed to the compliments.

"At the end of each session, we finish by sharing compliments, noticing positive things that happened in our group session. I am going to give each one of you a compliment about your work in group today."

The compliment circle provides an opportunity for self-reflection and performance evaluation, reinforcing children's efforts at social skill building and teamwork. First, model giving a compliment to each child. In later sessions, children will be invited to compliment themselves and each other. Model and reinforce compliments regarding performance during group activities—for example: "[Name], I liked the way you shared your ideas in the Line-Up challenge. You had a good idea that helped the team get started on that challenge." Proceed until each child has received a compliment, and then close the session.

SPECIAL ISSUES

1. Some children may feel anxious and remain aloof or quiet during this first session. Provide encouragement and reassurance, but do not pressure children to join in right away. Allow them to watch for a while if they need time to feel comfortable in the group setting.

2. Use this first session to assess the verbal and behavioral control skills of children in the group. If the session demands appear too advanced, consider using early elementary sessions or replacing some of the discussions with early elementary session activities.

3. A central goal of the first session is to establish a sense of comfort and security in the group context, so the guidelines emphasize desired behaviors and positive expectations. In some groups you may need to add "school rules" (e.g., no fighting, yelling, bathroom talk, or cussing). Ignoring behavioral infractions and praising appropriate behavior will be sufficient to control problem behaviors in many groups. However, if additional behavioral supports are needed, you can add rule prohibitions (e.g., No Fighting, No Put-downs, Take Care of Our Place), along with token rewards and response costs (see Chapter 4 on behavior management).

4. In the Group Juggle some children have difficulty catching or throwing the objects with control. If this occurs, encourage children to think of ways to help each other (e.g., by throwing more gently or by moving closer together). If put-downs occur, ask children to think of a positive, friendly way to make a suggestion—for example: "The important thing about these challenges is how the group is able to work together to be successful. We need a good suggestion about how all of you could work as a team to master this challenge."

5. If you are running groups in school, make a copy of each Friendship Tips page for each child's classroom teacher. This will keep the teacher informed of the group focus and activities, and help you work with the teacher to plan for generalization of skill use to the classroom, playground, and lunchroom.

SESSION 2. Having a Conversation: Asking Questions and Listening

GOALS

1. Review the conversation skills of a friendly face and telling something about yourself.
2. Introduce the conversation skills of asking questions and listening.
3. Practice conversation skills in structured activities.
4. Practice cooperation skills in collaborative group activities.

MATERIALS NEEDED

- Friendship Group Guidelines
- Category cards for friendship circle activities (Activity Page 2.1, see p. 342; one set)
- Game board and shapes for Shape Game (Activity Page 2.2, see p. 343; one per child)
- Bag and items for What Is It? game
- Categories for Game Show (Activity Page 2.3, see p. 344; one list)
- (Optional) Trail mix ingredients (e.g., pretzels, popcorn, raisins), bowl, spoon, plastic bags
- Friendship Tips Handout for Session 2 (Activity Page 2.4, see p. 345; one per child)

SESSION OUTLINE

- *Friendship Circle:* Conversation skill review, presentation, and practice (10 minutes)
- *Construction Station:* Listening games—Shape Game, What Is It?, Game Show (15 minutes)
- *Snack:* Collaborative trail mix (optional, 15 minutes)
- *Collaborative Challenges:* Toe-to-Toe, All Together (12 minutes)
- *Closing Circle:* Compliments, Friendship Tips, and assignment (8 minutes)

ADVANCE PREPARATION

- Hang Friendship Group Guidelines poster.
- Cut out category cards for Keep It Going and cut out the Shape Game pictures.

DETAILED SESSION CONTENT

Friendship Circle: Conversation Skill Review, Presentation, and Practice (10 Minutes)

Review the names of the coaches and children in the group, and then ask the children about their experiences using the skills presented last week.

"Last time we talked about telling about yourself and showing a friendly face when you are making a friend. Did you give it a try? How did it go?"

If some children did not try the skills, ask them to think about instances when it might have been a good time to start a conversation, and express the hope that they will give it a try in the coming week. Then introduce the idea that, after telling something about yourself, you need to keep the conversation going by asking questions.

"Once you have started a conversation by telling about yourself, you need to keep the conversation going. If you do all the talking yourself, it is not much of a conversation. A good conversation goes back and forth, with each person taking turns. Asking the other person questions is a good way to get the other person talking. I'm going to show you some examples, and I'd like you to tell me how you think I'm doing."

Hold out the "category cards" (see Activity Page 2.1) and have one of the children pick one. Ask the child to respond to the category card by telling about him- or herself—for example: If he or she picks the card that says "Favorite TV Show," then the child should tell the group his or her favorite TV show). Next, ask the child several follow-up questions, smiling and nodding as the child answers it—for example "When is that show on?"; "What is it about?" After a few conversational turns, stop the conversation and ask the children to reflect on what they saw. Ask them what they noticed you doing in order to keep the conversation going. Then hold out a category card to another child in the circle and do a similar demonstration. After the child has responded to the category, ask him or her a few follow-up questions. After that child has answered your questions, ask the children to comment again on what they saw you doing to keep the conversation going. For a final demonstration, offer a category card to a third child. However, this time, behave in a distracted fashion after you ask a follow-up question—looking away, checking the time or checking your phone, and then changing the subject by commenting on yourself. Ask the children how you did, and let the children explain what was wrong with your behavior. More specifically, ask the children to evaluate your listening and to compare what was different (and better) about the first two examples compared to the third one. Summarize the main points: After you ask a question, good listening is important too—showing a friendly face and looking at the person who is talking, so that he or she knows you are interested in what the person has to say.

"We're going to try a little game right now to see how well you can keep a conversation going on the same topic by asking questions and listening. One person will be 'it' and will draw a card from this pile. [Place the unused category cards in the center of the circle.] The person who is 'it' begins by reading the card and telling about him- or herself. Then we'll go around the circle. Each one of you will ask a question to keep the conversation going, and let the person who is 'it' tell more about him- or herself. The goal is to see how long we can keep the conversation going on the same topic, by letting each person in our circle take turns asking questions. We will try to get all the way around the circle, so everyone has a chance to ask a question. We'll see how much you can find out about each friend."

As children try this game, praise their efforts to tell about themselves, show a friendly face, ask questions, and listen carefully. If children get stuck, encourage them to see if their friends have any ideas about additional follow-up questions to ask. If children go off-topic, reinforce their effort in asking questions, but redirect them to think of a follow-up question that stays on the same topic.

End the activity by praising the children for specific examples of good conversation skills that you observed, and move on to introduce the listening game challenges.

Construction Station: Listening Games—Shape Game, What Is It?, Game Show Interviews (20 Minutes)

The next set of games provides children with fun ways to practice conversation skills. Three different games are described. Consider which games you have time for and will be the most engaging for the children in your group. The games are set up so that children can earn ingredients for a trail mix snack. Making this snack provides an opportunity for social problem solving and collaboration. However, if you do not want to use the snack activity, the listening game challenges can be played without the snack mix rewards.

Shape Game

Children play in pairs, sitting back-to-back. Each child has an identical set of shapes, a blank piece of paper, and a glue stick. One child takes the role of leader and begins to paste the objects on a piece of paper, instructing the other in how to make the same design with the shapes—for example: "Put the red heart in the middle of the page. Put the bird above the heart." The other child is the listener who follows the directions given by the leader in order to try to create the same picture on his or her page as the leader. The listener can ask questions for clarification, but cannot look at what the leader is doing. Upon completion, the two partners turn around and compare the pictures they made, to see how well they succeeded in creating identical patterns. The children can talk about how well (or poorly) they did and how they might cooperate better. Then they reverse roles and try again. If desired, they can earn snack ingredients for their efforts.

What Is It?

One child is given a brown bag with an object in it. The child must describe the object to the other children in the group, without using its name or showing the object to anyone. The other members of the group try to guess what the object is and can also ask questions about it. For example, the person with the bag might say: "It's long and thin. It has a point on the end. You can use it to write with. You can erase with it; it has an eraser at one end." The children try to guess during the sequence of clues, eventually guessing the correct answer—in this case, *pencil*. It is often best for the coach to go first and model how the descriptive process works in this game, prior to giving the children a turn. Once the children guess correctly, put a new object in the bag (without letting the children see it) and let the next person in the circle take a turn at describing it. Continue until all children have had a turn (or interest diminishes).

Game Show Interviews

Children break up into pairs and interview each other to find out information that will be needed for the Game Show (see the Game Show categories on Activity Page 2.3). They take turns asking each other questions and listening to the answers in preparation for the Game Show. If time allows, mix up the different pairs of children, so that each child has a chance to talk with several others in the group. Once the children have had a chance to talk with each other, hold the Game Show. The goal of the Game Show is to earn ingredients for a special snack by remembering things they've learned about each other. The coach acts as the host of the show, asking questions and judging answers. One at a time, each child in the group is called forward to sit in the "Hot Seat" for the show. The host asks the group three questions about the child that are drawn from the category list—for example: "What is his [her] favorite food?"; "How many brothers [sisters] does he [she] have?" The child sitting in the chair cannot give clues, but once his or her teammates have answered, he or she can agree (or disagree). Each child takes a turn sitting in the chair and having team members try to remember information about them. When running the Game Show, it is important to add a certain amount of "hype" to make the game interesting, fun, and challenging for the children. You may want to use a prop to indicate the host, such as a special hat or a pretend microphone. At the conclusion of the game, points can be turned in for the various ingredients in the trail mix or another group reward.

Snack: Collaborative Trail Mix (Optional, 15 Minutes)

In this activity, the group members put together a trail mix snack, using ingredients they earned during their Game Show. First, the children make a plan, discussing how they would like to organize the mixing and distribution of the trail mix. If you feel that a particular group is "out of steam" for this sort of problem solving at this point in the session, you can simply suggest a particular system, such as an assembly line organization. However, if children are able, let them practice communication and negotiation skills as they make a plan.

> "So, now you have earned these fine ingredients to put together a special Friendship Group trail mix for snack. Nicely done with your conversation and listening skills! We need some good ideas for how we can work together to use these ingredients to make a trail mix for everyone, and then divide it up. Who has an idea about how we can do this?"

Once children come up with a plan, let them mix the snack and then enjoy it, as you encourage and facilitate social conversation.

Collaborative Challenges: Toe-to-Toe, All Together (10 Minutes)

Two physical challenges are included here to balance the verbal demands of the session and provide a fun opportunity for teamwork. *Toe-to-Toe* is played as follows. Start with pairs, asking two children to sit holding hands, toe to toe. Their challenge is to stand up at the same time, connected with their toes touching. Once pairs have mastered the activity, see if they can master the challenge with a group of three or four, still touching toes. *All Together* is also played in pairs. Two children sit on the ground with their backs to each other. The partners reach behind their backs and link arms. When you call out "Go," the partners try to stand out without separating. Before each challenge, ask the children to make a plan—for example: "Who has an idea about how you can do this?"; "What do others think of that idea?"; "Does anyone have another idea of how to go about this challenge?" After children complete the challenge, ask them how they did it—for example: "What did you have to do to succeed?"; "When your plan didn't work the first time, how did you turn things around to succeed the second time?" Congratulate the children on their good teamwork.

Closing Circle: Compliments, Friendship Tips, and Assignment
(5 Minutes)

Join in a friendship circle and distribute the Friendship Tips Handout for Session 2.

> "Have you guys had a good time in our friendship group today? I really enjoyed spending time with you today, and I'm impressed with your conversation skills and teamwork! We are going to end our session by looking at the Friendship Tips and talking about how you can work on your friendships this week at home and school."

Review the handout with the children, highlighting the skills they worked on during the session. Read through the suggested practice activities for children to try at home, and let them know that you will be interested in hearing about their experiences with these skills when you all get back together next week. Then proceed to the compliments.

> "You may remember from last week that we finish Friendship Group by sharing compliments, noticing positive things that happened in our group session. Today I'm going to give each one of you a compliment about your work in group today, and I'm also going to ask you to share compliments with each other."

Begin by selecting one child in the group, giving him or her a compliment about a behavior or an effort that you observed during the session—for example: "[Name], you surprised me in the Game Show Interviews —you remembered so much about your friends! You were really a good listener today." Then ask if anyone else has a compliment to share about something positive they saw this child do during the session. Choose one child to give a peer compliment, and then move on to the next child in the circle. Proceed until each child has received a compliment from the coach and a compliment from one of the peers in the group. Then close the session.

SPECIAL ISSUES

1. On occasion, individual children will find it difficult to engage with the group (exhibiting withdrawal or intrusive, distracting behavior), because they feel insecure or anxious in this group setting. To help them settle in, make a particular effort to connect with them and provide a "secure base," attending carefully to those children, maintaining positive eye contact, and providing physical support (e.g., pat on the back) and extensive praise.

2. In general, do not worry if you do not complete all of the activities in this session. Several options are provided to let you choose activities that best suit particular groups. Some groups discuss topics much longer than others.

3. If you are concerned about using the physical challenges in your group, consider the option of the Make a Machine activity from Early Elementary Session 18. Another alternative is a group game such as Apples to Apples, Pictionary Junior, or Outburst Junior that offer structured opportunities to practice communication skills in a fun, game context.

SESSION 3. Initiating Interactions, Inviting Others, Joining In

GOALS

1. Review conversation skills (present a friendly face, tell something about yourself, ask questions, listen).

2. Introduce skills for initiating play: group entry and inviting others.

3. Discuss prosocial friendship qualities.

4. Practice extended conversations.

MATERIALS NEEDED

- Friendship Group Guidelines poster
- Materials for role plays: ball, paper, pencils, game rules (Activity Page 3.1, see p. 346; one per child)
- Paper, glue, decoration materials to divide, statements (Activity Page 3.2, see p. 347; one set per child)
- Up the Ladder game categories, tape
- Friendship Tips Handout for Session 3 (Activity Page 3.3, see p. 348; one per child)

SESSION OUTLINE

- *Friendship Circle:* Skill review, new skill introduction, group entry role plays (15 minutes)
- *Construction Station:* Friendship quality discussion and document making (15 minutes)
- *Snack:* Usual procedures (optional, 15 minutes)
- *Collaborative Challenges:* Up the Ladder game (10 minutes)
- *Closing Circle:* Compliments, Friendship Tips, and assignments (5 minutes)

ADVANCE PREPARATION

- Hang Friendship Group Guidelines poster, prepare small pieces of paper with numbers 1–5.
- Cut out friendship quality statements, create model friendship document.

DETAILED SESSION CONTENT

Friendship Circle: Skill Review, New Skill Introduction, Group Entry Role Plays (15 Minutes)

Review coach and child names; then ask about children's skill practice experiences:

> "Last time, we talked about asking questions to keep a conversation going, and showing a friendly and interested face when you are listening. Who gave it a try? How did it go?"

Ask children to tell about their experiences with asking questions and keeping the conversation going. If they did not try the skills, ask them to think about times when it might have been a good idea to ask questions in a conversation, and express the hope that they will give it a try in the coming week.

To introduce the next activity, remind the children that they have been working on making friends in the past two sessions by telling about themselves and asking questions. Note that having conversations is a good way to build friendships. But before you can have a conversation, you have to get together with another person. You have to invite someone to play with you, or you have to join in a game or activity that is already going on. Explain that today, they are going to work on joining in with others—inviting someone to play with them or asking to join someone else in his or her play. To do so, they are going to play a game that requires some playacting. As the coach, place cards with the numbers 1–5 facedown and mix them up (add more cards if there are more than five children in the group). Ask each child to draw a number. This number will indicate his or her role for the upcoming role-play scene. Explain that you will do one practice scene together to help them get comfortable with playacting, and proceed to read Scene 1.

Scene 1

> "Two friends [Players 1 and 2] are sitting on a bench during recess with nothing to do. [Have the children with the card numbers 1 and 2 pretend to sit on a bench and comment to each other that they are bored and have nothing to do.] A child [Player 3] walks by holding a ball. [Give Player 3 a ball and have him or her walk by the bench.] The challenge for Players 1 and 2 is to find a way to join together in play. Players 4 and 5—you are the judges. You are going to watch what happens, and see if they do a good job in inviting others to play and join in together. So, let's hear some ideas about how you could get a game going in this scene."

Let the players talk with each other about their ideas, and provide support, as needed. Suggest an intrusive alternative (e.g., "You could throw the ball at the kids on the bench") and encourage the children to tell you why that is a bad idea, emphasizing the take-home point (e.g., "You're right, it's better to ask"). They will suggest that one child ask another if he or she wants to play ball. Once they are ready, let them play out the scene. Ask the judges (Players 4 and 5) what they saw the children doing to join in, and how well they thought it worked—for example: "What kind of body language did you see when he [she] invited the friend to play?"; "Who did you see with a friendly face?"; "Do you have any suggestions for this group?" Have children choose new numbers for the next scene. Continue with new scenes until children's interest starts to fade. Then move on to the next activity, even if you have not finished all of the scenes. Other scenes:

Scene 2

All children are sitting at a table after lunch. Players 2 and 3 start to play Pig-in-a-Poke (also called the Dot Game). The others are just sitting there feeling bored. The challenge for the watchers is to find a way to join in the play. Player 1 is the judge.

Scene 3

Players 1 and 2 are riding on the bus, playing Rock, Paper, Scissors. Players 4 and 5 are sitting and watching; their challenge is to find a way to join in the play. Player 3 is the judge.

Scene 4

Players 2 and 3 are playing Tic-Tac-Toe at a table; Player 4 sits down near them, with the challenge of finding a way to join in the play. Players 1 and 5 are the judges.

Scene 5

Players 3 and 5 are tossing a ball back and forth. Player 2 walks up to watch, then tries to join in the play. Then Player 1 walks by and also tries to join in. Player 4 is judge.

After each scene, ask the judges and other children to evaluate the experience. Use varied questions to encourage them to reflect on their experience:

"What worked?"

"What did not work?"

"What was hard about that situation?"

"How did you feel when you were asking to play?"

"How did you feel when someone was asking to join in your game?"

"What did you do with your body language to show your interest and friendliness?"

"Would your solution work at your school?"

Note that the Friendship Tips for the day include ideas for how to join in an ongoing game, and can be introduced here if it seems helpful. To join an ongoing game, children are encouraged to follow these steps:

1. Look around. Who looks ready to include you?
2. Move closer and watch that person.
3. Say something nice about his or her game (e.g., "Nice move"; "That looks fun").
4. Ask if you can play.
5. If he or she says no, try again later or look around for someone else to play with.

Construction Station: Friendship Quality Discussion and Document Making (15 Minutes)

The next activity involves the construction of Friendship Qualities documents. The purpose of this cooperative craft activity is to encourage children to think about the qualities of a good friend and to practice communication skills (expressing their viewpoint and listening to their friends) as they talk about friendships. In addition, children are asked to give ideas and make a plan together to divide up materials to decorate their documents. To set up for this activity, have the children sit around a table. Give each child a blank page with "A good friend is . . ." written at the top. In addition, give each child a set of precut statements describing friendship characteristics (Activity Page 3.2), along with some blank strips of paper, in case they want to write down their own ideas. Children choose statements (or write statements) that they feel are important to friendships and glue or tape them onto these papers. Then they take turns showing the statements they chose to the rest of the group and describing why they selected those statements. It is often helpful to prepare one finished example of a Friendship Qualities document that includes some of the prepared statements (e.g., Activity Page 3.2) and some original written statements to show the children before they begin the task.

> "I'm excited to show you the activity I brought today. Each of you will have a chance to make your own Friendship Qualities document. [Show finished example.] You each have a paper that says at the top 'A good friend is. . . .' Your job is to think about the qualities that you think are important in a friend. You can write your own ideas on these slips of paper, or you can choose things that are already written. For example, this paper says 'Fun to be with' and this one says 'Cares about my feelings.' Those are things that some of you might feel are important qualities in a friend, and you might have your own ideas too. I'll give you time to make your selections and tape them on your paper, and then we'll all share our ideas. When you are done, we'll decorate these documents."

You may need to help some children read the statements or write additional ideas. As children work, praise their efforts, converse with them about their choices, and comment on their positive teamwork. Once the children have created documents, move ahead to share their ideas:

> "Your papers are looking great—you selected some really good ideas about friendship. We are going to go around the table and give each person a chance to share his or her ideas about friendship. You can show us your page and tell us about your choices and what you think is most important in a friend. We'll work on being good listeners."

Let children take turns describing the statements they chose and why they think those qualities are important in a friendship. Ask one or two follow-up questions; see if others have questions or comments. Then introduce the decoration materials. It is important to have some decorations that need to be divided (e.g., stickers, sequins, ribbons) so that children have something about which to negotiate and plan. As you hold these materials in your hands, so that children can see them, explain how you'd like the group to negotiate the division of materials:

> "To finish up these posters, I brought several things that I thought you could use to decorate your papers. I have these great stickers for you to use, and also this ribbon. I need your help in coming up with a plan for how we can divide up these materials so that everyone has some good decorations. Who has a good idea about how to do this?"

Encourage children to suggest some strategies for dividing up the materials. Ask them to listen to their friends, and give each child a chance to offer an idea. Then review the ideas and ask children to indicate which idea they feel is best. If children have trouble reaching a consensus and their interest starts to fade, choose one idea to try and let them know that you will remember the other idea(s) to try in the future. Let the children implement the plan and finish decorating their posters. Praise them for their teamwork and transition to the next activity.

Snack (Optional, 15 Minutes)

The usual procedures are followed. During snack time, encourage conversation among the children. When you notice children sharing information and asking each other questions, comment on their good conversation skills. If children speak primarily to the adults, bring other children into the conversation by asking if they had a similar experience or have a comment to share about the topic.

Collaborative Challenges: Up the Ladder Game (10 Minutes)

In this game, one person is "it" and stands at the front of the group. Four strips of tape should be place horizontally on the floor in front of the person who is "it," wide enough for the other children to stand along each strip of tape (creating the rungs of the ladder). The person who is "it" chooses a category card that identifies a topic area for conversation (e.g., school, this weekend, sports, holidays, chores, brothers and sisters, animals, trips, pets, wishes). The other children stand along the line of tape that is farthest away. They take turns asking questions to get more information from the person who is "it" about the category—for example: "What school do you go to?"; "What is your favorite subject?"; "What do you like least about your school?" The players raise their hands when they have a question in mind, and the person who is "it" calls on them. After they ask their question and get an answer, the question-asker is allowed to move forward one step to the next horizontal line closer to the person who is "it." Once a person reaches the top of the Ladder, by asking questions and stepping up each of the lines, that person becomes the next "it." The other players go back to the first line, and the new "it" draws a new category card.

Closing Circle: Compliments, Friendship Tips, and Assignments (5 Minutes)

For the closing activity, join in a friendship circle and distribute copies of the Friendship Tips Handout for Session 3. Go around the circle and let each child say what he or she liked best about the session. Give each child a compliment about his or her effort and accomplishments in the session, and also ask a peer to give the child a compliment. Review the Friendship Tips Handout for Session 3 and the practice "assignment" for the children to work on during the week.

SPECIAL ISSUES

1. The role-play activity and Up the Ladder game place demands on children's verbal and attention skills. Take care to pace these activities to keep children engaged. If needed, increase involvement by giving all children active roles in the role play (doubling up on roles) and reducing the steps in the Up the Ladder game from four to three to reduce the number of questions needed to progress and increase the rate of turnover in roles.

2. Note that these activities assume that the children attending the group have the basic skills needed to work together cooperatively—the skills of helping, sharing, and taking turns. If these tasks are too challenging for your group, consider using early elementary sessions to build basic skills before moving on to the more complex social skills in advanced elementary sessions.

SESSION 4. Practicing Conversations: Performance Review

GOALS

1. Review and consolidate the target conversation skills.

2. Self-evaluate to recognize gains and set personal goals to improve conversation skills.

3. Practice cooperation skills in the context of collaborative group activities.

MATERIALS NEEDED

- Poster: Friendship Group Guidelines
- Cards for the Conversation Charades circle game (Activity Page 4.1, see p. 349; one set per group)
- Poster board for Friendship Movie—Scene 1 list of ideas
- Recording and playback device: cell phone or digital camera
- Director's Checklist score sheet for movie planning/review (Activity Page 4.2, see p. 350; one per child)
- Soft objects for Group Juggle
- Friendship Tips Handout for Session 4 (Activity Page 4.3, see p. 351; one per child)

SESSION OUTLINE

- *Friendship Circle:* Conversation Charades, Talk Show Host introduction (15 minutes)
- *Construction Station:* Rehearse, tape, review Talk Show Host interviews (20 minutes)
- *Snack:* Usual procedures (optional, 15 minutes)
- *Collaborative Challenges:* Group Juggle extended challenges (5 minutes)
- *Closing Circle:* Compliments, Friendship Tips, and assignment (5 minutes)

ADVANCE PREPARATION

- Hang poster.
- Cut out Conversation Charades cards.

DETAILED SESSION CONTENT

Friendship Circle: Conversation Charades, Talk Show Host Introduction (15 Minutes)

Begin by touching base and asking children about their experiences using their friendship skills—for example: "It's good to see all of you. I'm interested in hearing how your week went. Last time we talked about inviting others to play and joining in play. Did anyone give it a try?" If children did not try the skills, ask them to think about times when they felt that they wanted to invite others to play or join in the play. Ask them to describe the situation and elicit suggestions from the group about what type of invitation or strategy might work in that situation. Express the hope that they will give it a try in the coming week. Then introduce the Conversation Charades game.

> "We're going to play Conversation Charades today. In this game, two children are actors and the rest of you are the judges. We'll take turns so everyone gets a chance to be actors and judges. One of the actors will choose a card from this pile [use the category cards from Session 2, Activity Page 2.1] and tell something about him- or herself. The other actor will choose a card from this pile [show the Conversation Charades cards], which tells the person how to act when he or she responds. Some of these cards have good ideas about how to keep the conversation going, such as this one: 'Look at the person and ask a question.' Some have ideas that are not so good, like this one: 'Look bored and tired.' The actor will read this card secretly and act out what it says. The judges will watch and guess what was on the card."

Ask for two volunteers to start things off. If any children have trouble reading, provide assistance. Let them each draw cards, and ask them to start the action. Let them talk for a few turns before asking the other children (the judges) to guess what was on the card. Once they guess correctly, ask them a few follow-up questions—for example: "What made you think that [Name] was acting interested?"; "How did that make his [her] partner feel?"; "How did it affect the conversation?"

Construction Station: Rehearse, Tape, Review Talk Show Host Interviews (20 Minutes)

The purpose of the interview recording is to provide children with the opportunity to practice conversation skills and then review their performance, in order to evaluate themselves and set personal goals. The task is set up as a TV "Talk Show" in which a host interviews an individual to learn more about them.

> "Have you ever watched a talk show on TV, where a host interviews a celebrity and asks questions about him or her? [Let children respond and get an example or two of talk shows with which they are familiar.] Today we are going to film our own talk show. This will give you a chance to show off your interview skills. One person will play the talk show host, asking questions and listening. The other person will play the celebrity who is being interviewed, answering questions about him- or herself. We'll take turns so that everyone has a chance to be the host and to be interviewed. How does that sound?"

Before starting to film the show, it is important to engage children in planning what they will say. Set the stage by identifying a seat for the host and one for the celebrity guest. If desired, tell children they can do a "dry run" rehearsal before you turn on the recorder. Alternatively, they can simply discuss their plan for the conversation or interview. Encourage them to brainstorm what topics the talk show host might ask the guest about. These might include things like hobbies, favorite movies or books, favorite sports or video games, pets, future plans,and the like. Use a blackboard or paper to record them so they are available during taping.

Show the Director's Checklist (Activity Page 4.2) and explain that, together, you will review the talk show to see how well it demonstrates a good conversation: showing a friendly face, asking questions, telling about yourself, listening carefully, and keeping it going with more questions. Once children have a plan and are ready to go, begin the taping process. Talk Show interviews should be short (2 minutes or so) to allow children to rotate so that each plays the part of host and guest.

After taping an interview, do a formal review with the group. Play the taped segment, referring children to the score sheets as you work through the items. After each segment, ask the host and guest how they thought they did on the different skills noted on the checklist, see if other children have thoughts, and give your input. The goal is to identify skills that are looking good and also ways to improve and refine skill performance. In some cases, children may want to redo their interviews to improve their segment. If they are interested in doing this, let them redo the taping to practice their skills, even if it means that you will need to skip the next game.

Snack (Optional, 15 Minutes)

The usual procedures are followed. Note that, if desired, you can watch and review the tapes together during snack.

Collaborative Challenges: Group Juggle Extended Challenges (5 Minutes)

The amount of time left in the session after taping the Talk Show Interviews and reviewing them varies from group to group. In some cases, you will need to proceed directly to the compliment circle, without a group game. In other cases, you may have time for one or two games. If time allows and the group enjoyed Group Juggle during the first session, consider playing it again with one or more of the following extensions. To start off, repeat the game as it was played in Session 1. Then ask the children if they are ready to try an extra challenge. Ask them how many things they think they can juggle at one time. Let the group pick a number (up to four), and let them try it. To get multiple objects going, start the first one in the usual way. Then, when it has moved forward by two or three catches, start the next object in the pattern. Continue until all objects are circulating. If time allows, add a speed challenge. Repeat the circle toss pattern with one object. Quietly time the task, and let the children know how many seconds it took them to complete the pattern. Ask the children how fast they think they could do it if they tried their best. Ask for input from around the circle to get various responses, and have the team agree on an initial time goal for which to aim. Encourage the children to share their ideas about how they can reduce their time—for example: "What can you do differently to finish the pattern more quickly?"; "How will you help each other be faster?" Let the group try their plan. In some groups, children will try to speed up too much and toss/throw wildly. If this happens, ask the children to think about what happened and why, and how they could reduce the risk of lost time due to wild throws in the next try. If the team succeeds, challenge the children to get very creative and think about the most efficient and fastest method for moving the ball through the sequence. How quick can they be? What could they do to improve their time? Note that it is possible for a group to get their time down to 10 seconds or so by repositioning team members so that they are standing as close as possible to each other, and lined up in the order of the pattern. If children do not consider reorganizing themselves when they are problem solving, ask a few questions to elicit flexible thinking—for example: "I wonder if getting up and moving around or changing the circle might help?" After the children complete their attempt, encourage them to reflect on their success with a few discussion questions—for example: "What did you do that was the most helpful in speeding up your time?"; "How did you think of that solution to the problem?"; "How did you work as a team in that challenge?"; "What worked for you?"

Closing Circle: Compliments, Friendship Tips, and Assignment (5 Minutes)

Going around the circle, give each child a compliment describing the efforts and skills he or she displayed during the session. Ask for a peer compliment for each child, and ask the child to give him- or herself a compliment about the efforts made in the taping—for example: "What contribution did you feel most proud of?" Then review the Friendship Tips Handout for Session 4 and the assignment for the week.

SPECIAL ISSUES

1. In some cases, children may feel shy about participating in the video. Let them double up with another child for his or her part for the first time, so the child does not feel stressed about playing the part alone. Let the child know that children often feel funny doing this the first time, but it gets much easier to do after gaining experience with it.

2. In some cases, children may get silly with the video, making goofy faces or loud noises in the movie. One way to handle this is to tell the children that after they make a serious movie, you will film them making a short silly movie. Choose this option only if you think the children will be able to make a short silly movie without becoming disorganized. If needed, remind them that the school rules hold and they cannot use bathroom talk or other impolite gestures in the movie. If you feel that the opportunity to film a short, silly segment will be disorganizing for the group, explain that you would like to show this movie to others and cannot show a silly movie. Express the hope that they are up to the challenge of making a good production, but film contingent on appropriate behavior.

3. Time management can be challenging in this session. Some groups will be highly engaged in the video construction and review and will spend most of the session working on this task. If so, do not worry about completing the Group Juggle.

4. If children seem shy about complimenting themselves, note:

"When you watch yourself on tape, it's easy to focus on the things you wish you had done differently. I don't want you to forget about all of things you did well! So, after I give each of you a compliment about the way you participated during the group, I'd like you to think of a compliment for yourself about how you talked or got along with others in our group during our movie-making today. It's always good to focus on what is going well, in addition to the things you'd like to improve."

Category Cards for the Discovery Circle Activity

Favorite food	Best carnival ride	Number of brothers and sisters
Your pets	Favorite TV show	What you like to do on Saturday
Best movie	Favorite sport	Silliest TV show
What you would buy with $1,000	Scariest movie you have seen	Best book

Friendship Discovery Poster

Total number of pets	Band everyone likes	Three foods no one likes 1. 2. 3.
Place everyone wants to visit	Good things about school: 1. 2. 3. 4.	Games everyone likes: 1. 2. 3.
Total number of brothers and sisters	Favorite summer activities: 1. 2. 3. 4.	Favorite after-school activities: 1. 2. 3.

Friendship Tips Handout for Session 1

Remember

When meeting and greeting others:

Show a friendly face.

Tell about you.

Try It Out

Practice telling interesting things about yourself to your family and close friends.

Practice showing a friendly face.

Self-Check

What interesting things did you talk about?

How much were you able to tell?

Did you smile and look the person in the eye?

Was the person friendly in response?

Category Cards for Keep It Going

Foods you like	A trip you took	Favorite TV show
Animals you like	Favorite school subjects	What you like to do after school
Things you don't like to do	Favorite holiday	Superhero power you wish for
Something that annoys you	Favorite sport	Your dream vacation

Pieces for the Shape Game

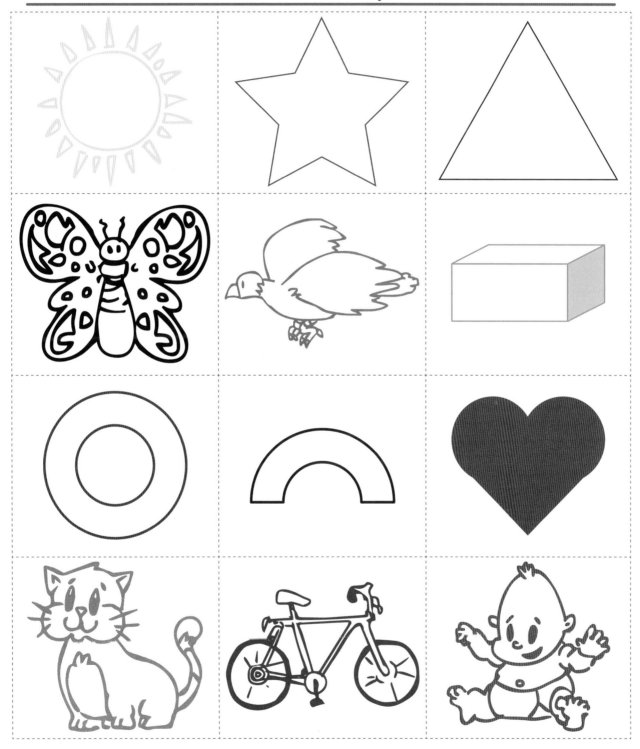

List of Categories for the Game Show

Number of brothers and sisters
Pets
Favorite movie
Favorite sport
Toppings you like on pizza
Favorite ice cream flavor
Grade in school
Birthday month
Favorite food
Least favorite chore
Secret talent

Friendship Tips Handout for Session 2

Remember

To talk with others:

Show a friendly face.

Tell about yourself.

Then keep it going:

Ask questions.

Listen.

Try It Out

Practice asking questions to get your family and friends to tell you more.

Self-Check

Did you ask questions about what the other person said?

Did you keep the conversation going with questions?

Did you show you were interested?

What did you find out?

Game Rules

Pig-in-a-Poke (also called the Dot Game or Dots and Boxes)

Begin by creating an empty grid of dots (three or four rows of four dots each). Players take turns, adding a single horizontal or vertical line between two open, adjacent dots. A player who completes a box by putting in the final line puts his or her initial in the box, earns 1 point, and takes another turn. The game ends when no more lines can be placed. The winner of the game is the player with the most points (i.e., the most boxes completed).

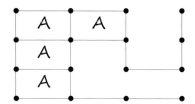

Rock, Paper, Scissors

Two players each make a fist with one hand and hold the other open, palm upward. At the same time, they tap their fists in their open palms once, twice, and on the third time form one of three items: a rock (by keeping the hand in a fist), a sheet of paper (by holding the hand flat, palm down), or a pair of scissors (by extending the first two fingers and holding them apart).

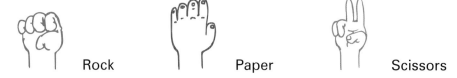

Rock   Paper   Scissors

If the same item is formed, it's a tie. For the other forms, the hierarchy is that rock smashes scissors, scissors cut paper, and paper wraps over rock.

Tic-Tac-Toe

Create a grid of nine boxes by making two vertical and two horizontal lines. Players take turns placing either an *X* or an *O* in an empty box. When three *X*'s or *O*'s in a row are attained (vertical, horizontal, or diagonal), the player wins.

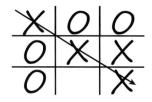

Words and Phrases for Friendship Qualities Discussion, with Blank Cards for Children's Ideas

Friendly	Helpful
Fun to be with	A good sport
Nice	Loyal
A good listener	Someone I can talk to
Caring	Honest

Friendship Tips Handout for Session 3

Remember

To be a part of the play:

Invite someone to play with you.

Ask if you can join in.

Try It Out

To join in someone's play:

1. Look around. Who is ready to include you?

2. Move closer and watch them.

3. Say something nice about their game ("That looks fun").

4. Ask if you can play.

5. If they say "no," try again later or look for someone else to play with.

Self-Check

Who did you invite to play? Did he or she say "yes"?

Did you try to join in to someone else's play? How did it go?

If he or she said "no," did you try something else?

Cards for Conversation Charades

Look interested, ask a question.	Smile and agree with them. Say "Me too."	Look bored and tired.
Look away, play with your clothes or shoes.	Smile. Nod.	Look angry. Tell them they are wrong.
Look at them. Smile. Ask for more information.	Interrupt. Talk when they are talking.	Look friendly, give a compliment.

Movie Planning and Review Guide

Director's Checklist

Talk Show Host: _____.

☐ Showed a friendly face.

☐ Asked questions.

☐ Showed good listening skills.

☐ Kept the conversation going with more questions.

Celebrity Guest: _____.

☐ Showed a friendly face.

☐ Showed good listening skills.

☐ Told about him- or herself.

☐ Kept the conversation going by answering questions.

Things to keep in the show that went well:

_____

_____

_____

_____

_____

Things to work on to improve the show:

_____

_____

_____

_____

_____

Friendship Tips Handout for Session 4

Remember

Talking with others builds friendships:

Start a conversation.

Ask a question. Listen.

Tell about you.

Keep it going with another question.

Try It Out

Where can you start a conversation?

> Before school starts.

> On the bus.

> At lunch.

> After school.

> On the phone.

Self-Check

How did you do? Did you start a conversation?

Did you keep it going by listening, telling about you, and asking a question?

UNIT II

Understanding and Respecting Others

SESSION 5. Friendly Competition: Good Sportsmanship and the Golden Rule

---

GOALS

1. Introduce and discuss the concept of the Golden Rule.

2. Introduce and discuss the concept of good sportsmanship.

3. Review strategies to cope effectively with competitive play (winning and losing).

4. Practice applying these skills in competitive and collaborative play.

MATERIALS NEEDED

- Posters: Friendship Group Guidelines, Golden Rule with cut-out words to tape on (Activity Page 5.1, see p. 372; one set per group)

- Pennant/flag materials: markers, glue, stickers, pictures (Activity Page 5.2, see p. 373; one set per group)

- Class Champion story and role-play guide (Activity Page 5.3, see pp. 374–375; one per group), name tags

- What to say when you win/lose ideas (Activity Page 16.1 from Early Elementary Session 16, see p. 210; one per group)

- Two cups, five dice, Fair Play Score Sheets (Activity Page 5.4, see p. 376; one per group)

- Friendship Tips Handout for Session 5 (Activity Page 5.5, see p. 377; one per child)

SESSION OUTLINE

- *Friendship Circle:* Check in, introduce the Golden Rule (10 minutes)
- *Construction Station:* Pennant decoration, Class Champion story and play (20 minutes)
- *Snack:* Usual procedures (optional, 15 minutes)
- *Collaborative Challenges:* Good things to say when you win/lose, dice games (10 minutes)
- *Closing Circle:* Compliments, Friendship Tips, and assignment (5 minutes)

ADVANCE PREPARATION

- Hang poster.
- Cut out headings and words for Golden Rule poster; paste on the headings.
- Cut poster board into pennant or flag shape; cut out pictures for pennant/flag decorations.
- Cut "good things to say" into separate statements
- Create blank page entitled: "Friendship Tips: Good Things to Say When You Win or Lose"

DETAILED SESSION CONTENT

Friendship Circle: Check In, Introduce the Golden Rule (10 Minutes)

Greet children and ask about their friendship experiences and skill use in the past week.

> "It's good to see all of you. I'm interested in hearing how your week went. Does anyone have a friendship story to share? Or a friendship problem they'd like to talk about? Did you try out any of the tips we talked about in Friendship Group?"

Let children share their experiences. If they bring up concerns or problems, ask whether any of the other children in the group have any thoughts about the concern or ideas about how to deal with it. If relevant, encourage them to apply the friendship tips and ideas from group. Then introduce the Golden Rule poster and ask the children to discuss it, as follows.

> "I brought a new friendship poster with me today. [Show Golden Rule poster.] At the top here it says 'The Golden Rule: Treat others as you want to be treated.' What does that mean to you? Can you give me some examples? [Let children discuss.] At the bottom it says 'To make a good friend, be a good friend.' What does that mean to you?"

After children have shared some thoughts, bring out the cut-out words that describe friendship qualities. Explain that you would like to personalize the poster and add words that these group members feel are especially important to them in their friendships. Go around the circle and let each child pick one or two words that he or she would like to add to the poster, asking the child to explain why he or she thinks that quality is important in friendships. Once the extra words have been added to the poster, tape it on the wall, and move to a table to construct the team pennant.

The pennant construction activity provides practice in several social skills, including inhibiting impulsive actions and planning before acting; expressing ideas in a group setting; recognizing, understanding, and tolerating different points of view; and using communication skills to resolve conflicts. To get started, pull out a large poster board cut in a triangle (pennant) or square (flag) shape and the decorating materials (pictures, stickers, markers, glue) and explain the task.

"Today, you are going to decorate a pennant [flag] for your friendship team. We want everyone in the group to be happy with the pennant [flag]. So, before you start, I'll give you time to share your ideas and listen to your friends, and make a plan for how you want to decorate the pennant [flag]. There are three things you should talk about: (1) what kind of a border you want around the outside of the pennant [flag], and who is drawing that; (2) which of these stickers or pictures you want on your pennant [flag], and who will put them on; and (3) what message you want to write on your pennant [flag], and who will write it. The message might be something like 'Go Team!' or 'We're Number 1!'"

Hold on to the materials as the children talk about their plan. Provide help, as needed, to facilitate their planning and discussion. Once they have a plan, let them begin the decoration process. Note that if you think that your group will find the planning discussion difficult, simplify by dropping one of the discussion elements (e.g., plan the pictures and words, drop the border). Once children have completed their plan and moved into the arts-and-crafts part of the activity, explain that they will put on a play later in the session and you want to review that story.

"After you are done with your team pennant [flag], I have a new challenge for you. I'm going to read you a friendship story and talk about it a little bit. Then, when you're done decorating, we'll put on a little play, and each of you will get to play a part in this story. What do you think about that? As I read through it, we'll talk about the characters and what you think they might be feeling, and you can think about what part you'd like to play."

The first time you read through this story with them, it is important to ask a few questions about how they think the characters are thinking and feeling, and why the children are behaving the way they are. The goal is to help them reflect on the challenges of competitive play and balancing a desire to win with an awareness of others' feelings. Some sample questions are included. When you read the story the first time, ignore the bolded lines that you will use when you role-play the story.

After you finish reading the story and the children finish decorating the pennant/flag, put on a play of "The Class Champion" story. Have children discuss and select the roles they want to play and give them name tags for their parts in the story. Note that the character names can be changed to be male or female (e.g., Tim/Tami, Daniel/Dana, Carter/Carli), and additional classmate names can be added so that every child has a specific role. If a child is very reluctant to take part, he or she can serve as the director and help organize the action. If desired, you can also bring small props (e.g., baseball hats, sweatbands) to help the children get into the spirit of the play. Once players are ready, begin the play by reading through the story again, section by section. Stop after reading each section to allow the children to dramatize their parts; suggested role-play actions are included in bold type, but children can also be encouraged to consider how they want to dramatize the story events. Remind them to think about what their characters are thinking and feeling in each scene. At the conclusion of the play, congratulate the children on their acting and ask them how it felt.

Snack (Optional, 15 Minutes)

The usual procedures are followed. Snack time provides a good opportunity to talk more generally with the children and to follow up with them about their feelings and friendship experiences in the context of competition. For example, you might explore their own experiences with competition or sports, whether they know anyone like Daniel, why they think competition sometimes brings out the worst in people, and what they think it means to be a good sport and a fair player.

Collaborative Challenges: Good Things to Say When You Win/Lose, Dice Games (10 Minutes)

Before bringing out the dice games, create a Friendship Tips poster using the statements and process from the Early Elementary Session 16 (Activity Page 16.1).

> "One of the things that can make competition really difficult is that it brings out strong feelings. When you win, it can be a real rush—very exciting. Have you ever felt that way when you win? When you lose, though, it can be a serious disappointment—very upsetting. Has anyone had that experience? In the face of those strong feelings, it's not that easy to stop and think about how your words might affect others. We're going to read through these ideas and decide which ones you think would be good things to say when you win or lose. Then, we'll tap them onto this Friendship Tips poster."

Bring out the suggested statements from Activity Page 16.1 (Early Elementary Session 16). Some of these are good thing to say when you win or lose because they help you express your feelings in words that won't hurt your friends' feelings. Let children take turns drawing the statements and putting the good things to say on a Friendship Tips poster. See if they have any additional ideas to add.

The purpose of the following dice games is to give children practice keeping their cool and using the Friendship Tips to maintain good sportsmanship in a competitive situation. These games work best if you divide children into dyads and triads, so they are not waiting a long time for their turns. Show children the Fair Play Score Sheet and explain that you want them to keep track of wins and also of good sportsmanship—good effort. Give them a copy of the "good things to say" tips, so they have it handy. As they play, provide praise and positive comments when you observe their efforts at fair play and good sportsmanship.

The dice games require five dice and a cup. For Five Up, children take turns shaking the five dice in a cup and then tossing them down. Each turn, they get to throw the dice three times. The goal is to get as many dice of one number as possible over the course of those three throws. So, the strategy is to keep out dice that match the same number each throw. For example, if they threw two 5's in the first throw, they might hold out the 5's and toss the other three dice again to see if they could roll additional 5's in the following turn. Children get a point for the largest number of matching die they roll (e.g., two of a kind is 2 points; three of a kind is 3 points). At the end of the game, the player with the most points wins.

The second variation of this game, Five Straight, also uses the dice in the same way, except that children try to get dice in a 1-2-3-4-5 sequence. Their score is the number of unique numbers they get. At the end of the games, ask the children how it went, and whether they used any of the "good things to say" tips, or if they used any other strategy to keep their cool when they won or lost.

Closing Circle: Compliments, Friendship Tips, and Assignment (5 Minutes)

For the closing activity, join in a friendship circle and distribute copies of the Friendship Tips Handout for Session 5. Review the handout with the children, highlighting the skills they worked on during the group. Read through the suggested practice activities for children to try at home (or let children take turns reading them aloud), and let them know that you will be interested in hearing about their experiences with these skills when you all get back together next week. Then proceed to the compliments.

> "One way to be a good friend is to notice when others are making positive efforts. We're going to share compliments today, and I'd like to ask you to focus your compliments on something you saw a team member do today that really showed a good effort at using the Golden Rule—treating others with consideration and kindness."

Proceed to go around the circle, so that each child receives a compliment from you, a compliment from a peer, and gives a compliment to him- or herself.

SPECIAL ISSUES

1. This session has a lot of opportunity for discussion. If the children in your group have less well-developed verbal skills and find these discussions very effortful, you may need to be energetic and supportive in helping children to voice opinions and contribute to plans. You will also need to monitor children's engagement, and may need to reduce (or skip) some of the discussion options in order to maintain their interest. If you are concerned about this issue with your group, use your judgment to modify some of the verbal demands to keep the session within an optimal level of difficulty for the group—and avoid a level of demand that elicits boredom or unresponsiveness.

2. A different kind of difficulty that can emerge in this session is that some children become highly engaged in the discussion topic and want to share extensive information about themselves and their experiences, whereas other children are less interested and become disengaged. In this case, the challenge for coaches is to keep the discussion moving forward, politely redirecting individual children if they monopolize the discussion or divert into detailed descriptions of their own experience—for example, you might say: "It's great to hear your thoughts on this, but I've noticed we're running short on time. I just want to make sure the others have a chance to put in their thoughts before we have to move on"; or "That is a very interesting story that would be fun to hear more about sometime, but I've noticed we've gotten off our friendship topic for today. I want to make sure we have a chance to finish this plan." In general, it is important for coaches to monitor the pacing of this group to maintain positive engagement for all members.

3. If competitive play is very challenging for children in your group and they need more practice, consider using some of the sessions from the Early Elementary Friendship Group Manual that spend more time building fair play concepts and practicing good sportsmanship skills.

SESSION 6. Cooperating and Negotiating: Work It Out, Make a Deal

GOALS

1. Introduce the problem-solving model with the Traffic Light poster.
2. Practice the steps of the problem-solving model.
3. Practice the skills of good sportsmanship, problem solving, and negotiation during play.

MATERIALS NEEDED

- Posters: Friendship Group Guidelines, Golden Rule, Traffic Light
- Role-play cards and balloons, cups or envelopes for hiding (Activity Page 6.1, see p. 378; one per group)
- Poster board and team mascot/motto pictures (Activity Page 6.2, see p. 379; one per group)
- Materials for Memory Tray, "platform" for All Aboard team challenge
- Friendship Tips Handout for Session 6 (Activity Page 6.3, see p. 380; one per child)

SESSION OUTLINE

- *Friendship Circle:* Introduce the Traffic Light poster with role plays (15 minutes).
- *Construction Station:* Team mascot and motto discussion (10 minutes)
- *Snack:* Usual procedures (optional, 15 minutes)
- *Collaborative Challenges:* Memory Challenge, Human Tangles, All Aboard (15 minutes)
- *Closing Circle:* Compliments with Pass the Yarn sharing, Friendship Tips (5 minutes)

ADVANCE PREPARATION

- Hang Friendship Group Guidelines, Golden Rule, and Traffic Light posters.
- Cut out role-play scenarios, place in balloons, cups, or envelopes.
- Prepare Memory Tray.

DETAILED SESSION CONTENT

Friendship Circle: Introduce the Traffic Light Poster with Role Plays (15 Minutes)

Greet children and check in about their friendship experiences and skill use during the past week.

> "It's good to see all of you. I'm interested in hearing how your week went. Who used some Friendship Tips? Tell us about your friendship experiences."

Let children share their experiences. Reinforce them for their efforts. If they bring up concerns or problems, see if any of the other children have input or ideas. Ask them whether any of the friendship tips or ideas from group might be used. Then introduce the Traffic Light poster.

> "I brought a new friendship poster with me today. [Show the Traffic Light poster.] At the top it says: 'When You Have a Problem—Work It Out.' Then there are three steps."

Read through the steps listed under the Red, Yellow, and Green lights. Explain that children can use these steps to work out a problem and make a deal with each other. Show them how to "Take 5" (see full explanation in Early Elementary Session 7).

> "I've noticed that when I have a problem, I feel upset. I can feel my heart beating faster in my chest. Have you noticed that? So I put my hand over my heart to steady it, and I take a deep breath and count to 5 to calm myself down. [Show how you breathe in through your nose for a count of 3, and out through your mouth for a count of 2.] I just blow some of the stress out, so I am ready to talk about my feelings and work out the problem."

Ask the children what they think of the Traffic Light poster. Find out if they have ever used something like this traffic light, and how it worked for them (or if not, how they think it might work for them). If they express doubts, let children know that today they will be trying out these steps to see how they work. Next, introduce the role plays (see Activity Page 6.1). For fun, cut the scenarios into small slips of paper and place them inside balloons that are then blown up, or place the slips inside cups or envelopes. Explain that each child will have a chance to take a turn. To do so, each child will select a team member as a partner, and then pop a balloon (lift up a cup; open an envelope) to find out what their problem is. Their task is to use the Traffic Light steps to role-play a problem-solving discussion to make a deal with each other and work out the problem.

Proceed with the role plays until all children have had a turn. As they work, remind them to enact each of the three steps on the Traffic Light poster (going to the red light, yellow light, green light). As they finish, ask them how they felt about their negotiation—and their solution. Reinforce their efforts and lead the group in clapping for each pair as they finish their role play. Then proceed to the table for a discussion of the team mascot and motto.

Construction Station: Team Mascot/Motto Discussion, Memory Challenge (15 Minutes)

This activity gives children "real-life" practice in listening, communication, and negotiation skills, as they engage in group decision making. Their task is to select an animal mascot that has qualities they admire as a team. The animal name will become their team mascot and the animal qualities will become the team motto. Introduce the idea like this:

> "I wanted to talk with you today about our Friendship Team. In some ways, we are a lot like other teams, like baseball teams or football teams, because we work together to get things done and we have fun together. I've been thinking that we need a name and a mascot. Did you ever wonder why teams pick certain names or mascots? [Let children respond.] Like the Chicago Bulls—why do you think they picked that name? What does a bull mean to you? What do you think about when you think of a bull?"

The goal of this discussion is to help the children recognize that team names and mascots are symbols designed to highlight qualities that team members admire. Use additional (and local) illustrations, as needed, to help them catch onto the concept and the variety of images that represent various sports teams (e.g., Miami Dolphins, Nittany Lions, Washington Huskies).

"Today, I'm going to give you a chance to pick an animal mascot and a motto for our Friendship Team. I brought some pictures of different animals with me today to give you some ideas. Some are real animals that you could see at the zoo, and some are mythical animals that you can't see but you can read about them in stories and myths. Different animals make us think of different kinds of qualities. For example, here is an elephant. Elephants are strong, powerful, and loyal. Today, we are going to try to pick an animal that makes you think about the qualities that your team has and the qualities that you all admire. The animal you pick will be your team mascot and the qualities that you admire in that animal will be your team motto. For example, if you pick the elephant, you will be the '[Location] Elephants' [using the city name for your location] and your motto will be 'We are strong, powerful, and loyal.'"

Show examples of animal pictures and qualities. The blank lines allow children to add qualities if they want to do so. Guide children in following the steps of the Traffic Light in talking with each other about the animal and motto they want to represent their team. The goal of this discussion is twofold: (1) to give children a chance to share their personal opinions about the qualities/goals they want to set for the team, and (2) to give children practice with interpersonal communication and negotiation around an issue about which they may have some strong feelings. In order to achieve these goals, it is important for the coach not to become too "task-oriented" or to try to be too "efficient" in getting the children to make a decision quickly. Indeed, the outcome of this discussion (e.g., which animal the children actually select) is immaterial. Instead, it is the *process* of the discussion that is important. Encourage each child to express his or her opinion about why he or she wants to have a particular animal as the team mascot. Don't rush children or let them move on to a decision process too quickly, without considering the different possible points of view. Once all viewpoints have been expressed and actively listened to, children should decide how they want to move forward toward making a decision.

If you are concerned about whether the children in your group can sustain attention in a large-group discussion, consider dividing the group into dyads (or triads). In each of these small subgroups, children talk with each other to find out which mascot they like and what motto they like and why. Together, their job is to agree on a first, second, and third choice. Then the dyads/triads come together (perhaps during snack) and list the three choices of their subgroups. They compare their "short lists" and look for areas of shared preference.

Prior experience with this task has shown that children often become quite affectively engaged with a particular choice, and negotiation can be difficult. Some groups become stonewalled in their decision process. If this happens, the coach may want to offer suggestions that allow for flexible problem solving. For example, in one group the girls wanted macaws as their mascot and the boys wanted tigers, and neither was willing to move from their preference. The group leader suggested that they could pick both animals to be the team mascots, becoming the Macaw–Tigers, which provided the team with a win–win solution to their problem.

Snack (Optional, 15 Minutes)

The usual procedures are followed.

Collaborative Challenges: Memory Tray Challenge, Human Tangles, All Aboard (15 Minutes)

Depending on the time left, proceed with one or more of the collaborative challenges.

Memory Tray Challenge Game

This game offers children a good opportunity to work together to master a challenge. The team is shown a tray with objects on it for 10 seconds, and then the objects are covered with a cloth. The team has a tray and a pile of similar objects in front of them. The children's task is to reconstruct the arrangement of objects on the tray from memory. After they finish, the cloth is removed from the first tray, so that they can check and see how many of the objects and positions they remembered correctly. Possible items to arrange on the tray include cup, fork, spoon, large paper clip, pencil, button, sticky note, eraser, pen, and so forth.

A good way to play this game is to begin with an easy initial challenge with just three objects. Each round, add one additional object, so that the number of objects and locations to be remembered increase gradually. As the task gets harder, encourage children to talk with each other to develop strategies for working together that might help them remember more objects. For example, children will often subdivide the tray, with some remembering what was on the right side, and others remembering what was on the left side. However, don't suggest this solution to them; instead, see if they can generate a strategy to work together on the task. Throughout the process, notice and praise the children for their use of problem-solving strategies and good teamwork.

All Aboard

The group is provided with a space or "platform" marked by one or two carpet squares taped together (or pieces of cardboard about the same size as carpet squares). This platform needs to be taped securely on the floor so that it will not slide around as children are stepping on it. The challenge for the children is to see if they can get their whole group to fit onto the platform. To be "on" the platform, each child needs to have at least one foot touching the platform but no feet touching the ground around it. Some children solve this by having team members hold a foot in the air to condense space on the platform, or by letting one member lift another member part-way up. The coach can encourage the children to talk with each other to plan how they might go about meeting this challenge before they start. Alternatively, since the trial-and-error learning pace of this task is fairly quick-paced, the task can be simply explained and the children left to their own devices to sort out how they will approach it. The coaches should provide spotting, to make sure that the children are safe physically as they try to cram onto this small space. If the task is accomplished easily at first, an extension activity is to make the platform smaller (by removing a carpet square or overlapping two squares to create a surface about the size of 1½ squares) and asking the team to try it again.

Note that the actual size of the "platform" needs to vary depending upon the size of the group. At a maximal level of skill, working effectively together, about eight children can find a way to fit onto one carpet square. You may want to give the group more space than that originally, decreasing the amount of space as the activity progresses, or you may want to start with the challenge of fitting onto one square. During a postplay discussion, ask the children "How did it go?"; "How did you work together?"; "What problems did you have at first?"; "What did you do to solve those problems?" Use reflective listening to underscore the comments of children who notice the importance of communication, planning, and cooperation skills in planning this task.

Human Tangles

In this game, all members of the group stand in a circle and take hold of the hands of two people other than those standing next to them. Then the members work together in an attempt to untangle themselves without letting go of hands. Discussion points include how they can help each other keep their grip, and how they can work together to sort out their tangles without hurting anyone's hands.

Closing Circle: Compliments with Pass the Yarn Sharing, Friendship Tips (5 Minutes)

Join in a friendship circle and distribute Friendship Tips Handout for Session 6. Review the handout, highlighting skills the children worked on during the session. Read through the practice activities, and let them know that you are interested in hearing about how it goes for them when they try out some of the activities. If you want to introduce variety into the compliment circle, try the Pass the Yarn activity (optional). Take a ball of yarn, hold onto one end, and then roll to someone else in the group, giving him or her a compliment. That child then gives him- or herself a compliment and, holding on to the yarn at one end, rolls the yarn ball to someone else, giving that person a compliment. You can also ask the children to identify a friendship idea they plan to try outside of the group. By the time everyone has had a turn, a spider web has been formed connecting all of the group members. Then the group members must undo the web, by each rolling the ball of yarn back to the person who threw it to him or her. Before doing so, they must remember at least one compliment that person received.

SPECIAL ISSUES

1. During the role plays, make sure that children practice the steps of the Traffic Light. Otherwise, children may quickly dispense with the problem without taking the time to practice calming down, defining the problem, coming up with alternatives, and considering the best plan. We want the children to practice the whole process because these steps provide a valuable foundation for future problem solving in more stressful "real-life" problem situations. Coaches may want to role-play the process first to model how to follow the steps of the traffic signals. For example:

> "First, I'll go to the red light and stop, calm down, and 'Take 5.' Let's try that together. [Demonstrate.] Now, I'll tell what the problem is and how I feel about it, and I'll let my friend do the same thing. [Demonstrate.] Now we're at the yellow light, so it's time to suggest an idea, and listen to my friend's idea. [Demonstrate.] I'm going to check to see if we have a good idea that will solve the problem and be fair for everyone. [Demonstrate.] Hurray, now we can say 'yes' to a good idea, and go to the green light and give it a try."

2. These discussion activities require verbal skills and attention control. If they are too challenging for your group, divide into pairs or triads, or consider using early elementary sessions, which practice problem-solving and negotiation skills with fewer verbal demands.

3. If your group needs more practice with fair play skills, consider using competitive games (board games that include group communication, such as Pictionary Junior, Outburst Junior, or Apples to Apples) for extra practice with the Fair Play Checklist (from Session 5).

SESSION 7. Understanding Different Points of View

GOALS

1. Help children consider and respect different points of view in a conflict with a friend.
2. Practice listening skills.
3. Apply the steps of the problem-solving model to manage friendship conflicts.
4. Practice the skills of good sportsmanship in collaborative play.

MATERIALS NEEDED

- Posters: Friendship Group Guidelines, Golden Rule, Traffic Light
- The story of "Joe and David," with feelings cards for discussion (Activity Page 7.1, see p. 381; two sets per group)
- Paper, pencils, clipboards, drawing designs (Activity Page 7.2, see p. 382; one set per group)
- Paper cups (one for each child) and poker chips for role plays
- Friendship Tips Handout for Session 7 (Activity Page 7.3, see p. 383; one per child)

SESSION OUTLINE

- *Friendship Circle:* "Joe and David" story illustrating different points of view (15 minutes)
- *Construction Station:* Back-to-back drawing for listening skill practice (10 minutes)
- *Snack:* Usual procedures (optional, 15 minutes)
- *Collaborative Challenges:* Round robin role plays, active games (15 minutes)
- *Closing Circle:* Pass the Yarn compliments, Friendship Tips, and assignment (5 minutes)

ADVANCE PREPARATION

- Hang posters.
- Cut out feelings cards and back-to-back drawings.

DETAILED SESSION CONTENT

Friendship Circle: "Joe and David" Story to Illustrate Different Points of View (15 Minutes)

Begin by checking in with children about their friendship experiences during the past week. Ask about their use of the problem-solving skills.

"It's good to see all of you. I'm interested in hearing how your week went. Who did something with a friend this week? Tell us what you did and how you used your friendship skills. [Let children respond.] Who had a chance to use the Traffic Light steps to solve a problem? [Let children respond.] It's great to hear how you are using our Friendship Group ideas to solve problems and enjoy your time with friends."

If children do not offer any examples of how they used the problem-solving steps, be prepared to give an example of how you used the Traffic Light steps to solve a problem with a friend, using an illustration that will be relevant to the children. You can also extend this conversation by asking children whether they have tried the problem-solving steps with their siblings or parents. If they did not use the Traffic Light this week, ask them each to think about when they could use it in the coming week. The goal is to encourage children to apply the Friendship Group ideas outside of the group setting, and to help them put in the effort needed to extend their positive peer experiences. Then present the Joe and David story.

"In our last meeting, we talked about using the Traffic Light steps to solve problems with a friend—like who is going first in a game, or how you will work together as a team. Today, I want to talk about another kind of friendship conflict—one that can be challenging to solve."

Note that, in order to make this story relevant to your group, decide ahead of time whether you want the story to be about two girls or two boys, and what sport you want to highlight. (This story is about soccer, but you can modify the story to be about an alternative sport, if desired.) To foster discussion, divide the group into two subgroups—one taking the perspective of one story character, and the other taking the perspective of the other story character. Give each subgroup a set of feeling words, cut up into cards. Review the feelings; check to see that the children can read the feeling words and know what they mean.

"While I tell you the story of what happened, you two are going to take the side of Joe, and you three are going to take the side of David. I'm going to ask you about their feelings. I will give each group a set of feelings to choose from. Here is what happened."

The Story of Joe and David

"Joe and David were good friends. They were on the local soccer team. They had been on the same team for years. This year, they were going to try out for the travel team. On Saturday, they went to the try outs together and both played well."

Let children select feeling cards to show how each of the boys felt during the tryouts. Let them share their choices and their thoughts. Remind them that Joe and David might have mixed feelings—for example, they might be excited about the travel team and worried about not making the team.

"The next Tuesday was soccer practice. David went, but Joe did not show up. David missed Joe—he did not have other good friends on the team. After practice, he called Joe. Joe told him that he had a soccer lesson with a private coach. He wanted to be good enough to get onto the travel team."

Let children select feeling cards to show how each of the boys felt after the phone call. Have them explain why they think their character felt that way. For example, if they think David felt worried about or angry at Joe, have them explain why. The goal is to encourage the children to recognize different points of view. If needed, ask additional questions to help them consider why Joe is working with a private coach and skipping team practice (e.g., he really wants to make it to the travel team; he is not satisfied with the regular team) and how this makes David feel (e.g., lonely, possibly jealous, worried).

> "On Thursday, David went to soccer practice. Joe was not there. David did not enjoy the practice. He wondered what Joe was doing. After practice, he called Joe. Joe did not answer and did not call him back. The next day, David saw Joe at lunch. Joe waved to David, but David ignored him and went to another table to eat with a different friend."

Let children select feeling cards to show how each of the boys felt at the end of the day, and let them explain. Ask them to describe the problem that has occurred between the friends, and what they think will happen next. If needed, ask additional questions to encourage them to explore the nuances of the story—for example, how did David feel when Joe did not come to practice? How did he feel when Joe did not call him back? Why did David ignore Joe and eat with someone else? How did Joe feel when David ignored him and walked away?

> "On Friday, David got a letter in the mail with the soccer team assignments for the year. David was on the local team—he did not make the travel team this year. He looked for Joe's name. Joe was on the travel team. David ripped up the letter. He decided he would quit soccer and find another best friend."

Let children select feeling cards to show how each of the boys felt about the team assignments, and let them explain their choices. Ask them what they think will happen to the boys' friendship. Ask them what they think the boys need to do in order to solve this problem that has come between them. Responding to the children's comments, note that the friendship could fall apart if neither of the boys takes the first step to talk through the problem. In addition, even though they can't fix the problem completely (Joe made the team and David didn't), they might keep their friendship going if they can understand the other's point of view and talk about their feelings.

The challenge for the children is to role-play a solution to this problem. First, let each subgroup talk about what its character could do to take the first step to resolve this conflict (e.g., what could Joe say if he called David; what could David say if he called Joe). Once they feel ready, let the children role-play the two conversations. In summarizing afterwards, point out that, in order to solve the problem, one of the friends had to decide to be the peacemaker—to take the first step to reach out and talk about the problem. And both friends had to listen to the other and respect the other's feelings. Note that some children may solve the problem by having Joe quit the travel team to stay on the team with David. If they do, ask them to think further about the problem—for example: "Was it wrong or unfriendly for Joe to try out for that team? Can the boys resolve the problem and stay friends even if Joe plays on the travel team?" Ask them to role-play a conversation in which Joe and David work things out, without requiring Joe to leave the team.

Construction Station: Back-to-Back Drawing for Listening Skill Practice (10 Minutes)

This fun activity provides practice in listening skills and in explaining a point of view. Each child gets a clipboard with a blank piece of paper, and they sit in a circle with their backs toward the center (so they cannot see what others are drawing). One child is the "art teacher" and is given a simple image to draw. He or she must give verbal instructions to the others on how to draw the image. When the children are done, all the children turn around to compare their drawings and see how well they matched the original image. Here is a sample introduction to this game:

> "Now we are going to play a game that will challenge your listening skills. You are going to take turns being an art teacher or art students. The art teacher is going to tell you how to draw a particular picture, and you will try to draw it exactly the way she [he] describes. The challenge is that you can't see what you are trying to draw; you have to listen very carefully to the art teacher's directions. You can also ask questions. When you are done, you'll all get to see the picture you were trying to draw. What do you think you will need to do to master this challenge?"

Children can rotate in the role of the "art teacher" until they tire of the task or you run out of time. At the end, ask children to reflect on the listening skills they used in the task.

Snack (Optional, 15 Minutes)

The usual procedures are followed.

Collaborative Challenges: Round Robin Role Plays, Active Games (15 Minutes)

Role Plays

Put the names of the role-play characters into a hat and let children pick their characters. (If you want to limit the number of role plays, let children pair up to play each character.) Set the stage by taping six small circles on the floor in a line in this order: red, yellow, green, green, yellow, red. For the first role play, the two characters each stand on a red circle, facing each other. As they complete each step in the role play, they move from the red circle (red light) to yellow circle (yellow light) to green circle (green light), where they solve the problem. Children who are not involved in a particular role play act as "coaches," giving suggestions as needed and cheering on the characters. Their group goal is to solve the problems and save time for games. Introduce the following role plays:

> "Here is your challenge. I have a set of friendship problems that need to be solved before we can play our game. I'm going to ask everyone to choose a child's name from this hat, and it will be your task to solve that child's problem. [Let children choose names out of a hat or cup. Choose the name of Keisha for yourself.] OK, I got the name *Keisha*, and I'll go first to show you how this works. My problem is with Maria—who got Maria? We each start by standing on the red circles, at the red light. Here is what happened: Maria invited two friends to a movie. But she did not invite Keisha. I'm going to be Keisha, and I am going to go to the red light, calm down, 'Take 5,' and tell what my problem is and how I feel. [Model the 'Take 5' deep breath.] 'Maria, I feel really upset that you invited friends to go to a movie and you did not invite me. I thought we were good friends, but now it seems that you like those other girls more than you like me.'

OK, now it is Maria's turn to calm down, 'Take 5,' and tell me her point of view. [Give your child partner Maria a chance to follow the red light steps. If she is not sure what Maria might say, let her ask the 'coaches' who are watching. Only if needed, help them generate Maria's point of view.] For example, Maria, you might say 'I wanted to invite you too. But my mom said I could only invite two people. I honestly did not think you would like this movie, because it was not your type of movie. I still want to be your friend.' We both explained our point of view on the problem, so we move to the Yellow Light. [Take a step forward onto your yellow circle, as your child partner Maria steps forward onto her yellow circle.] Now, I'm at the yellow light, so I need to give an idea about how to solve the problem. 'Maria, can we do something else together this weekend—something we both like? Maybe you can come over to my house.' [See if your child partner Maria has another idea, or if she things your idea will work to solve the problem. If she says 'yes' to your good idea, you both move to the green circle to try it out.] 'Let's go ask our moms.'"

At the end of each role play, ask the other group members for their input—for example: "How did that go?"; "Would it work out like that in real life?"; "Why or why not?" Then call the names of the characters in the next role play and repeat the process. The scenarios are as follows:

1. Maria invited two friends to a movie. She did not invite Keisha. One of the friends told Keisha, and Keisha felt upset and left out.

2. Jim had an extra cookie in his lunch. He asked the group around the lunch table, "Who wants this cookie?" John said, "I do!" Jim said, "Never mind" and put the cookie away. Then he left the table. John felt insulted.

3. Anna said she would help Don with his math homework. But when he called her that night, she said she couldn't talk to him because her favorite TV show was on. Don had to do his homework alone. He was angry that Anna said she would help, but then did not help.

4. David's class was going on a field trip. He asked Eric to be his bus buddy. Eric said "no" and walked away. David called after him, "Yeah, well I don't want to be your bus buddy either!"

As time allows, reward your group with an active game (two choices are described in the following sections) or, if you are in a small space, replay the dice game or a board game (Apples to Apples or Outburst Junior).

Growing Fish

To play this game, children need to know how to play Rock, Paper, Scissors. Review Rock, Paper, Scissors first to make sure all children know how it works. The game begins with a story about how a pond has gotten very, very crowded. It is too crowded, because there are too many eggs in the pond. There is just one way to help the eggs grow up and leave the pond, and the group's challenge is to try to "clean up" the pond by helping the eggs grow up. Here's how it works. Everyone in the group begins as an "egg." "Eggs" move around in crouched positions and say, in high-pitched voices, "Wobble, wobble." When two "eggs" meet each other, they play Rock, Paper, Scissors. The "winner" of the match becomes a "tadpole"; the other continues to walk around as an "egg" looking for other "eggs" with which to match. The "tadpoles" walk around, moving their arms like they are swimming, saying, "Swishy, swishy." When two "tadpoles" meet, they play Rock, Paper, Scissors. The winner of the match becomes a "frog." "Frogs" hop around saying *ribid*." When two "frogs" meet, they play Rock, Paper, Scissors, and the winner is then out of the pond. The goal in this game is to get the pond cleaned out. The pond is clean when there is just one egg, one tadpole, and one frog in it, and all the other extra eggs have grown up and left the pond. It is important to stress the fact that the goal is to have one of each species left in the pond (we don't want them to be extinct, just less overcrowded), so those left behind are not the "losers," but in fact part of the winning picture. Although this activity is pretty silly, it is designed to give children practice in good sportsmanship behaviors, as well as following a series of rules and listening and paying attention to each other as they play. To do well, the children have to attend to which type of creature they are and to seek out others like them to match.

Balloon Races

Divide the children into two teams. If there are unequal numbers, one of the coaches can play. Set up a simple course around a chair or pylon. Give each team a large spoon and a balloon. Each team member must try to carry the balloon on the spoon around the course and then transfer it to the next person on their team. They cannot touch the balloon with their hands or let the balloon touch the floor. If someone touches the balloon or allows it to touch the floor, that member of the team must return to his or her starting point and try again. The team whose team members carry the balloon around the course successfully first wins. This game requires a lot of composure under pressure. Team members can discuss strategies for success, and identify the best ways to support team members in the task. Encourage them to "Take 5" to keep their composure during this challenge.

Closing Circle: Pass the Yarn Compliments, Friendship Tips, and Assignment (5 Minutes)

For the closing activity, join in a friendship circle and distribute copies of the Friendship Tips Handout for Session 7. Let the children read through the handout with you. See if they have ideas about when they can try out the skills at school or at home, and let them know that you will be interested in hearing about their experiences with these skills when you all get back together next week. If desired, use the Pass the Yarn process for compliments, or simply go around the circle to share compliments.

SPECIAL ISSUES

1. In some groups, children will become actively engaged in the discussions of the friendship problems and the problem-solving process, and there will not be sufficient time to complete all the activities in the session. Do not feel concerned about this. The active games are fun for the children, but the problem-solving discussions are likely to be more useful in terms of building their social competencies. When children can imagine themselves facing the problem situations in the role plays, and they practice using the problem-solving steps to manage these conflicts, the process provides preparation for the generalization of these skills to real life. Therefore, do not worry if the role plays take most of the session, as long as the children remain engaged.

2. If the children in your group struggled with the basic use of the Traffic Lights steps to resolve conflicts in Session 6, consider slowing down the practice of these problem-solving steps by expanding this session. That is, replace the role plays in this session with some that are similar

to those in Session 6 to give the children in your group a chance to practice the basic application of the problem-solving steps, and use some of the games in this session. This format will provide a foundation for moving on to this session, in which more challenging friendship problems are tackled by applying the problem-solving steps.

SESSION 8. Practicing Social Problem Solving: Performance Review

---

GOALS

1. Review and consolidate the target negotiation and social problem-solving skills.

2. Self-evaluate to recognize gains, and set personal goals to improve skills.

3. Practice good sportsmanship and problem-solving skills in collaborative group challenges.

MATERIALS NEEDED

- Posters: Friendship Group Guidelines, Golden Rule, Traffic Light
- Poster board for Friendship Movie ideas
- Secret Mission goals for each child (Activity Page 8.1, see p. 384; one per child)
- Recording and playback device: cell phone or digital camera
- Director's Checklist for movie planning/review (Activity Page 8.2, see p. 385; one per group)
- Move the Marbles materials: newspaper, tape, marbles, and two bowls/buckets
- Friendship Tips Handout for Session 8 (Activity Page 8.3, see p. 386; one per child)

SESSION OUTLINE

- *Friendship Circle:* Check-in, movie planning, and secret missions (10 minutes)
- *Construction Station:* Rehearse, tape, and review the Friendship Movie (20 minutes)
- *Snack:* Usual procedures (or movie review) (optional, 15 minutes)
- *Collaborative Challenges:* Move the Marbles group construction challenge (10 minutes)
- *Closing Circle:* Compliments, Friendship Tips, and assignment (5 minutes)

ADVANCE PREPARATION

- Hang posters.
- Cut up cards and write out secret missions for each child.

DETAILED SESSION CONTENT

Friendship Circle: Check-In, Movie Planning, and Secret Missions (10 Minutes)

Begin by checking in and asking children about their friendship experiences.

> "It's good to see all of you. I'm interested in hearing how your week went. Tell us about your friendship experiences. Any good times with friends to share? Any challenges?"

Let children share their experiences. If they have positive experiences to share, ask them why they think the encounters went so well, with a focus on helping them identify efforts, thoughts, or behaviors of theirs that helped things go well. As the opportunity arises, reinforce their use of skills (and their efforts). If they bring up concerns or problems, ask other children for their thoughts and advice. Then remind them about the focus on problem solving introduced in the prior sessions and review the steps in the Traffic Light poster—for example: "Last time we met, we talked about using the steps of the Traffic Light to solve problems and make a deal with friends. Who remembers what you do first at the red light?" Proceed to review all three steps of problem solving with the children, encouraging them to give examples of what happens at each step, and responding to their comments to clarify and emphasize each step.

Next, introduce the Friendship Movie. As in Session 4, the purpose of this recording is to provide children with the opportunity to practice new skills and review their performance; the goal is to help them evaluate themselves and set personal goals. In this movie, the role plays focus on peer problems that occur in everyday peer interactions, and the problem-solving processes that can be used to resolve them.

> "Who remembers the Friendship Movie we made several weeks ago? [Let the children discuss that experience a little, remembering what they did and what they liked about it.] Today we are going to make another movie. The scene that we are going to film will show what you have learned about working out problems with your friends and classmates. How does that sound to you? [Allow children to respond, express opinions, ask questions.] The first thing we need to do is decide what kind of problem we want to show in our movie. We need to think about times when kids your age get into conflicts or have problems with their friends or classmates, and have to work things out. I have a few examples to share, but you can decide exactly what you want to do in the movie."

Using a blackboard, poster board, or paper, give a few examples to get the discussion started. Children can select more than one scene if they want to; the essential features are that the scene(s) allows everyone to be involved, provides an opportunity for the children to practice their conversation and problem-solving skills, and is similar to challenges the children face in their real lives. In each scene, there needs to be a problem that leads some of the children to feel upset (angry, disappointed, etc.), followed by the traffic signals steps of calming down and identifying the problem and feelings, generating alternatives and listening to others' ideas, selecting a solution and trying it out, and evaluating how the solution worked. The following scenes can be suggested to the children as initial ideas, but the goal is to encourage the children to share their own ideas about what kind of scene they want to do and how they want to set it up. (The planning of the movie itself is an opportunity for the children to practice collaborative problem solving.) Possible idea starters:

1. The class is going on a field trip and three (or five) friends want to sit together. But the children have to pair off for the bus seats (two to a seat). Someone will have to sit by him- or herself. They have to decide who gets to be together and who has to sit alone or with a different partner.

2. One of the group members is going to see a new movie on the weekend. He or she asked one friend to go. The other friends found out about it, and they are upset that he or she did not tell them about it or ask them to go.

3. The group members are part of a basketball league, but they play on different teams. One team is winning in the league and the other is losing. The members on the winning team are bragging about it at school and teasing the children on the other team.

In addition, as noted later, each child is given a "secret mission" for which the coaches specify a particular program skill on which to focus. Any of the skills covered in the program thus far or a particular social behavior or attitude that the child needs to work on can be selected.

Construction Station: Rehearse, Tape, and Review the Friendship Movie (20 Minutes)

Once children have selected the topic for their movie, it is important to engage them in planning what roles they will play and how they will set up the scene and show the problem-solving steps, following the Traffic Light poster. In many cases, it is helpful to do a "dry run" rehearsal before you record. Walk through the scene and brainstorm what children their age might feel, think, and say at each phase of the problem. Have them identify how they will display each phase of the Traffic Light problem-solving model within the movie. Use the poster board or a piece of paper to record the basic idea, so the children can refer to it as needed.

Show the Director's Checklist and explain that when the group reviews the videotapes, they will be looking for certain things that show a good problem-solving process: calming down, explaining the problem and your feelings, giving good ideas, listening to others and saying "yes" to good ideas, choosing a solution, and trying it out. Explain that each child will also be given a "secret mission" on which to focus in the movie. Distribute the "secret mission" cards and answer any questions that children have about them. These missions should be prepared in advance for all the children; identify a specific skill that each child needs to work on (e.g., "Sharing your good ideas" for a reticent child; "Listening to others and saying 'yes' to others' ideas" for a domineering child; "Joining in and staying a part of the team" for an inattentive child; "Remembering personal space so you don't crowd your friends" for a child who is intrusive). Once the children have a plan and are ready to go, begin the taping process. Friendship movie scenes can be short (3–5 minutes); they can include one long scene or be broken up into shorter scenes (2–3 minutes) and include the whole group or subgroups.

After taping, as you play the taped segments, bring out score sheets to which children can refer. Let children share their "secret missions" and what they were especially trying to illustrate in the movie. As you watch the movie together, ask the children to watch each of the actors for their implementation of the skills. After each segment, ask the children how well they felt they implemented the skills and their secret mission. Then ask for their assessment of the movie as a whole, and brainstorm ways that they might make the illustration of problem solving better. In some groups, children may have an interest in redoing the tapes. If they are interested in doing this, allow them to do so.

Snack (Optional, 15 Minutes)

Follow the usual procedures or lead the movie review. If you are having snack, you can also plan to show the movie and review the movie performances as children are eating.

Collaborative Challenges: Move the Marbles Group Construction Challenge (10 Minutes)

Move the Marbles is best done in dyads or triads. In a larger group, break into two smaller teams. For this challenge, children are given newspaper, tape, marbles, and a bowl or bucket. Their challenge is to work together to design and construct a pipeline that carries marbles from the table into a bucket. Extra points are given if the team can include turns and/or dips in its pipeline. For maximum benefit, engage the children in pre-challenge planning (e.g., "How are you going to work together to solve this challenge?") and in postplay review (e.g., "What did you do that worked well?"; "Where did you have problems working together?"; "How did you solve them?").

Closing Circle: Compliments, Friendship Tips, and Assignment (5 Minutes)

Finish by handing out and reviewing the Friendship Tips Handout for Session 8, and sharing compliments focused on children's efforts at learning and practicing the friendship skills during the session.

SPECIAL ISSUES

1. Groups will vary in terms of how much structure they need in order to succeed at making a video that illustrates their social problem-solving skills. In some groups (typically groups that contain older children with more well-developed verbal and social-cognitive skills), children will be actively engaged in suggesting common peer problem scenarios to role-play in their movies. In other groups (typically groups that contain younger children, or children with less well-developed verbal, attention, or social-cognitive skills), children will need more concrete direction from coaches regarding the peer scenarios to role-play. In some cases, the role-play scenarios listed in the manual will be too advanced, and coaches will want to use more concrete peer problems (such as role plays showing good sportsmanship and effective coping with competitive play). It is important to monitor the time spent planning the role plays. If you see that children are becoming disengaged or that their attention is beginning to wander from the task, provide additional structure and guidance to help them select appropriate scenarios for the role plays and to select roles, so that the group moves on to practicing the skills in the videos.

2. In some groups, children will be highly engaged in creating and making the videos and reviewing their performance. In other groups, children will be less engaged. In the latter case, children may need more direction from the coaches and may finish and review their videos relatively quickly. The collaborative challenge that follows the video in this session (Move the Marbles) can be quite time-consuming. If your group has spent considerable time and energy on the video, consider replacing this collaborative challenge with a structured game instead that is more time-limited (Pictionary Junior, Outburst Junior) and save this collaborative challenge for a later session.

Statements for the Golden Rule Poster

The Golden Rule

Treat others as you want to be treated.

To make a good friend, be a good friend.

Be honest	Respect others	Be kind
Care about others	Be fair	Cooperate
Be polite	Listen to others	Be cheerful
Be loyal	Have fun	Forgive

Pictures for Team Pennant/Flag Construction

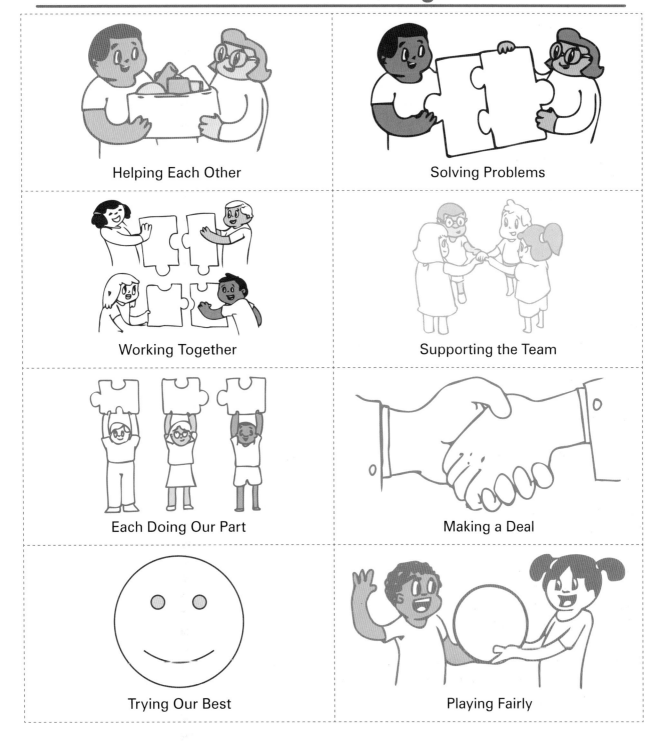

Helping Each Other

Solving Problems

Working Together

Supporting the Team

Each Doing Our Part

Making a Deal

Trying Our Best

Playing Fairly

"The Class Champion" Story and Role-Play Guide

Every year, the fourth grade at Jefferson Elementary School has a competition day in gym class. All of the fourth graders compete at three events: a softball throw, a long jump, and a quarter-mile race. Whoever wins is crowned the class champion.

Role Play: You are fourth graders talking about the gym class competition. You wonder who will win class champion. How are you feeling? What are you saying to each other?

This year, Tim is the favorite to win. He is the fastest runner in the fourth grade and a good jumper. But there is a new kid in school. Daniel looks just as strong as Tim. He looks like a pretty fast runner.

Ask a few questions here, such as "Do you have any competition like that at your school?"; "Have you participated in a competition like that?"; "What kinds of feelings do kids have when they are competing in something like that?"; "How many kids worry about how they will do or who will win?"

Role Play: Tim's friends tell him how they hope he wins. They express worries about Daniel, who might win. How do you feel? What will you say?

Tim's friends tell him that they hope he will win. One of Tim's friends is Carter. Carter is the smallest kid in the fourth grade and he has asthma. He cannot run very fast, but he tells Tim that he hopes he can finish all of the events, even if he doesn't win.

Some possible questions: "Do you know anyone like Carter, who is not very good at sports?"; "How does that person feel when there is a competitive race or game of some kind?"

Role Play: Carter says that he knows he can't win, but wants to finish all the events. The kids cheer him on.

The big day arrives—it is the competition day in gym class. The first event is the softball throw. Daniel throws the farthest, and he wins the event. Tim comes in second. The kids congratulate Daniel on his good shot. Daniel says, "Of course it's a good shot. I'm the best athlete in the whole school!"

Role Play: The kids take turns at the softball throw. Act out Daniel's win, the kids' comments, and Daniel's reply. Then act out the long jump, Tim's win, the kids' congratulations, and Tim's comments.

(page 1 of 2)

The next event is the long jump. Tim jumps the farthest and wins the jump. Daniel comes in second. The kids congratulate Tim, who says, "Thanks! I thought we all did a great job! I think Carter jumped farther than I've ever seen him jump before."

Possible questions: "What do you think of Daniel's comment?"; "How about Tim's comment?"; "How do you think the other kids in the class felt about what they each said when they won? Why?"

The last event is the half-mile run. At first, Tim is ahead, leading the whole pack around the track. But then, at the very end of the race, Daniel makes a sudden lunge and moves ahead of Tim to cross the line first, with a one-step lead. "Good race," said Tim, gasping out of breath, "You are a fast runner." "Yeah," said Daniel, "I knew I'd win."

Role Play: The race and the comments. How do the kids feel and react when they hear the boys' conversation?

Inside, Tim feels really disappointed. He had really expected to win, but he has lost the championship. He looks around to see how Carter is doing. All of the other kids have crossed the finish line and are waiting. Carter is moving slowly around the last loop.

Role Play: As these events play out, ask the others how they think the kids feel and react to the events. Daniel might be showing his medal and saying that he is now class champion. The classmates should be standing around watching what happens, and reacting.

Finally, Carter plods across the finish line. "Way to go, Carter!" Tim yells. "Yeah, nice job, Grandma," jokes Daniel, which makes the other kids laugh. "I made it!" Carter smiles. Then he whispers to Tim, "I'm sorry that Daniel beat you." "I know," says Tim. "I really wanted to win." Carter nods and says, "Win or lose, you're still the real champion."

Possible questions: "Who do you think was the class champion in the story? Why?"; "What was the difference between the way that Daniel and Tim handled the competition?"

Good Sports Score Sheet

Directions: Use this score sheet to keep track of points and good sportsmanship.

Game 1	Player 1	Player 2	Player 3
Wins Track points here			
Good Sport Track effort here			

Game 2	Player 1	Player 2	Player 3
Wins Track points here			
Good Sport Track effort here			

Friendship Tips Handout for Session 5

Remember

Treat others how you want to be treated:

Cooperate.

Talk it out.

Be a good sport.

Give a compliment.

Try It Out

Join in a group activity or game.

1. Be a team player:
   Give your ideas and listen to others. Work it out.

2. Be a good sport:
   Express yourself *and* be kind to others.

Self-Check

How did you do? Did you join in—were you able to give ideas and listen to others?

How did you handle a win? How did you handle a loss?

Problem Scenarios to Role-Play

1. A friend has come over to your house. He wants to play on the computer, but you want to go outside. Work out this problem with your friend.

2. At lunch, one of your classmates asks to sit next to you. You were saving that seat for your friend. Work out this problem with your classmate.

3. At night, you want to watch your favorite show. Your little brother/sister is watching TV and won't let you change the channel. Work out this problem with your little sibling.

4. You are at a friend's house, and she keeps hiding from you because she thinks it is funny. You are not having any fun, and you don't want her to hide from you anymore. Work out this problem with your friend.

Animal Mascots and Mottos

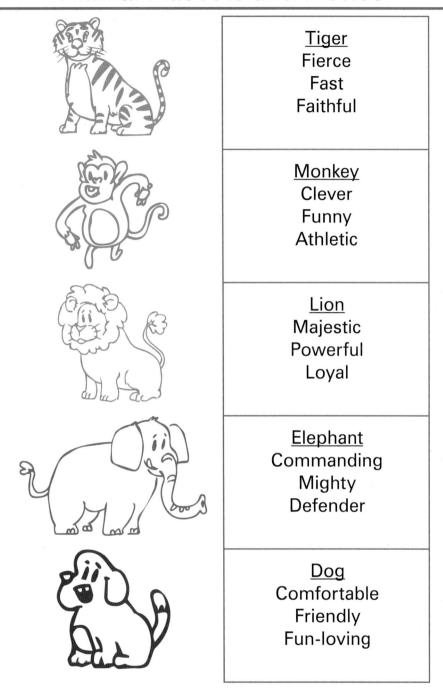

Tiger
Fierce
Fast
Faithful

Monkey
Clever
Funny
Athletic

Lion
Majestic
Powerful
Loyal

Elephant
Commanding
Mighty
Defender

Dog
Comfortable
Friendly
Fun-loving

Friendship Tips Handout for Session 6

Remember

When you have a problem:

Work it out, make a deal.

Try It Out

Next time you have a problem, try using the steps in the Traffic Light poster.

 1. Stop, calm down, "Take 5." Tell what the problem is and how you feel.

 2. Give an idea.
Listen to the other person's idea.
Say "yes" to good ideas.

 3. Give it a try. Did it work?

Self-Check

When you had a problem . . .

    Did you use the Traffic Light steps?

    Did you stop, calm down, "Take 5," and say the problem?

    Did you give an idea and listen to the other person's idea?

    Did you work it out and solve the problem?

Feelings Cards for the Joe and David Story

Sad	Happy	Surprised
Jealous	Lonely	Frustrated
Proud	Confused	Worried
Angry	Excited	Scared

Cards for Back-to-Back Drawing

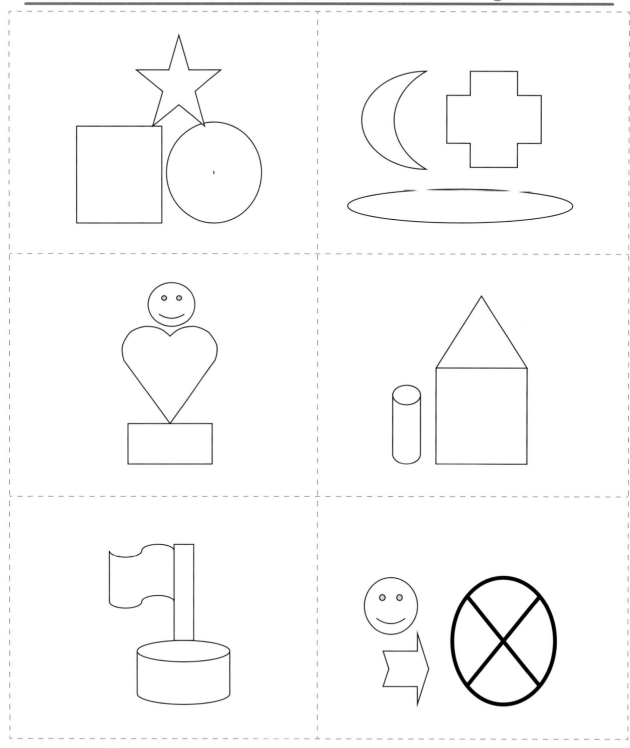

Friendship Tips Handout for Session 7

Remember

When you have a difficult problem with a friend:

Be a peacemaker and take the first step to work out the problem.
Share your feelings and listen to the other person's point of view.
Be creative and try to find a solution that works for both of you.

Try It Out

Next time you have a problem, try using the steps in the Traffic Light poster.

1. Stop, calm down, "Take 5." Say the problem and how you feel. Listen to the other person to understand his or her point of view.

2. Give an idea. Listen to the other person's idea. Is it a good idea? Would it work for both of you?

3. Say "yes" to good ideas. Give it a try. Did it work?

Self-Check

Were you a peacemaker? Did you take the first step to solve the problem? Did you follow the Traffic Light steps?

Did you listen carefully and respect the other person's point of view?

How did it work for you?

Cards for Secret Mission Activity

Secret Mission

Secret

Name: _____

Your secret mission is to: _____

_____

_____

_____

_____

Secret Mission

Secret

Name: _____

Your secret mission is to: _____

_____

_____

_____

_____

Secret Mission

Secret

Name: _____

Your secret mission is to: _____

_____

_____

_____

_____

Director's Checklist

Actor: _____

☐ Showed a friendly face.

☐ Took time to calm down.

☐ Explained the problem clearly and calmly.

☐ Listened to the other person's point of view.

☐ Offered ideas to solve the problem. Listened to ideas.

☐ Worked together to solve the problem.

Actor: _____

☐ Showed a friendly face.

☐ Took time to calm down.

☐ Explained the problem clearly and calmly.

☐ Listened to the other person's point of view.

☐ Offered ideas to solve the problem. Listened to ideas.

☐ Worked together to solve the problem.

Actor: _____

☐ Showed a friendly face.

☐ Took time to calm down.

☐ Explained the problem clearly and calmly.

☐ Listened to the other person's point of view.

☐ Offered ideas to solve the problem. Listened to ideas.

☐ Worked together to solve the problem.

Friendship Tips Handout for Session 8

Remember

Treat others the way you want to be treated:

Be friendly. When you have a problem, stay calm.

Take the first step to work things out.

Explain the problem and how you feel.

Listen to the other person's point of view.

Cooperate and work out a solution together.

Try It Out

When can you use your problem-solving skills?

1. When you are frustrated or upset at home.
2. When you are frustrated or upset at school.
3. When you have a problem with a friend.
4. When you are upset about the way someone is treating you.

Self-Check

How did you do?

If the problem solving did not work, what went wrong?

If the problem solving worked, what did you do to help solve the problem?

Coping with Social Stress

SESSION 9. Managing Stress: Keeping Your Cool

GOALS

1. Introduce and practice the skill of recognizing and labeling social stress.
2. Discuss deep breathing and other strategies for managing stress and calming down.
3. Practice collaboration and good sportsmanship during competitive and collaborative play.

MATERIALS NEEDED

- Posters: Friendship Group Guidelines, Golden Rule, Traffic Light
- Scenarios for the "stress test" (Activity Page 9.1, see p. 401; one set per group)
- Three colors of poker chips
- "Key pad" pasted on top of the Magic Box (Activity Page 9.2, see p. 402; one per group)
- "Stress ball" materials in box: balloons, salt or corn meal, funnel, permanent marker
- Role-play scenarios to practice "Take 5"
- Ingredients for a cooperative snack mix, in separate bags (optional)
- Prepared card deck for Iceman
- Friendship Tips Handout for Session 9 (Activity Page 9.3, see p. 403; one per child)

SESSION OUTLINE

- *Friendship Circle:* Stress test, "Take 5" deep breathing, and Magic Code (15 minutes)
- *Construction Station:* Construct stress balls, practice "Take 5" in role plays (15 minutes)

- *Snack:* Cooperative snack (optional, 15 minutes)
- *Collaborative Challenges:* Play a game of Spoons and/or Iceman (10 minutes)
- *Closing Circle:* Compliments, Friendship Tips, and assignment (5 minutes)

ADVANCE PREPARATION

- Hang posters.
- Cut out scenarios for "stress test."
- Prepare the Magic Code for the box. Cut out the "key pad" and paste it on top of the box.
- Make a model stress ball and place all materials for making stress balls in the box.

DETAILED SESSION OUTLINE

Friendship Circle: Stress Test, "Take 5" Deep Breathing, and Magic Code (15 Minutes)

Check in with children about their friendship experiences during the past week. Reinforce them for their efforts and use of skills. If they bring up concerns or problems, ask the other children if they have ideas to share. See whether any of the Friendship Tips could be applied.

Next, introduce the focus on *keeping your cool* in stressful social situations. Begin by noting that, at one time or another, everyone experiences social situations that make him or her feel uncomfortable. Sometimes things happen that make children feel worried, nervous, embarrassed, and unsure about what to do or say. Other children feel angry or hurt, for example, when they are left out by others or feel that they have been treated unfairly. Explain that everyone feels stressed in some social situations, but people differ in the way they react. Then introduce the "stress test" activity and pass out poker chips, explaining as follows:

> "In Friendship Group, we have been talking a lot about how to improve your friendships—how to make new friends and get along with the friends you have. I've been very impressed with how well you are learning these friendship skills and with the quality of your teamwork in our group! Today, I want to talk about another kind of social challenge: managing stressful social situations when you are with someone you don't know very well or someone who is not your friend. Everyone feels stressed at times, but not always for the same reason or in the same way. Today, we are going to do a 'stress test' with these poker chips to find out more about what stresses us out."

One color at a time, pass out three white, three blue, and three red poker chips (or colored pieces of paper, or other tokens) to each child. Explain that each color represents a different kind of feeling (e.g., white = feeling worried and nervous; blue = feeling sad, disappointed, or hurt; red = feeling angry, frustrated). As you introduce each color chip and label the feelings it represents, ask children to define the feeling (e.g., what it means to feel that feeling, what kinds of situations in which they feel that way). See if they can show each feeling with their faces and bodies, and describe what happens inside when they feel that way (e.g., worry feels like the heart racing, palms sweating). Then explain how the "stress test" works.

"Now we are going to play a game with these chips. I am going to pass around a basket while I sing a little tune. When I stop singing, whoever has the basket will draw a piece of paper and read the social situation. You will each have a chance to put in some chips to show how you would feel in that situation. You can put in white if you would feel nervous or worried, blue if you would feel sad or hurt, and red if you would feel angry or frustrated. You can put in one chip if you would feel that way a little bit, two chips if you would feel that way a medium amount, and three chips if you would feel that way a lot."

Let the children know that you will pick the first paper to show them how it works, and pick a scenario out of the basket. Read the scenario and describe how you would feel in that situation, putting some chips into the center pile. Model a response in which you put two or three chips of one color in (e.g., saying "I would feel very anxious"), and one chip of a second color (e.g., saying "And a little bit angry if that happened to me"). Go around the circle, letting each child put in chips to describe how he or she would feel in that same situation. Then send the basket around and start the game. Continue until each child has had a chance to pick a scenario, and/or as long as the children remain interested. After each scenario is read, the child who picked the scenario should respond first, but then all of the children should have a chance to put in chips to describe their personal feelings if they had the experience. As children go around the circle and share their feelings, comment on the similarities and differences in the way that different children respond to the various social stressors. You can also comment on the total pile of chips in the center at the end of the discussion—for example: "It looks like that would be pretty stressful for everyone; look at all the worried chips in our pile." After each scenario, children should take back their chips to prepare for the next scenario. Possible scenarios are listed on Activity Page 9.1; feel free to modify or add scenarios to suit your group.

After the "stress test," introduce the Magic Code challenge. Before starting this activity, identify a sequence of five numbers that represents the Magic Code, but keep this sequence hidden from sight. In this activity, children take turns pushing the numbers on the "key pad," one by one. As long as a child is pushing the buttons in the right order (i.e., matching the Magic Code), he or she is allowed to proceed. But as soon as a child hits a number that is in the wrong order, you give a "beep" and it is the next person's turn. Children need to work together, watching what works at each turn in order to learn the correct sequence. They win the challenge after each child has pressed the right sequence of numbers. Teammates are encouraged to help each other.

"In this Magic Code challenge, you will need to work as a team. Each one of you will take a turn pushing the numbers on this 'key pad' one by one. If you guess a number correctly, you will get to try the next number. If you guess wrong, I will go 'beep' and it will be the next person's turn. I'm going to let [Name] take one turn, so you can see how it works. [Let a child take a turn.] So, he got the first number right [wrong], which means the first number in the code is [is not] that number. The next person who takes a turn needs to remember that. You can help each other and work together as a team."

Check to see that children understand how the activity works, and then let them try the challenge. After the group finishes the game and masters the code so that they can open the box, ask them how they did it—for example: "How did you work as a team to figure out the code?"; "What did you do to help each other learn the code?" Praise their teamwork and problem-solving skills. Then open the challenge box to retrieve the materials to make stress balls.

Construction Station: Construct Stress Balls, Practice "Take 5" in Role Plays (15 Minutes)

Making the stress balls provides children with the opportunity to work with their hands as they engage in further discussion of managing stress. Particularly for children who find extended discussion difficult, the construction activity makes it easier. Explain to the children that sometimes it helps to have something to do with your body to calm down when you feel stressed. That's why stress balls were developed—they give us a little ball to hold in our hands and squeeze to reduce our stress. (Plan to make one stress ball ahead of the group to show them as a model.) The directions are as follows:

1. Use a deflated balloon, blow it up slightly, and pull on it to stretch it out.
2. Insert a funnel into the opening of the balloon
3. Fill the balloon with salt or corn meal until it forms a little ball.
4. Tie the end of the balloon into a tight knot.
5. If desired, use a permanent marker to draw a "face" on the stress ball.

The end product is a ball one can hold in one's palm and squeeze to reduce stress. As children work on their stress balls, introduce the idea of "Take 5," as follows:

"When you notice that your body is feeling stressed, it is a signal that you need to do some problem solving. You need to figure out why you feel stressed, what the problem is, and what you can do to solve it. But sometimes that is easier said than done. I want you to watch what happens to me when I get into a stressful situation."

Pick an anxiety-provoking situation to role play, such as one from the list above or another one of your choice. Role-play yourself in the situation, and show how you begin to freeze, worry, sweat, feel your heart racing, and so forth.

"Can you see why it is hard for me to solve this problem? [Let children respond.] Right, when I am in a situation like this, I am too upset to think straight. All I can think about is how embarrassed I feel and how I wish I could disappear. Have you ever felt that way? [Let children respond.] But I have found a little trick that really helps me calm down when I feel like this. Here is my trick. [Demonstrate "Take 5": Breathe in through your nose as you count quietly for three counts and then breathe out again for two counts.] Now I feel better. Did you see what I did? [Let children respond.] Yes, I took a deep breath. Watch, I'll do it again. [Do "Take 5" again, showing the children how you are counting out the deep breath.] I took a deep breath and blew out some of my stress, so I feel better. Now that I am calmer, I can focus on solving the problem. I've heard that actors and athletes do this too—they use deep breathing to calm down and stay focused."

As soon as the children have completed making their stress balls, explain that you will give them a chance to try out the "Take 5" strategy in some challenge situations. Each child takes a turn. You read a challenge situation from the list, and the child must role-play the situation, demonstrating two things: (1) how he or she would use the "Take 5" breathing strategy to calm down, and then (2) what ideas he or she would have to solve the problem (following the steps of the Traffic Light poster).

The other group members should help play parts in the role play, and they can also help the child think of solutions to the problem if needed. If you are having a snack time, you can add a prize for completing a role play successfully, with each child earning a special ingredient to contribute to the cooperative snack mix. You can select challenge scenarios for these role plays from the following list or make your own:

1. It is time for you to give your oral history report in front of the whole class. You go up to the front, but then you get nervous and forget what you planned to say. (Have the group members pretend to be the class in this role play.)

2. At lunch, you see your friend sitting with two other kids. There is one open chair at their table. You go over and start to sit down, but the other kid says: "Sorry, it's saved. You can't sit there." You look around and don't see anyone else you know. (Have the group members play the peers seated at the table.)

3. You are asked to solve a math problem at the board. It is a difficult problem. You finish and step back, and a kid calls out "Wrong!," making some other kids giggle. You look at the problem again, but you're afraid you don't know the answer. (Group members can play the class, and one can call out "Wrong!")

4. You got a new haircut. When you get on your bus, a kid says "What happened to you?!" You can't tell if it is a joke or an insult. (Group members can play kids on the bus.)

5. You see some kids from your class playing soccer after school, and you ask if you can join in. The players look at each other. Then, one says, "I don't think so, no." (Group members can play the soccer players.)

Snack: Cooperative Snack (Optional, 15 Minutes)

Follow the directions for preparing the collaborative snack that are provided in Advanced Elementary Session 2. The goal is to give the group additional practice in collaborative planning, negotiation, and social problem solving. Once the mix is made and distributed, encourage general conversation, looking for opportunities to promote peer interaction and to praise the use of conversation skills.

Collaborative Challenges: Play a Game of Iceman and/or Spoons (10 Minutes)

If time allows, the games of Iceman and Spoons are options. Both of these games foster practice in managing stress, staying calm, and showing good sportsmanship in competitive play.

Iceman

To play Iceman, children sit in a circle. This game is particularly fun if it is played in a semi-darkened room, but you will have to consider safety issues in your location as well as the characteristics of children in your group to determine whether semidarkness would be safe or overly arousing for the children. From a deck of cards, select enough cards for each person in the group to pick one. Include the Queen of Spades, but no other royalty cards. Have the children sit in a circle. Mix up the cards and then let each player in the circle draw one card. Privately, each player looks at his or her card and then hides it from sight. The player who has received the Queen of Spades is the Iceman. To play the game, children look around the circle, trying to look each other in the eye. When the Iceman looks someone right in the eye and winks one eye at them, that person is frozen. The goal of the Iceman is to freeze as many people in the circle as he or she can before his or her identity is discovered. The goal of the other players is to figure out who the Iceman is without being frozen themselves. Once someone thinks he or she knows who the Iceman is, that child can make an accusation. If the accusation is correct, that round of the game ends and the game begins again. If the accusation is not correct, the person who made it becomes frozen and the game continues. Before starting the game, it is a good idea to make sure that all of the children in the group can wink and that they know the difference between a wink and a blink.

Spoons

Another game that fits this session is Spoons, described in Early Elementary Session 15.

Closing Circle: Compliments, Friendship Tips, and Assignment (5 Minutes)

Join in a friendship circle and distribute copies of the Friendship Tips Handout for Session 9. Review the tips, highlighting the skills the children worked on during the session, and discussing the practice activities for them to try at home. Try to elicit a commitment regarding what they plan to try during the week (and when and how). Finish with compliments, asking children to focus on compliments that highlight the friendship skills each person demonstrated during the session.

SPECIAL ISSUES

1. Sessions like this one that focus on difficult peer situations can induce negative affect and leave some children feeling disengaged from the group. For that reason, there are positive group activities placed between the more serious discussion activities (e.g., Magic Code, cooperative snack, games at the end). Use your judgment regarding the pacing of the group. If children become disengaged after a few role plays, move along into the next activity.

2. In some groups, children will discuss stressful personal experiences. If this happens and you feel that the examples are also relevant to other group members, use the children's examples for discussion and role play, as these will often be more meaningful than hypothetical examples. Do not worry about how many examples you cover; deeper discussion of a few is often more meaningful than a superficial discussion of a large number of examples.

3. If you have a younger group and you want to include a more concrete practice activity to use with the "Take 5" introduction, consider including the physical challenges in the Early Elementary Session 10 (calming down to balance objects on spoons.)

4. If the session is held at school, consider adding some guidelines about taking the stress balls back to class (e.g., put them in your backpack; do not take them out in class).

SESSION 10. Appraising Social Situations: Be Aware, Think Positive

GOALS

1. Notice the way that your thoughts about others affect your feelings and behaviors.
2. Encourage perspective taking, considering different points of view.
3. Discuss the value of positive thinking on your behavior and social experience.
4. Practice positive thinking.

MATERIALS NEEDED

- Posters: Friendship Group Guidelines, Golden Rule, Traffic Light, Positive Thinking
- White and blue chips, Points of View pictures (Activity Page 10.1, see p. 404; one set per group)
- Positive thinking role plays (Activity Page 10.2, see pp. 405–406; one set per group)
- Materials for game or group challenge of choice
- Friendship Tips Handout for Session 10 (Activity Page 10.3, see p. 407; one per child)

SESSION OUTLINE

- *Friendship Circle:* Check-in, Points of View game, Magic Code replay (15 minutes)
- *Construction Station:* "Think positive" cartoon construction and role plays (10 minutes)
- *Snack:* Usual procedures (optional, 15 minutes)
- *Collaborative Challenges:* Game choice or group challenge (15 minutes)
- *Closing Circle:* Friendship Tips, compliments, and assignment (5 minutes)

ADVANCE PREPARATION

- Hang posters.
- Cut out positive and negative Points of View scenario cards and put in color-coded envelopes.
- Prepare Magic Code box, with poster and role-play scenarios inside, and choose new secret code.
- Cut out the four positive thinking role-play scenarios to put inside box.

DETAILED SESSION OUTLINE

Friendship Circle: Check-In, Points of View Game, Magic Code Replay (15 Minutes)

Check in with children about their friendship experiences during the past week, reinforcing their efforts to use friendship skills and to improve their friendships. Review "Take 5."

> "During our last meeting, we talked about stressful social situations—situations that make you feel nervous, worried, or upset. We also talked about how to calm down and keep your cool when you feel stressed. Who remembers how to 'Take 5'?"

Encourage children to discuss and demonstrate the steps for "Taking 5" to calm down. Ask them to give an example of how they used the strategy during the past week. Find out if they used any other strategies to "keep their cool" when stressed. Then introduce the idea that some social situations are stressful because they are confusing—you are not sure why people are acting the way they are and whether they like you or not. Give an example, such as the following:

> "I had an odd experience this week, and I still don't know what to make of it. I saw some friends of mine talking at the mall, and so I went over to say 'Hi.' When they saw me, they stopped talking and looked uncomfortable. I said 'Hi' and they said 'Hi' back. But then I felt funny and so I just said 'See you later' and walked away. I wonder why they stopped talking when they saw me. Some negative thoughts went through my mind. Were they talking about me? Were they keeping a secret from me? I still don't know."

Ask the children if they have ever had an experience like that, when they just weren't sure what to think about the way someone treated them. If they answer affirmatively, ask them to share their examples. Reflect that sometimes it is hard to tell why people treat you the way that they do, and introduce the Points of View activity. Explain that children divide into two teams and take turns discussing pictured events that are interpreted in two different ways: either with positive thinking or with negative thinking. Ahead of time, you will cut out two versions of the scenario cards on Activity Page 10.1 to create positive thinking cards (put into white envelopes) and parallel negative thinking cards (put into envelopes coded with a blue dot). For each turn, you will hold a blue poker chip in one closed fist and a white poker chip in the other, and let the teams take turns picking a fist, indicating whether they will get the white or blue envelope. Based upon their different points of view, they each address three questions: (1) What is the main story character thinking?; (2) How does the main story character feel?; and (3) What will the main story character do? The purpose of this activity is to help the children discover how their thoughts about others affect their feelings and behaviors.

> "I have a game for you called *Points of View*. On each turn, you will open an envelope and read about an event. Your team has to answer three questions about the event in the picture: (1) What is the story character thinking?; (2) How does he or she feel?; and (3) What will her or she do next?"

Hold your fists out to let the first team members pick a poker chip, and give them the first story scenario envelope (white or blue version, depending on their pick); give the other team members the opposite version. Give each team a few minutes to confer on how to answer the questions. Then let the two teams take turns telling their stories. Take a few notes on a blackboard or flip chart to compare the thoughts, feelings, and actions in the white versus blue scenario. Ask the children to reflect on how differently the two stories ended. Ask them to explain why the stories ended so differently, with such different feelings and actions by the main character. Let the teams try a few more rounds, as long as they remain engaged. After each set of stories, ask the children to reflect on why the stories ended so differently, and point out that the way they think about an event can really change how they feel and how they act. Note that the characters who were positive in their thinking felt better, acted friendlier, and had a better time than the characters who were worried about how the others felt about them and got stuck in negative thinking. Note that, in real life, it is sometimes confusing and hard to know why people treat you the way that they do (as in the example you gave earlier in the session when you saw your friends at the mall)—you don't always know whether they like you or they don't, and whether they are being friendly or mean. Reflect that, when you are not sure what the other kids are thinking or feeling about you in a situation, it is best to think positive and hang in there, to see if your situation can have a positive ending.

If your group enjoyed the Magic Code Challenge game in Session 9, repeat it here to provide a brief and enjoyable practice in group collaboration and problem solving. However, to increase the challenge, let the children know that you have a new code this time, and they must figure it out by working together *without talking with each other—just by watching and giving each other nonverbal cues.* Inside the box, let the children discover the Positive Thinking poster and the materials for the following cartoon and role-play activity.

Construction Station: Think Positive Cartoon Construction and Role Plays (10 Minutes)

Note that you want to talk some more about positive thinking, and review the Positive Thinking poster with the children. Have them read through it, and ask them what each line means to make sure that they understand the main points—for example: "What does it mean 'Don't sweat the small stuff?' Who has an idea about what that means in your friendships or social situations?" Then ask them why they think there are pictures of athletes on the poster. Let them answer, and reinforce the key concepts.

> "That's right. Athletes can't afford to get distracted by worries about their performance or whether their fans are cheering or jeering. They have to concentrate their efforts and focus on the task at hand. Sometimes athletes spend time before a game or a competition going over their plan in their head and imagining themselves doing well. That's because positive thinking helps them put in their best effort. Positive thinking can help in social situations too."

Introduce the next activity, which involves the social scenarios with cartoon captions. Divide children into teams again. Give each team a different social scenario. In the first scenario, there are already cartoon captions with examples of positive and negative thinking provided. Give each team a chance to talk over the scenarios and how they want to do the role plays. Then have one member from Team A role-play the scene as it would go with the positive thinking and have another member from Team A role-play the scene as it would go with the negative thoughts. The members of Team B must guess which is which (i.e., which role play represents positive vs. negative thinking), and they must also try to guess one of the positive and negative thoughts. Then switch around so that members of Team B do their role plays while members of Team A guess. (Note that some of the scenarios have empty captions so that team members can write in their own ideas of positive and negative thinking.) Continue to run through a second (or third) round of role plays if the children are positively engaged. After each team guesses which role play is which, ask a few follow-up questions for discussion—for example: "How could you tell which actor was thinking positively?"; "What made you think that actor was thinking negatively?"; "How would you respond if you saw someone behave that way?"; "What kind of thinking is better for making friends and why?"

Snack (Optional, 15 Minutes)

The usual procedures are followed.

Collaborative Challenges: Game Choice or Group Challenge (15 Minutes)

Select a game or group activity that you think your group would enjoy and that provides an opportunity to practice the friendship skills on which they have been working. Consider replaying the dice games (Advanced Elementary Session 5) or the Iceman or Spoons game from Session 9. Alternatively, consider giving your group a challenging construction task, such as the Marshmallow and Spaghetti Bridge construction activity described in Early Elementary Session 22.

Closing Circle: Friendship Tips, Compliments, and Assignment (5 Minutes)

Review the Friendship Tips Handout for Session 10 and assignments for the week, then share compliments. At this point in the program, compliments should be focused on efforts children are making to implement the friendship skills. Model compliments that focus on positive efforts (e.g., "I liked the way you remained calm and listened to your friends' ideas during the bridge construction challenge") and ask for specific compliments (e.g., "I would like to hear compliments about any positive thinking and good problem solving you saw in the group today").

SPECIAL ISSUES

1. Children who have been rejected by peers often become insecure in social situations. They may show insecurity by withdrawing socially, or alternatively, by intrusive and demanding behavior. Fears of social exclusion can become self-fulfilling, because both approaches (anxious withdrawal or demanding intrusiveness) alienate peers. For this reason, we encourage children to "think positive" when they face ambiguous social situations, rather than assuming the worst.

2. Some children in the 8- to 9-year-old age range struggle cognitively with the task of taking different perspectives. If this difficulty occurs in your group, focus children's attention on the concrete "take-home" point of the session, which is to use positive thinking in situations in which you are uncertain of peer intentions.

SESSION 11. Coping with Teasing and Bullying: Take Time to Plan

GOALS

1. Define and discuss bullying, and explore how it makes children feel.

2. Discuss strategies for coping with teasing and bullying.

3. Practice problem solving and planning skills to cope with teasing and bullying.

MATERIALS NEEDED

- Posters: Friendship Group Guidelines, Golden Rule, Traffic Light, Positive Thinking
- Bullying stories, signs for Vote with Your Feet discussion, tape
- List of bullying problems and response options (Activity Page 11.1, see pp. 408–409; one per group)
- Pieces of paper with letters on them to spell words
- Newspaper, duct tape or masking tape, book for team bridge building
- Friendship Tips Handout for Session 11 (Activity Page 11.2, see p. 410; one per child)

SESSION OUTLINE

- *Friendship Circle:* Check-in, bus problem, bully response discussion (15 minutes)
- *Construction Station:* Vote with Your Feet discussion of coping strategies (10 minutes)
- *Snack:* Usual procedures (optional, 15 minutes)
- *Collaborative Challenges:* Team bridge building (15 minutes)
- *Closing Circle:* Friendship Tips, compliments, and assignment (5 minutes)

ADVANCE PREPARATION

- Hang up posters.
- Prepare signs: avoid, ignore, join together, tell them to stop, tell an adult

DETAILED SESSION CONTENT

Friendship Circle: Check-In, Bus Problem, Bully Response Discussion (15 Minutes)

Check in with children, asking them about their friendship experiences during the past week. Ask about their use of the problem-solving skills, and reinforce their efforts to initiate friendship activities and use the problem-solving skills to resolve conflicts. Then use the following story to initiate a discussion of different ways to respond to teasing or bullying.

"Today I want to share a problem with you and see if you have any suggestions that might help. There is a child I work with who is about your age. He has a tough problem, and I'm not sure what the best solution is. I thought you might have some ideas for him. He rides the bus to school and he has a problem at the bus stop and on the bus. When he gets to the bus stop, there are some kids there who push him around and sometimes take his things. One time they took his backpack and tossed it in the mud. When he gets on the bus, he likes to put on his headphones, listen to his music, and read his book. But these kids take his book and toss it around. They pull his headphones out. It's upsetting to him, and he doesn't really know what to do about it. I thought you might have some ideas, since you are about his age and you ride the bus. What are your thoughts on this?"

The goal of this discussion is to elicit children's thoughts about and reactions to bullying. Being teased or bullied is a very challenging peer experience because it is typically very distressing and there is no single optimal solution. Depending upon the situation, the seriousness of the behavior, and the presence of other children or adults, different strategies are called for and different approaches are effective. Adults often want to offer standard suggestions (e.g., "Tell the bus driver"), but depending on the situation, these suggestions may not be effective and may even lead to increases in bullying. Hence, the goal is to encourage a problem-solving approach, in which children take time to calm down and think, generate multiple possible solutions, and then develop a plan to try the solution that seems optimal in a given situation. The idea is that children will be most effective at dealing with bullying if they can approach it with this sort of flexible, problem-solving approach.

In many cases, the "bus problem" story will elicit considerable discussion from children as they offer suggestions—things they think the child should or should not do in the situation. In other cases, you may need to ask questions or offer suggestions to elicit further discussion—for example, "He decided not to read on the bus anymore, so they can't take his book. What do you think of that solution?"; "What do you all think about telling the bus driver—what would happen if he did that? Would it work?" In this discussion, it is important to allow the children to voice their opinions. However, if a dangerous solution is offered, such as using violence, reflect on the negative consequence that could have for the child—for example: "You think he should get a rock to protect himself? You are thinking that he might be feeling pretty desperate to stop the teasing. But I don't think arming himself with a rock is a good solution. First, I don't think it would work because there is more than one kid teasing him, and second, he could get into a lot of trouble if he threw a rock. We want to think of a solution that will work and will not get him into trouble." As the discussion comes to a close, summarize some of the key points the children have made. Use words that correspond to the major categories of problem-solving efforts that will be used in the upcoming Vote with Your Feet activity. These categories of possible solutions are: avoid, ignore, join together, tell them to stop, tell an adult.

"I want to summarize some of the different ideas you had about what someone can do when he or she is being teased or bullied in a way that is upsetting. One idea I heard was to *avoid* the bully. For example, [Name] suggested that he could stand farther away at the bus stop and wait until after the other boys got on, and then sit away from them. That would be avoiding the teasing situation. Another idea I heard was to *ignore* the bully. [Name] thought that if he just pretended to ignore the boys and act as if they didn't bother him, they might stop. [Name] suggested *joining together* with a friend or relative to go to the bus stop. She thought that my friend would be safer if he had someone with him. And, he could also *tell the bullies to stop*, which sometimes works. Another idea was to *tell the bus driver*. Those are all good ideas, and

I am going to share them with my friend. He will have to think about which one he thinks will work best in his situation."

Thank the children for their excellent discussion of a difficult topic and then explain the Vote with Your Feet discussion.

Construction Station: Vote with Your Feet Discussion of Coping Strategies (10 Minutes)

To set up for this activity, tape the signs describing different ways to respond to teasing or bullying to a wall, and place a piece of masking tape on the floor leading up to each sign (so that there is a line that leads to each sign). Explain that there is no single best way to respond to bullying or teasing, because the best solution depends upon the situation and what the person feels comfortable doing. In this game, you will describe some teasing or bullying situations, and they will *vote with their feet* by standing on the line next to the strategy they think is best. If they can provide a good reason for their answer, they can earn "letters" that they will use later in a challenge activity (e.g., to spell out the contents of snack, or, if you do not have snack time, that spell out some other relevant words, such as *friends* or *teamwork*).

Select examples of bullying from the list provided (Activity Page 11.1) or make up your own scenarios. It is not necessary to present all of these problems. Instead, select three or four based upon the interests of your group. If there are naturally occurring events that better describe the sorts of challenges children in the group experience, adapt or replace these stories with provocation situations that are likely to be most common for the children in each group. For the activity, read the problem example and the different response options. Then ask children to Vote with Their Feet to choose one of the options (e.g., avoid, ignore, join together, tell them to stop, or tell an adult). They may also want to add another option. Once children have gone to stand on a line connected with the solution they think is best, ask them to explain what they would do and why. If they give a reasonable answer, give them a letter, and move on to the next problem. At the end of the activity, children will have earned letters. Their team challenge is to put the letters together to spell words. Give them a few hints, as needed, to help them sort out the words together.

Snack (Optional, 15 Minutes)

The usual procedures are followed.

Collaborative Challenge: Team Bridge Building (15 Minutes)

For this collaborative challenge, the group can work together to make one bridge, or it can be divided into two subgroups, depending on the size of the group (a good group size for this activity is three or four). The challenge is to use newspaper and duct tape to design a bridge that is strong enough to support a book. First, the children in each team are asked to follow the steps of the Traffic Light poster and talk with each other to make a plan before they get their materials. Once they have a working plan, you can give them their materials and they can work together to carry out their plan and put the bridge together. Once they are done with the bridge, they should indicate that they are ready to test it. Coaches "test" the bridge to see whether it can hold a book. If it does not hold the book, children have a chance to work on the bridge some more to see if they can revise their plan. The goal of this activity is to encourage practice in teamwork, communication, and problem solving.

Closing Circle: Friendship Tips, Compliments, and Assignment (5 Minutes)

After joining in a circle, distribute copies of the Friendship Tips Handout for Session 11. Review the points on the handout, highlighting the skills they worked on during the group, and discussing how children can practice at school and at home. Share compliments.

SPECIAL ISSUES

1. In some groups, children will share their own personal experiences with bullying. It is often of more value to children to talk about their personal situation and experiences rather than to discuss the examples provided in the manual. When possible, encourage the children to share their own experiences and concerns and use their examples for the problem-solving discussion. In this case, do not worry about skipping the scenarios provided in the manual.

2. On occasion, you will find that one or two of the children in the group become disengaged during the discussion of the bus problem or other bullying scenarios, even though other children are engaged and want to keep talking. Typically the disengagement occurs for children who have limited verbal or attention skills and find sustained discussion to be challenging. If you anticipate that it may be a problem in your group, plan ahead. Consider giving this child a set of jobs (e.g., coloring the posters to be used in the Vote with Your Feet activity) to help sustain the child's involvement with the group. If it is necessary to remove the child from the discussion in order to maintain the discussion opportunity for other children, have the co-leader provide the inattentive child with another activity (e.g., preparing the snack or setting up materials for the next activity), so that the leader can continue the discussion with the other children.

3. On occasion, children describe experiences of bullying and victimization that require individual follow-up because of the seriousness of the allegations. Be prepared for the possibility that you may need to have a follow-up discussion with a child and his or her parents or teachers if you feel that the child is in danger or requires adult help.

4. The collaborative bridge-building challenge can be quite time-consuming, and generally requires at least 15 minutes. If you do not have time because the bullying discussion was extensive, play an alternative game. A good option is to have some group board games (e.g., Apples to Apples Junior, Pictionary Junior) on hand as an alternative if there is insufficient time for the bridge-building activity.

Scenarios for the Stress Test

You have to give a speech in front of the class.
You fall over the ball at a soccer practice. Other kids laugh.
It is the first day of summer camp. You don't see anyone you know.
You are waiting to buy a movie ticket. A group of kids cuts into the line in front of you.
You are asked to read a poem out loud in front of the class.
You are carrying your lunch tray and someone knocks into you. Your milk spills.
You have your bathing suit on and you are walking to the pool. You hear a group of kids laughing at you as you walk by.
You give the wrong answer in class, and you think you hear someone laugh.
Someone you don't know sits down next to you on the bus.
A group of kids from your class are talking about going to a movie on Saturday. You ask, "What movie?" One of them looks at you and says, "This is a private conversation."

"Key Pad" for the Magic Code Game

Directions: The coach should identify a sequence of numbers that represents the Magic Code, but keep this sequence hidden from sight. The children take turns pushing the numbers on the key pad, one by one. As long as the child is pushing the buttons in the right order (i.e., matching the Magic Code), he or she is allowed to proceed. But as soon as the child hits a number that is in the wrong order, the coach says "beep" and it is the next person's turn. The children need to work together and watch each other. They need to learn from each person's turn, and help each other learn and remember the correct sequence. The team has won the challenge after each child has pressed the right sequence of numbers to open the box. Help from teammates is encouraged—working together is the goal of the exercise!

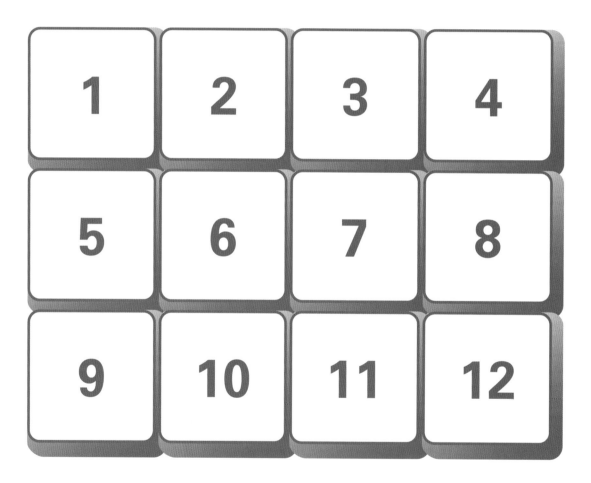

Friendship Tips Handout for Session 9

Remember

Everyone feels stress.

First, "Take 5" to calm down.
Then try to solve the problem.

Try It Out

Notice your feelings. When do you feel stressed?
What helps you to calm down?

"Take 5" deep breathing

Thinking positive thoughts

Listening to music

Taking a walk

Spending time with your pet

Talking about your feelings and the problem

Doing something to take your mind off it

Self-Check

Did you notice your feelings when you felt stressed?

Did you "Take 5" or something else to calm down?
How did it go?

Were you able to calm down and solve the problem?

Pictures for Points of View Activity

Directions: Make a set of "positive thinking" scenario cards using columns 1 and 2; make a second set of "negative thinking" scenario cards using columns 2 and 3. Both sets include the picture of the event, but then include either a positive thinking or a negative thinking interpretation.

White Team: Positive Thinking	Picture of Event	Blue Team: Negative Thinking
The girls are having fun splashing in the sprinkler, and they want me to join in.		The girls are splashing water at me because they don't want me to join in.
We are practicing karate kicks together. By accident, she came too close and actually hit me. She did not mean to.		She is practicing her karate kicks on me. She hit me and it hurt. She wanted to hurt me because she doesn't like me.
I see some girls sharing a secret. They are not telling me because it's something between them and they don't think I would be interested.		I see some girls sharing a secret. They are not telling me because they don't like me. They are making fun of me or saying something bad about me.
We're all rushing to get to the bus to go home. I'm a fast runner so I'm ahead of the others.		We're all rushing to get to the bus to go home. The other kids are running more slowly than me because they don't want to sit with me on the bus.
The boys are going to build a snowman. They might want me to help them.		The boys are going to build a snowman. I'm sure they don't want me to help.

Positive/Negative Thinking Role Plays

SCENE 1: You are watching some classmates playing basketball at the gym. You would like to join in the game.

Actor 1: Positive Thinking
They will probably let me play.
They look friendly.
It will be fun.
I can ask if I can join in.

Actor 2: Negative Thinking
They will probably say "no."
They will laugh at me.
I'm no good at basketball.
I look stupid standing here.

Show yourself watching the basketball game. Show how you feel. Then, show us what you do next. Help us guess what you are thinking by watching your body language when you decide if you will join in, and how you will go about it.

SCENE 2: You want to go to the movies with a classmate this weekend. You would like to call someone up to invite him or her.

Positive Thinking
This person will want to go with me. I am fun to be with. I know what to say on the phone.

Negative Thinking
They won't want to go with me. They have better friends. I don't know what to say on the phone. They will think I am strange.

Show yourself holding your phone. Show how you feel. Then show us what you do next. Help us guess what you are thinking by watching your body language when you decide if you will call your friend, and what you say to your friend when you call.

(page 1 of 2)

SCENE 3: You are waiting for a friend to call you. The friend said he or she would call you tonight, but the friend has not called yet. It is getting late.

Positive Thinking
My friend got busy or forgot.
That's OK, it's not a problem.
I can wait some more.
Or I can call them.

Negative Thinking
My friend doesn't like me anymore.
I can't trust them.
They don't care about my feelings.

Show yourself waiting for a phone call. Show how you feel. Then show us what you do next. Help us guess what you are thinking by watching your body language if you decide to call your friend, and what you say.

SCENE 4: You tripped on the way into the classroom and almost fell down. Some classmates saw you trip and laughed.

Positive Thinking
That was funny, I am laughing too.
It could happen to anyone.
We can have fun laughing about it.
It is all in fun.

Negative Thinking
They think I am clumsy.
They are making fun of me.
They are mean.
I am embarrassed.

Show yourself tripping and almost falling down. Show how you feel. Then show us what you say or do next. Help us guess what you are thinking by watching your body language and seeing what you say to the classmates who are watching.

Friendship Tips Handout for Session 10

Remember: Think Positive

Focus on the positive.

Make a good effort.

Tell yourself that you can do this.

Don't sweat the small stuff.

Try It Out

When you feel stressed:

Notice your feelings. "Take 5" to calm down.

Consider the situation. Think positive!

Use the problem-solving steps:

What different things could you do?

What would work best?

Self-Check

Did you "Take 5" or something else to calm down?

Did you control your negative thoughts?

Were you able to calm down, think positive, and solve the problem?

Problem Examples for
Vote with Your Feet Discussion

Problem 1: A bully is waiting at the front corner of the school building. He told you that he was going to beat you up this afternoon. He is bigger than you, and you have heard that he is very mean. What should you do?

Avoid—Plan to sneak out of the school and get on the bus before he finds you.

Ignore—Pretend you did not hear him. Just ignore him and look the other way.

Join together—Ask a friend to walk to the bus with you so you are not alone.

Tell the bully to stop—Tell him you are not afraid of him, and you are not going to fight.

Tell an adult—Tell the teacher what the bully said.

Problem 2: You get on the school bus. You are in your seat, waiting to leave, when you see a kid giving you a dirty look. The kid looks mean and starts walking over to you. What should you do?

Avoid—Calmly turn and look out the window.

Ignore—Pretend you did not see him or her and don't react.

Join together—Move to a seat next to a friend, or turn around to talk with a friend.

Tell the kid to stop—Tell him or her that you don't like the way he/she is looking at you.

Tell an adult—Tell the bus driver.

Problem 3: You are in the bathroom at the sink and a kid from your class bumps you from behind, so that you get water all over your shirt. What should you do?

Avoid—Leave the bathroom as quickly as you can.

Ignore—Pretend you are not bothered by it.

Join together—Move over to where other kids are standing.

Tell the kid to stop—Tell the kid you don't like getting wet. Ask him/her not to do it.

Tell an adult—Go and tell the teacher.

(page 1 of 2)

Problem Examples for Vote with Your Feet Discussion *(page 2 of 2)*

> <u>Problem 4</u>: You are playing kickball with a group of kids. You kick, but it's not a very good kick. One of the kids yells out, "Ha-ha, Baby can't kick!" What should you do?

Avoid—Say that you don't want to play anymore and go find someone else to play with.

Ignore—Just ignore the comment and pretend you didn't hear it.

Join together—Go stand by your friend, so he or she can cheer you up.

Tell the kid to stop—Tell him/her the comment wasn't funny and you don't appreciate it.

Tell an adult—Find the playground monitor and report what happened.

> <u>Problem 5</u>: You are carrying your lunch tray and bump into a table so that your milk spills onto the kid sitting there. The kid looks really mad and says, "You jerk! What's wrong with you?!" What should you do?

Avoid—Just tell the kid that you are very sorry and leave.

Ignore—Just ignore the kid, say nothing, put your head down.

Join together—Look for your friends and go sit with them.

Tell the kid to stop—Tell the kid it was an accident and you didn't mean to do it.

Tell an adult—Tell your mom what happened.

Friendship Tips Handout for Session 11

Remember: Take Time to Plan

If you are being teased or bullied:

"Take 5" to calm down.
Use the problem-solving steps:
What different things could you do?
What would work best?
Tell yourself that you can do this.

Try It Out

Avoid.
Ignore.
Join.
Tell the person to stop.
Tell an adult.

Self-Check

Did you "Take 5" or do something else to calm down?
Did you take time to plan?

What ideas did you consider?

What idea did you try?

How did it go? What did you learn?

Responsible Decision Making

SESSION 12. Generating Alternatives: Social Problem Solving

GOALS

1. Review the skills targeted in the program.
2. Provide practice in flexible thinking and generating multiple solutions for social problems.
3. Provide applied practice in using the skills in the context of collaborative games.

MATERIALS NEEDED

- Posters: Friendship Group Guidelines, Golden Rule, Traffic Light, Positive Thinking
- Dear Problem Solvers letters, placed into sealed envelopes (Activity Page 12.1, see pp. 424–425; one set)
- Quiz props: poker chips, bowl, rewards (optional), list of problems (Activity Page 12.2, see p. 426; one)
- For Team Newspaper Race: several sheets of newspaper
- Friendship Tips Handout for Session 12 (Activity Page 12.3, see p. 427; one per child)

SESSION OUTLINE

- *Friendship Circle:* Check-in, Dear Problem Solver letters (15 minutes)
- *Construction Station:* Skill review with Challenge Quiz Bowl (15 minutes)
- *Snack:* Usual procedures (optional, 15 minutes)

- *Collaborative Challenges:* Giants, Wizards, and Elves; Team Newspaper Race (10 minutes)
- *Closing Circle:* Friendship Tips, compliments, and assignment (5 minutes)

ADVANCE PREPARATION

- Hang posters.
- Prepare Dear Problem Solvers letters and put them in envelopes.
- Cut up Quiz Bowl Challenges.
- Prepare "cheat sheet" for Giants, Wizards, and Elves.
- Cut newspaper into half sheets.

DETAILED SESSION CONTENT

Friendship Circle: Check-In, Dear Problem Solvers Letters (10 Minutes)

Check in with children about their friendship experiences during the past week, reinforcing their efforts to use friendship skills and to improve their friendships. Find out who used "Take 5" breathing to "keep their cool," who used positive thinking to cope with a problem, and who made a plan to solve a problem. Praise their efforts to join in, be a better friend, and be a peacemaker in their schools and communities. Introduce the Dear Problem Solvers letters.

> "During our last few meetings, we've been talking about tips for how to handle different kinds of social problems. Today I am hoping that you will be able to help some other children with their friendship problems. These letters describe problems that children posted on the Web, hoping that someone could give them good advice. I'm going to pass them out in a few minutes."

Show children the letters, each sealed in an envelope. However, before you pass them out to the children, pass out the Friendship Tips Handout for Session 12 (Activity Page 12.3) to provide a brief review of the key Friendship Group concepts for them to use as they give advice.

> "To help you give advice, I brought this Friendship Tips sheet. Let's take a quick look at it. Who remembers when we talked about the Golden Rule? [Let children respond.] What is it? [Let children respond.] How about the Traffic Light—how do you use it to help you with social problems? [Let children respond.] Then there is this idea: Keep your cool. Who can show me how to 'Take 5'? [Let children respond.] Who can remind us about positive thinking? When is that useful to a friendship? [Let children respond.] And what about this last one—what does it mean to 'take time to plan'? [Let children respond.] OK, fantastic. I think we are ready to apply these ideas to some friendship problems. Who wants to read their letter first?"

Let the first volunteer select and read a letter. Ask that child for a suggestion for the letter writer, reminding him or her that they can use the Friendship Tips handout to help them give advice. Then ask other children in the group if they have ideas for the letter writer. As needed, refer to the Friendship Tips page to encourage children to think about how the skills might be applied in the specific situation faced by the letter writer. If children give just one solution to the problem (e.g., "Just say you're sorry"), ask them what else the letter writer could do. If the children do not refer to core skills (e.g., the use of the problem-solving steps), then ask them directly how they would apply those steps in the letter writer's situation—for example: "Do you think it would help 'Mad to Be Left Out' to learn how to 'Take 5'? How would it be helpful? How could 'Mad to Be Left Out' use the Traffic Light problem-solving steps?" If children are interested in these letters, go around and let each child select and discuss a letter. If interest begins to diminish, discuss two or three letters and then save the others for discussion at snack.

Construction Station: Skill Review with Challenge Quiz Bowl (15 Minutes)

A central feature of social competence is the ability to control the impulse to react immediately when faced with a social problem, instead of taking the time to consider alternative responses. Impulsive reactions are often overly aggressive or passive, and therefore not the ideal responses to social problems. This next activity is designed to give children practice at generating multiple possible responses in the face of various types of common social challenges. It is set up as a "game show" activity, with the children working together as a team to earn points by generating multiple alternative responses to each scenario. Consider providing small rewards (e.g., pencils, erasers) for the team if it can earn enough points at this game. To set up for the game, have all team members stand behind a table. If possible, give them a "buzzer" to push when they have an answer to give (e.g., a black dot taped on the table, a small bell push). Then introduce the game:

> "Now, it is time for the Challenge Quiz Bowl. You will all be contestants, and so you will stand behind this podium. [Show children where they stand and the 'buzzer' they will use to respond.] I am the host for the Quiz Bowl, and so I will read you the questions. Your job is to give as many good answers as you can. You will get 1 point for each good answer. [Indicate the poker chips at your table and show how you will put one into the bowl to recognize each good answer.] If your team can earn enough points, you will each earn a prize. Before we start officially, I'll give you a practice question so you can see how the game works."

> Read a sample question: "You are about to sit down at lunch and your friend stops you and says, 'You can't sit there today, I'm saving it for someone else.'" Explain that the children need to give ideas about what someone could do or say in that situation. Let the children know that they will earn a point for every different answer they can think of. Creative thinking is good, but only reasonable answers will earn a point. Encourage children to use the "buzzer" if they have an idea, and then call on them and listen to their idea, tossing a poker chip in the bowl for each reasonable idea they generate. If they generate only one or two ideas, add a few more ideas to model different responses. Summarize their responses and ask them which response they think would be the best one to use and why. Give them a poker chip for providing a rationale for the best response choice, and then move on to start the game officially. Continue until children tire of the activity. As the game progresses, praise the children for their creative thinking and for coming up with several different ways to respond to social challenges. Comment on the value of considering different ideas about how to respond, and summarize some of the strategies that they chose as most often effective. At the end of the game, tally up the points the team earned and let them know you will give them their reward at the end of the session.

Snack (Optional, 15 Minutes)

The usual procedures are followed. During snack, encourage general conversation, looking for opportunities to encourage peer interaction and to praise the use of conversation skills. If desired, discuss more Dear Problem Solver letters, or ask children whether they have experienced any of the events in the Dear Problem Solvers letters or the Challenge Quiz Bowl. If they have, ask them to share what happened and how they responded. If the problem was not resolved, ask them and the other children to problem-solve about what else could have been done in that situation.

Collaboration Challenges: Giants, Wizards, and Elves; Team Newspaper Race (10 Minutes)

Giants, Wizards, and Elves

This game is similar to Rocks, Paper, Scissors, except that children work in small teams and must decide together what role to take in each round. The three roles to choose from are (1) giants (stand tall with arms over head, fingers curled, growling); (2) wizards (stand slightly bent, hold arms out with fingers extended and ready to cast a spell, hissing); and (3) elves (squat down, with arms pulled in and hands in front, calling out "Watch out"). The hierarchy is that wizards win over giants (by casting spells on them); giants squish elves (by sheer size); and elves win over wizards (by outsmarting them). Before starting the game, have the whole group practice each of the poses, and review the hierarchy of poses. In each round, the small teams (dyads or triads) huddle and decide which role to take. The teams take their places, and the coach gives a signal to begin. The two teams enact their selected roles, and the coach announces the winner of the round. Then the small teams huddle again to decide their role for the next round. This is a very quick-paced game, and gives children practice in negotiating with their partners and handling competition effectively. After five rounds, you can announce a team winner and rearrange the teams for another game.

Team Newspaper Race

The team must race to a designated turning point and back, but can step only on newspapers. Each person is given one half sheet of newspaper. For them to move forward as a group, they need to come up with a plan in which they alternate the use of each person's newspaper sheet. To start, one or more team members need to put their newspaper down on the ground, so that all team members can stand on it. Another team member can place their newspaper in the front of the group, in the direction of the finish line, so the team can step forward onto it. As the team moves forward, they can "re-cycle" the newspaper sheets they have already stepped on and left behind them, by moving them to the front to reuse. There are two ways to make this a race. If you have a small group, the team can race itself, by trying the task two to three times and trying to beat their time. If you have a larger group, you can divide them into two subgroups who race each other.

Alternatives

If you have a very small group or a space that does not allow for these active games, consider a dice game or card game used in earlier sessions, or an alternative published game (e.g., Apples to Apples Junior; Outburst Junior)

Closing Circle: Friendship Tips, Compliments, and Assignment (5 Minutes)

In this session, the Friendship Tips handout was used at the start of the session. Check to see that children have this handout to take home with them, then share compliments. Focus compliments on specific efforts that children exerted to implement friendship skills, and ask children for compliments about friendship skill demonstration—for example: "Let's focus on [Name]. I thought [Name] did an excellent job of using the problem-solving steps in his advice to the letters. Who saw [Name] using one of our Friendship Group ideas during the Quiz Bowl or group game today?"

SPECIAL ISSUES

1. You will want to give some thought to how many Dear Problem Solvers letters to use, and which ones to select. If you think that this will be a highly engaging activity for your group, you can give each child a letter and ask him or her to lead the problem-solving discussion to generate a response. If you think that your group will have trouble sustaining interest in a long discussion, you can pair children up, giving each pair a letter around which to lead a problem-solving discussion. Choose the examples you think are most relevant to the children in your group.

2. If, for any reason, you have a group member who is not be comfortable as a contestant in the Challenge Quiz Bowl activity, this child can be given a role of moderator, perhaps collecting the poker chips in the bowl for good answers, calling out the names of contestants who push the "buzzer" and are ready to answer, and so on.

3. Some children will want to play the Giants, Wizards, and Elves game as individual players, rather than working with a partner. Working with partners requires them to negotiate which role to take in each round, providing them with more skill practice than playing as an individual. However, after playing the game in small teams or partner pairs, the children can be allowed to play as individuals in a second round if they have a strong preference to do so.

SESSION 13. Performance Review: Consolidating Friendship Skills

GOALS

1. Review, practice, and consolidate the friendship skills targeted in the program.
2. Self-evaluate to recognize gains and set personal goals to improve skills.
3. Practice skills in the context of a collaborative group challenges.

MATERIALS NEEDED

- Posters: Friendship Group Guidelines, Golden Rule, Traffic Light, Positive Thinking
- Friendship Tips Handout for Session 13 used for movie planning (Activity Page 13.1, see pp. 428–429; one per child)
- Blackboard or poster board for listing movie ideas
- Recording and playback device: cell phone or digital camera
- Director's Checklist for movie scoring and review (Activity Page 13.2, see pp. 430–431; one per child)
- Materials for the maze (carpet squares or colored paper, answer key)

SESSION OUTLINE

- *Friendship Circle:* Check-in, "How to Make and Keep Friends" movie planning (10 minutes)
- *Construction Station:* Rehearse and tape movie; review, score, and discuss (20 minutes)
- *Snack:* Usual procedures (optional, 15 minutes)
- *Collaborative Challenges:* The Maze Team Challenge (10 minutes)
- *Closing Circle:* Friendship Tips, compliments, and assignment (5 minutes)

ADVANCE PREPARATION

- Hang posters.
- Make the maze.

DETAILED SESSION CONTENT

Friendship Circle: Check-In, "How to Make and Keep Friends" Movie Planning (10 Minutes)

Begin by checking in with children about their friendship experiences during the past week. Mention that this is the second to last group session. Then introduce the "How to Make and Keep Friends" movie. As in Sessions 4 and 8, the purpose of the movie recording is to provide children with the opportunity to practice and consolidate the friendship skills on which they have been working. This is the final video, and hence the goal is to practice the skills that they have been working on throughout the program. To accomplish this goal, children are asked to develop two movie segments designed to give other children their age the best advice they can about how to make friends (Part 1) and how to solve problems with friends (Part 2). The schedule involves a general planning discussion for Part 1; rehearsing and filming of Part 1; scoring, review, and discussion of Part 1; and then a repeat of those three steps with Part 2.

> "Who remembers the friendship movie we made several weeks ago? [Let the children discuss that experience a little, remembering what they did and what they liked about it.] Today, we are going to make a final movie about what you've learned about friendship. During Friendship Group, we've talked about a lot of friendship ideas, including how to make new friends and how to manage social stress and conflicts. The goal of this movie is to give advice to other children your age about friendship. There will be two parts to this movie, and the first part is called 'How to Make Friends.' How does that sound? [Let children respond to this general idea.] Has anyone seen a 'how-to' show—for example, a how-to-cook or how-to-garden show? How was it set up?"

Let children discuss the format of a "how-to" show, and as needed, explain that the goal is to give advice to other kids about how to make a new friend. To help them plan, explain that you will review some of the tips from Friendship Group with them. First, they will make a plan for the movie. They will decide how they want to share those tips in their movie and how they will demonstrate the skills. The focus of the first part of the movie is to give advice and demonstrate how a student can make friends after he or she moves to a new school.

Distribute page 1 of the Friendship Tips Handout for Session 13 for children to consider in developing Part 1 of the movie. Go around the circle and let each child take a turn at reading through a tip in one of the boxes. Then explain to the children that they need to plan the scene(s), and think about how they want to use these tips in their movie. Use a blackboard or poster board to record the children's ideas about which skills they want to demonstrate and how they will set up Part 1 of the movie. Be prepared to give the children suggestions and advice if they need it. An essential part of this movie-making process is demonstrating how to start a conversation with someone you just met, and illustrating how you can join in an ongoing activity. The context for showing a new student how to accomplish these social tasks may vary (e.g., during lunch, on the bus, at recess) depending on the ideas of the children in the group. You can help the children decide by asking questions—for example: "Where do you want to demonstrate the skills for starting a conversation?"; "Who will be involved in this scene?"; "Will you have a narrator explaining the tips, and if so, how will that work?" Make sure that everyone has a role. It may be best to do two short scenes for each part of the movie to make sure that all of the children are actively involved.

Construction Station: Rehearse and Tape Movie; Review, Score, and Discuss (20 Minutes)

Once the group has a plan for Part 1, children will need to do a "dry run" rehearsal, where they block out how they are going to stage the scene(s) and who is going to take which part. It is a good idea to plan a narrator for each scene who can present the Friendship Tips, but in some cases, children will have other creative ideas about how to do this. Before you turn on the recorder, have the children walk through each scene; brainstorm with them what children their age might feel, think, and say at different points in the movie; and ask how the Friendship Tips can serve as a guide. Write notes, as needed, on the planning poster board, so the children remember their plan while you are filming. Then film the first scene(s) showing how to make friends.

Next, review and discuss Part 1 of the film with the children. Show the Director's Checklist and explain that when the children review the movie, they will be looking for how well the Friendship Tips were explained, and how well the actors did with their demonstrations. As you watch the movie together, ask the children to pay attention to each of the actors' implementation of the skills. After each segment, ask the children how well they felt they implemented the skills. Then ask for their assessment of the movie as a whole, and brainstorm ways in which they might better illustrate how to problem-solve in this kind of situation. In some groups, children may have an interest in redoing the tapes. If they are interested in doing this, allow them to do so.

When you are ready, explain that the second part of the movie is called "How to Work Out Friendship Problems," and the goal is to illustrate how students can use the steps of the Traffic Signals poster to resolve problems with friends.

> "Great teamwork planning the first part of the movie—you have a great plan! Now, we need to plan the second part or our movie, which is called 'How to Work Out Friendship Problems.' In this part, you will need to give advice and demonstrate how a student can solve a problem with a friend at school. [Distribute page 2 of the Friendship Tips Handout for Session 13.] Let's review the Friendship Tips for solving problems, and then you'll be able to plan how you want to include and demonstrate these skills in your movie."

Proceed to review the tips, going around the circle and letting each child read through one of the tips. Explain that the children first need to decide what kind of problem they want to show in the movie. Children can generate their own problem or choose from one of these options:

1. A friend talked about you behind your back.
2. Some kids in the class tease you because you wear glasses, calling you "four eyes."
3. Your best friend started sitting with a group during lunch, but those kids say there is no room at their table for you.
4. You are always picked last for teams because you are not very good at sports.

Encourage children to talk about how they want to give advice in the movie and how they want to demonstrate the process of problem solving, writing their ideas down on a blackboard or poster board. Their goal is to illustrate a problem that leads a child to feel upset (angry, disappointed, etc.), followed by the Traffic Light steps of calming down and identifying the problem and feelings, generating alternatives and listening to others' ideas, selecting a solution and trying it out, and evaluating how the solution worked. Then follow the same steps as for Part 1: Rehearsing Part 2, tape Part 2, and then review Part 2 using the Director's Checklist. Ask the children how well they felt they implemented the skills. Then ask for their assessment of the movie as a whole, and brainstorm ways that they might better illustrate how to problem-solve in this kind of situation. In some groups, children may have an interest in redoing the tapes. If they are interested in doing this, allow them to do so.

Snack (Optional, 15 Minutes)

The usual procedures are followed. After the snack is served and while the children are eating, it is also a good time to watch and score Part 2 of the friendship movie.

Collaborative Challenges: The Maze Team Challenge (10 Minutes)

This game is similar to the Magic Code game used earlier in the program, but children must discover the correct pathway by trial and error, walking through the maze. The game requires good attention skills, turn taking, and impulse control, and it fosters the practice of communication, planning, and collaboration skills. Most groups really enjoy the challenge. To prepare for the maze, tape colored pieces of paper or different-colored carpet squares onto the floor to create a multicolored grid. (It is important to secure these with tape, so that children don't slip on them.) For yourself, draw a small grid on paper and create a secret pathway through the spaces by drawing a route on the small grid that corresponds to the large grid on the floor (keep this "key" hidden from the children). A good size is 5×5 (25) squares, but if you are worried about the team's capacity for this game, you can begin with a grid that is 4×4 (16) squares and then expand the maze for the second try (the greater the number of squares in the grid, the harder the maze).

Explain to the children that they will need to work as a group to find the correct way through the maze. To do so, they will each take turns stepping onto the grid. Each person moves one block at a time. If a child's choice is incorrect, the coach "beeps" him or her out of the maze. If the choice is correct, the child moves onto a second block in the maze. The children need to work as a group, using a trial-and-error method, in order to discover the hidden path through the maze. The goal is to get the entire group across the maze using the correct pattern.

The rules and procedures of the game are as follows:

1. Only one person can move at a time. A person takes a turn by beginning to walk from square to square in the maze, waiting at each step to hear if the choice is correct. If there is a "beep," then the last step is not in the correct sequence—which means that the person's turn is over, and he or she must return to the line.

2. Teammates must stay in line and proceed taking their turns in a line. No one can take a second turn in the maze until everyone else in the team has taken a turn.

3. The correct path includes only moves to squares directly adjacent to each other (e.g., children never have to "jump over" squares to get to the next move).

4. Teammates can help each other with gestures and movements, but they cannot step onto the maze when it is not their turn.

5. Once a person has successfully reached the other side, he or she may not reenter the maze, but may encourage and help other team members to follow his or her successful path through the maze.

6. When the group is finished, all members will be on the other side of the maze.

7. (Optional) Children may not talk during the maze activity.

This game challenges children to focus their attention on the group, regulate their behavior, and support each other. Coaches can engage the group members in a planning discussion prior to the activity to encourage them to think of ways they can help each other with the challenge. Importantly, coaches should lead a postplay review after the children complete the maze challenge to discuss positive features of their group performance and areas for improvement. Possible discussion questions after the game is over include "How did you communicate with each other?"; "How did you help each other figure out the pattern?"; "How was teamwork important for this challenge?" Consider letting children talk the first time they try this activity, and then increasing the challenge by telling them that they cannot talk on a subsequent round of the game with a new maze challenge.

Closing Circle: Friendship Tips, Compliments, and Assignment (5 Minutes)

Finish by sharing compliments focused on children's efforts at learning and practicing the friendship skills during the session. It is a good idea to call children's attention to the fact that this is the second to last group session, and that you are planning some special activities for the final session. As you give your compliments, look for opportunities to comment on progress that you have seen the children make over the course of the program.

SPECIAL ISSUES

1. Groups will vary in terms of how much structure they need in order to succeed at making this final video. Based on past experience, plan to provide more structure and guidance or, alternatively, to give children more room for creative input.

2. If you think your group will find it difficult to plan two different parts for the movie, one option is to divide the group into triads/dyads, and let each subgroup plan and enact one part of the movie. If you select this option, you may want to plan some activity for the triad/dyad to do while the other subgroup is taping their video.

3. The amount of time that different groups spend on movie making can vary widely. It is a good idea to have additional group games of choice (games played or skipped in prior sessions) in case you have extra time at the end of this session.

SESSION 14. Celebrating Friendships: Setting Personal Goals, Making a Positive Change

GOALS

1. Review the skills covered in Friendship Group.

2. Share favorite memories.

3. Set personal goals.

4. Promote feelings of self-efficacy for future friendship experiences.

MATERIALS NEEDED

- Posters: Friendship Group Guidelines, Golden Rule, Traffic Light, Positive Thinking

- Poster board and statements for "Goals and Plans" discussion (Activity Page 14.1, see pp. 432–433; one set)

- "My Friendship Goals" page for Memory Books (Activity Page 14.2, see p. 434; one per child)

- Book decorations, affirmation pages, covers (see Early Elementary Session 26; one per child)

- Materials for the choice of games

- Certificates of participation (see Early Elementary Session 26; Activity Page 26.4, see p. 314, one per child)

SESSION OUTLINE

- *Friendship Circle:* Discussion of group memories, goals, and plans (10 minutes)

- *Construction Station:* Memory Book construction (15 minutes)

- *Snack:* Usual procedures (optional, 15 minutes)

- *Collaborative Challenges:* Favorite game(s) or challenge(s) (10 minutes)

- *Closing Circle:* Coach affirmations, Memory Book distribution (5 minutes)

ADVANCE PREPARATION

- Hang posters.
- Prepare materials for the Memory Books.
- Prepare the "Goals and Plans" blackboard or poster board.
- Prepare a list of games or challenges for the final activity choice.

DETAILED SESSION CONTENT

Friendship Circle: Discussion of Group Memories, Goals, and Plans (10 Minutes)

Begin by checking in and asking children about their friendship experiences in the past week. Introduce the topic of group closure and the plan to construct Friendship Group Memory Books.

> "Today is a special day for us because it is our last Friendship Group. I have a lot of mixed feelings about today. It makes me sad to think that this is our last meeting as a group. I know I'm going to miss seeing you. But I'm also happy and grateful that I got to know each of you this year and had such fun times learning with you. In honor of our last day, we are going to make Friendship Memory Books to remember the things we did together. It is always sad to say goodbye to a friend, but the feelings of friendship can go on and on, even when we are not together. Our Memory Books will help us remember each other and the fun times we had."

Let children share their feelings about the last session if they choose to do so. Ask children to share a favorite memory from the group sessions, and then present the goals and plans activity.

> "In addition to looking backward and thinking about what we enjoyed together in Friendship Group, we are also going to look forward today and think about the friendship experiences that are waiting in the future. Each one of you has ideas about good things you hope will happen with friends in the coming year and also ideas about friendship problems you want to solve. So today we are going to do a group activity about friendship goals and plans. It will help you create your personal friendship goals and plans for your Memory Book."

Reveal the blackboard or poster board, explaining that you have listed several friendship goals (see page 1 of Activity Page 14.1). Go around the circle and ask each child to pick a goal from the list, read it, and explain what it means to him or her. Ask the children if they have any other friendship goals that they would like to list and write down the additional goals that they mention. Once children have finished listing goals, bring out the basket with the cards noting various Friendship Group skills. Explain the discussion task ask follows:

> "Each one of you will have a chance to select three goals to write in your Memory Book as reminders of what your personal friendship goals are. In addition, it is important to have specific plans, so that you know what you are going to do in order to reach your goals. I have some plans in this basket that come from the Friendship Tips we've talked about together in our group. I'm going to hum a little tune while we pass this basket around. When I stop, whoever is holding the basket is going to draw a card and read the plan on that card. Then you are going to tape the card on the poster board under the column labeled 'Plans.' You are also going to draw a line from one of the goals over to this plan, to show how the plan can help you reach a goal. Don't worry, because we will all chip in to help if you have questions or want advice from the group."

Proceed with this activity. Children may want to draw lines from the plan to several different goals, which is fine, because many of the skills that are listed on the planning cards are good strategies for working toward more than one goal. There are no right or wrong answers; the important point is to ask children to explain their reasoning—for example: "Why did you choose that connection?"; "How would doing *X* help you reach the goal of *Y*?" At the end of this activity, the hope is that children have thought about the concept of friendship goals and considered their personal goals, and also that they understand that using different Friendship Tips from the group sessions will help them reach their personal friendship goals.

Construction Station: Personal Goal Setting, Teammate Affirmations (15 Minutes)

To construct the Memory Books, children should first complete a personal goals page for themselves. Introduce this personal goals page follows.

> "I am going to give each of you this page that says 'My Friendship Goals' at the top. You can put your name on it. We'll include it in your Memory Books. Who would like to read what it says in the box? [Let someone read.] What do you think that means? Where it says 'Figure out what goals you want to reach,' what do you think about? How would you make a plan to reach your goals? During our time together in Friendship Group, we've talked a lot about friendships—how to make friends, be a good friend, and solve friendship problems. As part of your Memory Book, you each have a chance to think about yourself and your friends. On these first two lines, there is a space for you to write down some things that you do well in your friendships—things you are already good at in terms of getting along with others. Next, there is a space for you to write down two things that you would like to improve in your friendships or in the way you get along with others. Finally, there are lines for your plans: what you intend to do next to take the first step toward reaching your goals. There are no right or wrong answers. This is an opportunity for you to put down your personal feelings about your strengths, your goals, and your plans for your friendships."

Answer any questions children have and let them work at their own pace to fill out these pages. Some children may need your help either to decide what they want to write or to write down their ideas on the paper.

As children finish, introduce the affirmation pages:

> "These blank pages have space for us to write affirmations for each other. Each one of you will make an affirmation page for each of the other team members, describing something you admire about the friendship skills and efforts of each teammate. These pages will get stapled together with a front and back cover page to make the Memory Book. Then you'll have a chance to autograph each others' books and decorate the front of your books."

If you feel that children in your group need more structure to create affirmations, provide them with some sample sentences that they can use (e.g., "I really liked the way you _____" or "You are good at _____"). In addition, if needed, provide children with the prewritten affirmations that they can copy or cut and paste for their teammates.

> "Next, we're going to make pages for each other to include in the Memory Books. Here, I have some blank pages. You will want to choose one to write on for each of your friends. Put your name and a friend's name at the top, and write a friendly comment describing something you appreciate about him or her."

Provide help, as needed, to make sure that each child is able to complete an affirmation page for each team member. Sometimes coaches will need to help one or children write, or offer to cut and paste a message of their choice to keep the process moving along. If some children finish early, they can decorate the colored page that will become the front page for their memory book. As children finish, collect their pages and staple the Friendship Group Memory Books together, inserting their Certificate of Participation with the coach's/coaches' affirmation(s). To summarize, the books should include (1) colored title page at the front, (2) the child's goal page, (3) affirmation pages from the teammates, (4) a Certificate of Participation with coach's/coaches' affirmation (prepared in advance), and (5) colored page at the back.

Snack (Optional, 15 Minutes)

The usual procedures are followed. This can be a good time to talk with children about what they learned in Friendship Group that was most helpful to them. You can ask them how they have used the friendship ideas in their friendships at school or home. You can also ask if they have suggestions for you—things to do more of (or less of) in future Friendship Groups to make them helpful for children. If desired, a special snack can be served in celebration of the group's accomplishments.

Collaborative Challenges: Favorite Game(s) or Challenge(s) (10 Minutes)

To help children choose a final game or group challenge activity, present them with a list of possibilities and let them vote. (Prepare this list ahead of time by considering the games and challenges that were favorites and bringing the needed materials with you.) If there was insufficient time to do the maze in the prior session, it is also a good activity for the final session. Be prepared to review the game procedures and rules.

Closing Circle: Coach Affirmations with Certificates, Memory Book Distribution (5 Minutes)

At the final compliment circle, distribute the Memory Books to each child. Display each child's Certificate of Participation, with the coach's/coaches' affirmation(s) and clap for each child. If time allows, children can also read through and share some of the affirmations they received from their friends.

SPECIAL ISSUES

1. Groups vary in the amount of time they spend discussing group memories. For groups that have been together for a longer period of time, and for children with more advanced verbal skills, the discussion and peer affirmation activities (e.g., Memory Book construction and discussion) can fill the whole session. For other groups, the discussions will be shorter and more perfunctory, and there will be more time for group games.

2. In some groups, it may be possible to include a presentation or "reception" for parents in this final group session. This option allows children to receive recognition from their parents for their accomplishments in this program. In some cases, coaches may also have the opportunity to meet privately with parents and give them feedback on the child's progress in the group, as well as suggestions for follow-through activities that parents can support at home.

Dear Problem Solvers Letters

Dear Problem Solvers,

I got in a big fight with my two friends. I wanted to watch my TV show and they said "no." I got mad and told them to go home. Now they aren't my friends anymore. What should I do?

—Lonely

Dear Problem Solvers,

This year I moved to a new school. I don't like it here. The kids ignore me. I don't have a single friend. Sometimes I think they hate me, because they never ask me to play. I don't know what to do.

—New Kid

Dear Problem Solvers,

Two boys in my class always cheat and it makes me really mad. So we fight. They start the fights, but I get into trouble. What can I do?

—Blamed

(page 1 of 2)

Dear Problem Solvers,

This kid in my class bothers me and my friends. He follows us around. He always wants to play with us. We tell him to leave us alone, but he doesn't. What should we do?

—Bothered

Dear Problem Solvers,

These kids in my class tell secrets. I think they are talking about me. It makes me really mad. I tell them that they must tell me what they are saying, but they don't. They just laugh.

—Mad to Be Left Out

Dear Problem Solvers,

I got put in the low reading group. Now some kids in the class make fun of me. They say I am stupid. What should I do?

—Not Stupid

Dear Problem Solvers,

I play a lot of sports and I do not like to lose. If we lose, I get mad at my team. The coach said I was a "poor sport" and made me sit on the bench for a whole practice. What should I do?

—Wants to Win

Questions for the Challenge Quiz Bowl

1. You are about to sit down at lunch and your friend stops you and says, "You can't sit there today. I'm saving it for someone else."

2. You get in line to take the bus home. Two kids you know are already in line. They turn around and one says, "Why are you always following us?"

3. On the telephone, a friend tells you that another friend said that he (she) doesn't like you because you think you are better than everyone else.

4. A friend wants to copy your homework, but you think that is cheating.

5. You are playing a board game with a friend, and you see the friend cheat. He (she) takes a card, looks at it, puts it back, and chooses a different card.

6. You ask a friend to go to a movie with you, but the friend says that he (she) is busy. You go to the movie with your mom, and see your friend there with another kid.

7. You see your friend sitting alone and writing. You sit down next to your friend and say, "Hi." Your friend says, "I need some privacy right now."

8. You walk toward your friend, who is telling jokes to a group of kids. Your friend sees you and says, "No, not you. You never laugh at my jokes."

9. You get a new haircut. Your friend sees you and says, "Wow—that is funny looking."

10. You ask your friend to work with you on a class project, but he (she) says, "No, because last time you did not do any work."

Friendship Tips Handout for Session 12

The Golden Rule
Treat others how you want to be treated.
To make a good friend, be a good friend.
Cooperate. Talk it out. Be a good sport. Give a compliment.

When You Have a Problem—Work It Out, Make a Deal

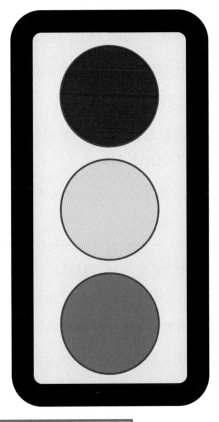

- Stop, calm down.
- Take a deep breath.
- Say the problem and how you feel.
- Listen to the other person.

- Give an idea.
- Listen to their idea.
- Is it a good idea?
- Would it solve the problem?

- Say "yes" to good ideas.
- Give it a try.
- Did it work?

Keep Your Cool
"Take 5" deep breathing

Positive Thinking
Focus on the <u>positive</u>.
Tell yourself that you can do this.
Don't sweat the small stuff.

Take Time to Plan
Think of different things you can do. Choose the best idea.

Friendship Tips Handout for Session 13

HOW TO MAKE FRIENDS

<u>Start a Conversation</u> • Show a friendly face. • Ask a question. Listen. • Tell about you. • Keep it going with another question.	<u>Join In</u> • Look around. • Who is ready to include you? • Move closer and watch. • Say something about the game. • Ask if you can play. • If not, try again later. Or try someone else.
<u>Treat Others as You Want to Be Treated</u> • Offer to help, cooperate. • Be cheerful and kind. • Be a good sport. • Give a compliment.	<u>If You Are Stressed, Keep Your Cool</u> • "Take 5" deep breathing. • Think positive thoughts. • Talk with someone about your feelings and the problem.

(page 1 of 2)

How to Work Out Friendship Problems

<u>Keep Your Cool, Think Positive</u>

- Focus on the *positive*.
- Take 5 to calm down.
- Make a good effort.
- Tell yourself: You can do this.
- Don't sweat the small stuff.

<u>Use the Traffic Light Steps</u>

- Stop, calm down.
- Say the problem and how you feel.

- Give an idea.
- Listen to the other person's idea.
- Say "yes" to good ideas.

- Try it out.

<u>Treat Others as You Want to Be Treated</u>

- Be a peace-maker.
- Take the first step.
- Be creative.
- Find a solution that works for both of you.

<u>Take Time to Plan</u>

- What could you do?
- Avoid.
- Ignore.
- Join together.
- Tell an adult.
- Tell the other person to stop
- What would work best?

Director's Checklist

How to Make Friends

Overall evaluation:

☐ Did the movie show how to start a conversation?

☐ Did the movie show how to join in?

☐ Did the movie show how to treat others the way you want to be treated?

☐ Did the movie show how to manage stress and keep you cool?

Did the actors:

☐ Show a friendly face?

☐ Ask questions?

☐ Show good listening skills?

☐ Tell about themselves?

☐ Keep the conversation going with more questions?

What you liked the best:

_____

_____

_____

_____

_____

_____

_____

_____

(page 1 of 2)

How to Solve a Problem with a Friend

Overall evaluation:

☐ Did the movie show how to keep your cool and think positive?

☐ Did the movie show how to use the Traffic Light steps?

☐ Did the movie show how to treat others the way you want to be treated?

☐ Did the movie show how to take time to plan?

Did the actors:

☐ Show a friendly face?

☐ Take time to calm down?

☐ Take time to plan and think positive?

☐ Explain the problem clearly and calmly?

☐ Listen to the other person's point of view?

☐ Offer ideas to solve the problem?

☐ Make a deal and say "yes" to good ideas?

☐ Work together to solve the problem?

What you liked the best:

_____

_____

_____

_____

_____

_____

_____

_____

Cards for Goals and Plans Poster Board

Directions: Create two columns on the poster board, listing *Goals* at the top of one column and *Plans* at the top of the other. Before the session, cut out the Goals cards and tape them in the Goals column, including a few blank ones for children to fill in. Cut out the Plans cards and place them in a basket or bowl. Children will take turns pulling out a Plans card, describing what it means, taping it into the Plans column on the poster board, and drawing a line to the goal(s) that the plan will help reach. The purpose is to help children link the Friendship Group skills (plans) with their future friendship goals.

Goals Cards

Make new friends.	Have more fun with friends.
Be kinder to others.	Argue less, be a peacemaker.
Get along better with others.	Be confident. Worry less about what others think of me.
Be a better friend.	Stop the bullying.

(page 1 of 2)

Plans

Show a friendly face. Give a compliment.	Make an effort to join in. Get close, watch for your chance, ask if you can play.
Start a conversation: Ask a question, tell about you.	Don't tease when you win. Don't cheat when you lose.
Treat others as you want to be treated: Offer to help, cooperate.	Consider your options: Avoid, ignore, join together, tell an adult, or tell the other person to stop.
Don't sweat the small stuff. Think positive thoughts.	When you are upset, do something to calm down ("Take 5," share your feelings).
<u>Use the Traffic Light:</u> ● Stop, calm down. ○ Talk it out, make a deal. ◐ Try your plan.	Reach out and take the first step to solve a problem. Find a solution that works for both of you.
	Tell yourself: You can do this.

My Friendship Goals

Name: _____

Goal Setting

Be the person you want to be.

Figure out what goals you want to reach.

Make a plan to reach your goals.

Take the first step in your plan.

My Strengths as a Friend:

1. _____
   _____

2. _____
   _____

My Friendship Goals:

1. _____
   _____

2. _____
   _____

My Plans:

1. _____
   _____

2. _____
   _____

References

Bierman, K. L., & the Conduct Problems Prevention Research Group. (1997). Implementing a comprehensive program for the prevention of conduct problems in rural communities: The Fast Track experience. *American Journal of Community Psychology, 25,* 493–514.

Bierman, K. L., Greenberg, M. T., & the Conduct Problems Prevention Research Group. (1996). Social skills training in the Fast Track Program. In R. Peters & R. J. McMahon (Eds.), *Preventing childhood disorders, substance use, and delinquency* (pp. 65–89). Thousand Oaks, CA: SAGE.

Bierman, K. L. (1986). Process of change during social skills training with preadolescents and its relation to treatment outcome. *Child Development, 57,* 230–240.

Conduct Problems Prevention Research Group. (1992). A developmental and clinical model for the prevention of conduct disorders: The Fast Track Program. *Development and Psychopathology, 4,* 509–527.

Conduct Problems Prevention Research Group. (1999a). Initial impact of the Fast Track prevention trial for conduct problems: I. The high-risk sample. *Journal of Consulting and Clinical Psychology, 67,* 631–647.

Conduct Problems Prevention Research Group. (1999b). Initial impact of the Fast Track prevention trial for conduct problems: II. Classroom effects. *Journal of Consulting and Clinical Psychology, 67,* 648–657.

Conduct Problems Prevention Research Group. (2002a). The implementation of the Fast Track program: An example of large-scale prevention science efficacy trial. *Journal of Abnormal Child Psychology, 30,* 1–18.

Conduct Problems Prevention Research Group. (2002b). Evaluation of the first 3 years of the Fast Track prevention trial with children at high risk for adolescent conduct problems. *Journal of Abnormal Child Psychology, 30,* 19–36.

Conduct Problems Prevention Research Group. (2010). Fast Track intervention effects on youth arrests and delinquency. *Journal of Experimental Criminology, 6,* 131–157.

Conduct Problems Prevention Research Group. (2011). The effects of the Fast Track intervention on the development of conduct disorder across childhood. *Child Development, 82,* 331–345.

Conduct Problems Prevention Research Group. (2015). Impact of early intervention on psychopathology, crime, and well-being at age 25. *American Journal of Psychiatry, 172,* 59–70.

Hill, L. G., Lochman, J. E., Coie, J. D., Greenberg, M. T., & the Conduct Problems Prevention Research

Group. (2004). Effectiveness of early screening for externalizing problems: Issues of screening accuracy and utility. *Journal of Consulting and Clinical Psychology, 72,* 809–820.

Kusche, C. A., & Greenberg, M. T. (1994). *The PATHS curriculum.* Seattle: Developmental Research and Programs.

Lavallee, K. L., Bierman, K. L., Nix, R. L, & the Conduct Problems Prevention Research Group. (2005). The impact of first-grade "Friendship Group" experiences on child social outcomes in the Fast Track program. *Journal of Abnormal Child Psychology, 33*(3), 307–324.

Lochman, J. E., & the Conduct Problems Prevention Research Group. (1995). Screening of child behavior problems for prevention programs at school entry. *Journal of Consulting and Clinical Psychology, 63,* 549–559.

McMahon, R. J., Slough, N., & the Conduct Problems Prevention Research Group. (1996). Family-based intervention in the Fast Track Program. In R. Peters & R. J. McMahon (Eds.), *Preventing childhood disorders, substance use, and delinquency* (pp. 90–110). Thousand Oaks, CA: SAGE.

Index

Note: *f* or *t* following a page number indicates a figure or a table.